Social Determinants of Health among African-American Men

Henrie M. Treadwell
Clare Xanthos
Kisha B. Holden

EDITORS

T0337850

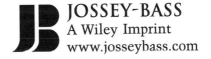

JOSSEY-BASS
A Wiley Imprint
www.josseybass.com

Library of Congress Cataloging-in-Publication Data

Social determinants of health among African American men / Henrie M. Treadwell, Clare Xanthos, Kisha B. Holden, editors.—1st ed.
         p. ; cm.
   Includes bibliographical references and index.
   ISBN 978-0-470-93110-3 (pbk.); ISBN 978-1-118-22134-1 (ebk.); ISBN 978-1-118-23518-8 (ebk.); ISBN 978-1-118-25982-5 (ebk.)
   I. Treadwell, Henrie M. II. Xanthos, Clare, 1969- III. Holden, Kisha B., 1971-
   [DNLM: 1.   African Americans–United States. 2.   Men's Health–United States. 3.   Health Status Disparities–United States. 4.   Socioeconomic Factors–United States. WA 300 AA1]
      362.1089'96073—dc23
                                                                        2012022688

Printed in the United States of America

FIRST EDITION

PB Printing   10 9 8 7 6 5 4 3 2 1

Contents

Figures and Tables

Figures

Tables

Foreword

Robert M. Franklin

In one of the most important books of the 20th century, Carter G. Woodson wrote these words: "This book, then, is not intended as a broadside against any particular person or class, but it is given as a corrective for methods which have not produced satisfactory results." Woodson sought to prepare readers for the truth telling and hope-filled corrective advice that would follow in his justly famous classic, *The Miseducation of the Negro*.

Once again, we encounter a book, this book, which speaks truth to power and speaks empowerment to a segment of the population that has been neglected, feared, misunderstood, and poorly treated in the nation's health system—African-American men. The brilliant editors of this volume have collected searing and insightful essays from some of our best and brightest minds who are working to improve health prospects for black men. Reading these chapters, you may feel that the ghosts of Du Bois and Woodson are peering over your shoulder. That is, each chapter is a scholarly tour de force of analysis that drives the theme that much of the unhealthiness, pathology, and morbidity we observe within the black male population and the black community generally is socially determined, not the result entirely of the choices of the individuals themselves. This is an important analytic perspective to appreciate in the context of policy debates and moral arguments that easily lapse into blaming poor people for poverty and victims for their condition. But Du Bois and Woodson, eminent scholars that they were, are also infusing the advocacy and activist spirit that you will detect in these pages. This book has an attitude, a high temperature, and an impatience for the status quo that commends it to all who wish to learn and then act to move the needle of change.

Fortunately, the nation is beginning to rediscover the unfinished agenda of improving life prospects for boys and men of color. As a nation we appear to go through waves of heightened interest and alarm in this issue that drives the public will to act. But then, for various reasons interest subsides. Decades ago, the nation was stirred by the moral leadership and rhetoric of Dr. King and Presidents Kennedy and Johnson to eradicate poverty and racism. But, as the war in Vietnam loomed and drained resources and will, the national effort was derailed. Years later, the nation focused on the crisis facing black men with the rise of a so-called underclass of permanent high unemployment and high rates of incarceration. At the same time, America witnessed the potential for self efficacy during the Million Man March. But once again, 9/11 and wars in Iraq and Afghanistan derailed these good efforts.

Now, an African-American man is president of the United States. If orchestrated wisely, this happy circumstance could increase public empathy for African-American men. In addition, a growing number of wealthy foundations are investing money to improve the plight of boys and men of color. And, a variety of national reports have been released documenting and lamenting the unsustainably dismal performance of schools in equipping many black boys and men for productive lives. Collective interest once again appears to be rising and our potential for producing change is great. Into this exciting and unpredictable socio-cultural and political environment, this book arrives. And, it is well suited to instruct, challenge, correct, and mobilize a more holistic effort to improve the plight of men, for their own health benefit and that of entire families and communities.

As president of Morehouse College, the nation's sole elite liberal arts college for educating African-American men, I am especially sensitive to threats to the well-being of the black male population. Our graduates like Dr. King, Surgeon General David Satcher, HHS Secretary Louis Sullivan, Julian Bond, and many others have devoted their lives to leading change for black men and all people. That is one reason this book has arrested my attention and why I think it will be so important for future discussions of this population. This current generation of college, public health, and medical students has an opportunity to increase public awareness, drive the public discussion, and generate new policies and programs to improve black male health. This book will be critical to informing that process.

This book could be, as Woodson said, a methodological corrective and a call to action for politicians and pastors, public health and corporate leaders to support a new perspective on why many black men are not yet thriving. But, we have the wherewithal to change directions. We should find assurance and hope in the words of the poet Goethe, "At the moment of commitment, the entire universe conspires for your success."

Preface

African-American men's health is in a state of crisis: African-American men not only have the lowest life expectancy and highest mortality rate among all other racial, ethnic, and gender groups in the United States, they are also confronted by staggering health care inequities in virtually all disease areas and medical services. The key message of this volume is that the *health status* of African-American men is underpinned by their corresponding *social status*. African-American men face some of the greatest social challenges in this country (e.g., low socioeconomic status, discrimination, mass incarceration). This volume shows how these social challenges—described in this book as social determinants—are inextricably linked with the health inequities affecting African-American men.

Since its inception in 1998, Community Voices of Morehouse School of Medicine has provided leadership in the field of men's health, with a particular focus on health disparities affecting poor men of color. In recent years, Community Voices has recognized the necessity of adopting a broader approach to addressing health disparities among men, that is, the need to address the underlying social determinants of health and mental health among men. In this vein, two policy briefs were released relating to social determinants of health and mental health among African-American men and boys, followed by an article in the *Journal of Men's Health* titled "Social Determinants of Health among African-American Men" (Xanthos et al., 2010). This book evolved naturally from discussions around these publications, and the appreciation of social determinants as pivotal factors in the physical and mental health inequities affecting African-American men.

Social Determinants of Health among African-American Men is ground-breaking in that it is the first book to apply the concept of social determinants of health to the health of African-American men. Indeed, currently, social determinants of African-American men's health tend to be overlooked in public health literature; much of the existing literature on African-American men's health is informed by a "health behavior framework," which focuses on African-American men's personal responsibility for their health status (e.g., unhealthy diet, lack of exercise, failure to participate in health screenings). Although the health behavior framework is undoubtedly important, it fails to acknowledge the critical role that social factors play in the health of this vulnerable population. So exploring the social determinants of health among African-American men allows us to reconceptualize the debate on African-American men's health by drawing attention to the impact of social factors on health and thus extending the debate beyond health behavior (Gadson, 2006).

Furthermore, this book is timely; in recent years, social determinants are increasingly recognized as having a pivotal influence on health, and are a critical issue in the public health debate, as evidenced by the spate of publications and initiatives launched by the Centers for Disease Control (CDC) and the World Health Organization (WHO) over the past few years.

In short, this volume enables students, faculty, researchers, policy makers, and professionals to identify, discuss, and evaluate the root causes of health inequities affecting African-American men as well as solutions for addressing these socially determined inequities. We also hope that *Social Determinants of Health among African-American Men* may serve to reinvigorate the debate around African-American men's health, and generate progress in the research and policy arena.

Organization of This Book

The book begins with an introduction to the social determinants of health among African-American men, and lays the foundation for the book. Following the introductory chapter, the book contains four key sections, which are subdivided into chapters. Part One, "Social Determinants of Health Status," (Chapters 2, 3, 4, 5, 6, and 7) deals with the direct impact of social factors (e.g., racism, low socioeconomic status, incarceration) on the health and mental status of African-American men.

Frequently the existing literature blames and stigmatizes African-American men for their unhealthy lifestyles without considering wider social factors that underpin unhealthy behavior. Part Two, "Social Determinants of Health Behavior" (Chapters 8, 9, and 10), considers these social factors that influence African-American men's health behavior, and health and mental health status.

Unequal health care is a significant social determinant of health among African-American men. Part Three, "Social Determinants of Health Care" (Chapters 11 and 12), shows how health care provider factors and health system factors contribute to health inequities affecting African-American men in the general population (Chapter 11) and within the correctional population (Chapter 12).

Part Four, "Addressing Social Determinants of Health Inequities" (Chapters 13, 14, 15, 16, and 17), describes and discusses policies and programs that address the social determinants of health among African-American men. Although this section specifically focuses on strategies to address health inequities affecting African-American men, all chapters contain sections on policy recommendations that correspond with each chapter.

Finally, to facilitate academic engagement, each chapter contains a list of study objectives, a list of discussion questions, and a list of key terms.

References

Gadson, S. L. (2006). The third world health status of black American males. *Journal of the National Medical Association*, *98*(4), 488–491.

Xanthos, C., Treadwell, H., & Braithwaite-Holden, K. (2010). Social determinants of health among African-American men. *Journal of Men's Health*, *7*(1), 11–19.

For our brothers, sons, husbands, fathers, uncles, nephews and cousins, not to mention our dear friends . . . whose voices have been muted by a system that is not yet ready to embrace social justice for all, in what we hope is the greatest democratic nation in the world. We speak with and for you. We stand with you. A wonderful day is coming because you are here and we are here with you. We will not rest until you are safe.

Acknowledgments

The editors would like to take the opportunity to acknowledge the people who have helped to make this book possible. We wish to express our appreciation and gratitude to the chapter authors for their collective efforts in producing an edited volume, which covers some of the most important social determinants of health among African-American men in the twenty-first century while simultaneously offering viable strategies for reducing socially determined health disparities among this population.

We would like to thank Timothy A. Akers, Sherman A. James, Stephen M. Rose, Jonathan VanGeest, and Raymond A. Winbush, who provided valuable feedback in the early stages of the manuscript's conception. Kyrel Buchanan, Keon Gilbert, Daphne Watkins Jacobs, and William Wiist provided thoughtful and constructive comments on the draft manuscript.

We are also grateful to Jossey-Bass for giving us the opportunity to publish this book. In particular, we would like to thank Andy Pasternack, senior editor, for supporting this important project, guiding us through the publication process, and bringing it to fruition; and Seth Schwartz, associate editor, for his advice, help, and professionalism.

The Editors

Henrie M. Treadwell, PhD

Dr. Treadwell is a research professor, Department of Community Health and Preventive Medicine at the Morehouse School of Medicine. Her major responsibilities include management for *Community Voices*, an informing policy initiative funded by the Kellogg Foundation. She focuses on special programs to facilitate reentry into community of boys and men of color. Dr. Treadwell is co-editor of "Health Issues in the Black Community (2009)" and serves on the editorial board of the *Journal of Men's Health*. Dr. Treadwell founded the Soledad O'Brien Freedom's Voice Award, an award to recognize individuals implementing significant work to improve global society. She was appointed in 2009 to the Georgia State Board of Corrections by Georgia's governor, Sonny Perdue, and she was recently appointed to the Georgia Criminal Justice Coordinating Council Advisory Committee.

Dr. Treadwell served for 16 years as program director at the W. K. Kellogg Foundation. Dr. Treadwell has a BA from the University of South Carolina, which she entered as a result of a desegregation lawsuit. She was the first African American to graduate post-Reconstruction and the first ever African-American woman graduate. Dr. Treadwell completed doctoral studies at Atlanta University and postdoctoral studies at the Harvard School of Public Health.

Clare Xanthos, PhD, MSc

Clare Xanthos, PhD, MSc is a social scientist whose research interests focus on social determinants of health and health care inequities. She is a research assistant professor at Morehouse School of Medicine, within the Department of Community Health and Preventive Medicine and the Satcher Health Leadership Institute; and a MSCR Fellow at the Clinical Research Center, Morehouse School of Medicine.

During her employment at the Morehouse School of Medicine, Dr. Xanthos has been involved in a wide range of projects relating to social determinants of health/health inequities issues. She authored two important policy briefs relating to social determinants of health and mental health among African-American men and boys. In addition, she is the lead author of a groundbreaking article titled "Social Determinants of Health among African American Men" published in the *Journal of Men's Health.*

Dr. Xanthos received her PhD in social policy from the London School of Economics and Political Science (LSE), where she was the recipient of several scholarships/awards. Additionally, she holds a master's degree in housing studies and a bachelor's degree in social sciences. Dr. Xanthos has lived and worked in several countries, including the United States, Barbados, and the United Kingdom.

Kisha B. Holden, PhD

Kisha B. Holden, PhD, is co-director of Community Voices: Healthcare for the Underserved and associate professor within the department of psychiatry and behavioral sciences and the Satcher Health Leadership Institute at Morehouse School of Medicine. She earned undergraduate, master's, and doctoral degrees from Howard University in counseling psychology; and completed a postdoctoral fellowship at Johns Hopkins University in the school of medicine and school of public health. She recently earned a master of science in clinical research degree from Morehouse School of Medicine. She has received funding from the American Psychological Association, National Institute of Mental Health, and National Institute on Drug Abuse Research to conduct clinical and translational research concerning mental health disparities, depression among African Americans, and innovative approaches to improve integration of mental and behavioral health care into community-based primary health care settings. Dr. Holden has co-edited two books, published in several peer-reviewed journals, and contributed book chapters to notable publications regarding health disparities. She is committed to encouraging mental health and well-being for ethnically and culturally diverse families, establishing successful mental health prevention and intervention approaches, and building the evidence base and strategies for mental health policy change.

The Contributors

Angela Glover Blackwell, JD
Founder and Chief Executive Officer
PolicyLink
Oakland, CA

Robert F. Belli, PHD
Professor of Psychology
Chair, Survey Research and Methodology
University of Nebraska, Lincoln

Jean J. Bonhomme MD, MPH
Department of Psychiatry
Morehouse School of Medicine
President, National Black Men's Health Network

Lisa Bowleg, PhD
Associate Professor
Drexel University School of Public Health

Qiana R. Cryer-Coupet, MSW
Doctoral student
Jane Addams College of Social Work
University of Illinois at Chicago

Jodi Drisko, MSPH
Principal, Parametrix Group, LLC

Robert M. Franklin, PhD
President, Morehouse College

Louis F. Graham, DrPH, MPH
University of Michigan School of Public Health

Derek M. Griffith, PhD
Associate Professor of Medicine, Health and Society
College of Arts and Sciences
Director, Center for Research on Men's Health Disparities
Vanderbilt University

Wizdom Powell Hammond, PhD, MPH
Assistant Professor
Department of Health Behavior and Health Education
UNC Gillings School of Global Public Health

Rhonda Conerly Holliday, PhD
Research Associate Professor
Department of Community Health and Preventive Medicine
Morehouse School of Medicine

John Van Hoewyk, PHD
Survey Research Center
Institute for Social Research
University of Michigan, Ann Arbor

Sherman A. James, PHD
Susan B. King Professor of Public Policy and Professor of Sociology
Community and Family Medicine
African and African American Studies
Faculty Affiliate Duke Population Research Institute
Sanford School of Public Policy

Jonetta L. Johnson, MPH
PhD candidate
Department of Health Behavior and Health Education
University of Michigan School of Public Health

Elisabeth Kingsbury, JD
Former Senior Researcher
Community Voices: Healthcare for the Underserved,
Morehouse School of Medicine

David J. Malebranche, MD, MPH
Associate Professor
Emory University Division of General Medicine

Nandi Marshall, MPH, CHES, DrPH(c)
Academic Researcher/Instructor
Co-PI Quality Improvement Initiatives
The State Coordinating Center for GA Public Health PBRN
Jiann-Ping Hsu College of Public Health
Georgia Southern University

Harold W. Neighbors, PhD
Research Professor and Director
Program for Research on Black Americans
Institute for Social Research
University of Michigan, Ann Arbor
Professor
Health Behavior and Health Education
School of Public Health
University of Michigan, Ann Arbor

Leda M. Pérez, PhD
Vice President, Health Initiatives
Collins Center for Public Policy

Susan D. Phillips, PhD
Research Analyst
The Sentencing Project
Washington, DC

Robert Pope, PhD, RN, MSN
University of California, San Francisco
School of Nursing
Department of Physiological Nursing
John A. Hartford Scholar
SAMHSA MFP Fellow

Trivellore E. Raghunathan, PHD
Chair and Professor of Biostatistics
Institute for Social Research
University of Michigan
Research Professor
Joint Program in Survey Modeling
University of Maryland

David Satcher, MD, PhD
Director, Satcher Health Leadership Institute
Poussaint-Satcher-Cosby Professor of Mental Health
Morehouse School of Medicine
16th Surgeon General of the United States

Arjumand A. Siddiqi, ScD
Assistant Professor
Dalla Lana School of Public Health
University of Toronto

David S. Strogatz, PHD
Director, Center for Rural Community Health
Bassett Research Institute
Cooperstown, NY

Adewale Troutman, MD, MPH, MA, CPH
Professor
Department of Community and Family Health
Executive Director
Public Health Practice and Leadership
University of South Florida
College of Public Health
Tampa Florida

Daphne C. Watkins, PhD
Assistant Professor
School of Social Work
University of Michigan

Elizabeth M. (Liz) Whitley, PhD, RN
Director Community Voices/Community Health Grants
Denver Health
Denver, CO

David R. Williams, PHD
Florence and Laura Norman Professor of Public Health
Professor of African and African American Studies and Sociology
Harvard School of Public Health

Chapter 1

Introduction to Social Determinants of Health among African-American Men

Clare Xanthos
Henrie M. Treadwell
Kisha B. Holden

Learning Objectives

- Acquire an overview of the health inequities affecting African-American men.
- Appreciate the significance of socially determined health inequities faced by African-American men.
- Understand the concept of "social determinants of health status" with reference to African-American men.
- Understand the concept of "social determinants of health behavior" with reference to African-American men.
- Understand the concept of "social determinants of health care" with reference to African-American men.
- Gain an awareness of potential strategies for addressing socially determined health inequities faced by African-American men.

• • •

This chapter is an introduction to the **social determinants of health** among **African-American men**, and lays the foundation for the book.[1] It starts by presenting an overview of the serious **health inequities** affecting African-American men, and then describes why this volume is needed. Next, it considers the social determinants of health among African-American men in relation to health status, health behavior, and health care, subdividing this concept into three interrelated components—the **social determinants of health status**, the **social determinants of health behavior**, and the **social determinants of health care**. Finally, suggestions are offered for addressing these **socially determined health inequities** affecting African-American men. These consist of recommendations for research and programs that address the social determinants of health among African-American men, social policies that tackle social and environmental issues affecting African-American men's health, and health policies that promote **health equity** among this and other vulnerable populations.

The Health Status of African-American Men

African-American men have the lowest life expectancy and highest mortality rate among all other racial, ethnic, and gender groups in the United States. The life expectancy of black men is 70 years as compared with 76 years for white men, 76 years for black women, and 81 years for white women (National Center for Health Statistics, 2007). African-American men's mortality rate is 1.3 times greater than white men, 1.7 times greater than American Indian/Alaska Native men, 1.8 times greater than Hispanic men, and 2.4 times greater than Asian or Pacific Islander men (Henry J. Kaiser Family Foundation, 2007). To cite some examples:

- With regard to cardiovascular disease, African-American men's mortality risk for stroke is 60 percent greater than white men (Office of Minority Health, 2008a). Additionally, among 30- to 39-year-olds, the likelihood of African-American men developing kidney failure as a result of hypertension is approximately 14 times greater than their white counterparts (USRDS, 2005). Moreover, the mortality rate for heart disease among African-American men is 30 percent greater than their white counterparts (Office of Minority Health, 2008b).

- With respect to cancer, black men in the United States suffer significantly greater rates of prostate cancer than their male counterparts worldwide (Zerhouni, 2002). In addition, African-American men's chances of developing lung cancer are 37 percent greater than white men (American Lung Association, 2007). Also, oral (mouth) cancer occurs far more frequently among African-American men than other population groups in the United States (NIDCR, 2008). The disparities in the survival rates for oral cancer are striking, with only 36 percent of African-American men surviving five years or more as compared with 61 percent of their white counterparts (National Institute of Dental and Craniofacial Research, 2010).

- Among African-American men, the death rate for diabetes is 51.7 per 100,000 as compared to 25.6 per 100,000 among white men (Office of Minority Health, 2008b).

- African-American men are more than seven times more likely to develop AIDS, and more than nine times as likely to die from AIDS as their white counterparts (Office of Minority Health, 2008b).

- Among young African-American men, the mortality rate for homicides is 84.6 per 100,000 of the population compared with 5 per 100,000 of the population for their white counterparts (Henry J. Kaiser Family Foundation, 2006). To put it another way, the mortality rate for homicides among young black men aged 15 to 19 is 46 times greater than young white men (National Urban League, 2007). Homicide-related mortality rates are not as high among older African-American men, but the rates among the 25-to-44 age group are still overwhelming (61 per 100,000 of the population) as compared with 5.1 per 100,000 among their white counterparts (Henry J. Kaiser Family Foundation, 2006).

Why This Book Is Needed: Social Determinants of Health and African-American Men

As has just been demonstrated, the health inequities affecting African-American men are staggering when compared to other racial, ethnic, and gender groups in the United States. Although there have been considerable efforts in recent years to tackle **health disparities** (Mullins, Blatt, Gbarayor, Yang, & Baquet, 2005), serious inequities persist, especially with regard to African-American men, who continue to face worse health outcomes than other racial, ethnic, and gender groups in the United States. At the same time, it is becoming increasingly clear that social determinants or social factors (e.g., low socioeconomic status, poor neighborhood conditions, discrimination, reduced access to quality education, reduced access to employment, incarceration, reduced access to quality health care) have a major impact on the health inequities affecting this population (Xanthos, Treadwell, & Braithwaite-Holden, 2010).

Although the social determinants of health are increasingly recognized as a critical issue in the public health debate, this topic has been largely neglected in much of the public health literature relating to African-American men. Indeed, the literature on African-American men's health has often been informed by a "health behavior framework" as opposed to a "social determinants of health framework." Research and programs relating to African-American men's health often concentrate on individual **health behavior** (e.g., unhealthy diet, lack of exercise, failure to participate in health screenings) (Gadson, 2006). What is missing from this framework is a recognition of African-American men's often difficult life circumstances. African-American men typically face more life adversity (e.g., reduced access to quality education, reduced access to employment, disproportionate rates of incarceration) than less vulnerable population groups (see Gehlert et al., 2008). In addition, African-American men are among the most **underserved populations** in the United States with regard to access to quality health and mental health services, which similarly contributes to their poor health outcomes (see Smedley, Stith, & Nelson, 2003). Although health behavior determines health to a certain degree, it is important to acknowledge that negative social and environmental factors play a critical role in negatively impacting the health of vulnerable minorities such as African-American men. As such, ascribing the health inequities affecting African-American men to health behavior only is not an adequate explanation (Gadson, 2006). Indeed, the health behavior framework can be problematic in that it can lead to "blaming the victims" for their unhealthy behavior, without taking into account the social and environmental factors that cause poor health (see Raphael et al., 2003). Exploring the social determinants of health allows us to reconceptualize the debate around African-American men's health by drawing attention to the critical impact of social and environmental factors on health.

In this volume, we seek to fill this gap by moving beyond a simple examination of health disparities among this population; we highlight the *social determinants* **of health inequities** affecting African-American men, and offer solutions to address these socially determined inequities. Further, the concept of social determinants of health is subdivided into three interrelated components—"social determinants of health status," "social determinants of health behavior," "social determinants of health care"—to allow for a comprehensive understanding of this issue among African-American men. In this vein, the book introduces students, faculty, researchers, policy makers, and professionals to the following major areas:

- The social determinants of health status among African-American men
- The social determinants of health behavior among African-American men
- The social determinants of health care among African-American men
- Addressing the social determinants of health inequities affecting African-American men

These themes are reflected in the subsequent chapters in this volume and are discussed next.

Social Determinants of Health Status

African-American men are exposed to a multitude of social and environmental conditions that have the potential to affect their health status, including both physical and mental health (Xanthos, 2008, 2009). For the purpose of this chapter, the focus is on three key social determinants of health that are particularly relevant to African-American men: **low socioeconomic status**, **racial discrimination**, and **incarceration**. These should not be seen as discrete factors; there is significant interplay between them, as is apparent in the following discussion. No list can be exhaustive, so these three social determinants encompass a broad array of some of the most significant stressors and negative life events affecting African-American men's health.

Low Socioeconomic Status

African-American men are disproportionately impacted by low socioeconomic status (SES). First, African Americans are three times more likely to live below the poverty line (approximately 25 percent of African Americans) than their white counterparts (National Urban League, 2007). Indeed, African-American men are paid less than 75 percent of what their white counterparts are paid; 9.5 percent of African-American men are unemployed as compared with 4 percent of white males. Additionally, African-American men are more likely to be in lower-income jobs as compared with their white counterparts (National Urban League, 2007). Due to lower incomes when compared with other racial/ethnic groups, African-American men are often forced to reside in disadvantaged communities, with poor neighborhood conditions (e.g., crime, substandard housing, crowding, noise pollution) (Adler & Snibbe, 2003) and environmental hazards (Bullard, 1990).

Concurrently, the relationship between low SES and poor health is well documented (Baum, Garofalo, & Yali, 1999; Marmot & Shipley, 1996). It has been suggested that the conditions associated with low SES lead to stress, and that in turn, stress leads to poor health outcomes (Baum et al., 1999). As such it is clear that reduced access to socioeconomic opportunities among African-American men is an important social determinant of health.

Finally, it is important to note that the relationship between SES and race is complex. For example, socioeconomic status is an important factor in explaining racial inequities in health, but by itself it is not an adequate explanation because racial disparities in health persist among populations with similar socioeconomic backgrounds (Williams, 1999). In addition, racial discrimination can have a harmful impact on health due to its negative influence on socioeconomic status (Williams, 1999). The following subsection seeks to shed some light on this issue.

Racial Discrimination

Racial discrimination is a significant aspect of life for African-American men; they must deal with everyday racism (e.g., proactive police surveillance, workplace tensions) as well as institutional racism (e.g., employment discrimination). In the interests of brevity, we highlight three important discrimination-related issues faced by African-American men and boys: reduced access to quality education, reduced access to employment, and disproportionate rates of incarceration.

First, African-American male students face significant educational inequities when compared to their white counterparts (Schott Foundation, 2006). Black boys are generally more likely to attend the poorest and most segregated public schools as compared with other racial, ethnic, and gender groups in the United States (Schott Foundation, 2006). In addition, underfunding of schools in African-American communities is a serious problem; in 2007, funds allocated per black student represented just 82 percent of funds allocated per white student (National Urban League, 2007). Moreover, it has been argued that school policies and practices play a role in the disproportionate levels of expulsion, suspension, and special education placement among African-American boys (Monroe, 2005; Salend, Duhaney, & Montgomery, 2002). As such there is a resulting achievement gap between black males and other racial, ethnic, and gender groups, which is well documented (Roderick, 2003; Schott Foundation, 2006; U.S. Department of Education, 1995).

Second, as noted earlier, there are significant employment inequities among African-American men and their white counterparts (9.5 percent of African-American men are unemployed as compared with 4 percent of white males) (National Urban League, 2007). Pager's study (2003) demonstrated staggering employment inequities among African-American men and white men. Among African-American men without criminal records, only 14 percent received callbacks for jobs as compared with 34 percent of white men without criminal records. Furthermore, the study found that white men with criminal records (17 percent) are more likely to receive callbacks for jobs than African-American men without criminal records (14 percent).

Third, inequities in incarceration are another important discrimination-related issue faced by African-American men and boys. (For a detailed discussion on incarceration, see the following section.)

Concurrently, there is now significant literature suggesting that racial discrimination leads to negative health outcomes (see, for example, Geronimus,

Hicken, Keene, & Bound, 2006; Krieger & Sidney, 1996; Taylor et al., 2007). To be sure, Geronimus et al. (2006) note that racism-related stress may cause disproportionate physiological deterioration and in turn greater morbidity and mortality among African Americans. This suggests that racial discrimination is a significant social determinant of health among African-American men.

Incarceration

Incarceration is a stark reality for many African-American men. First, discrimination and reduced access to socioeconomic opportunities such as education and employment can leave African-American men with few positive life options and a vulnerability to involvement in situations that could potentially lead to incarceration. To be sure, the term "school-to-prison pipeline" has been used to describe the increasingly recognized link between the exclusionary discipline practices in schools and incarceration (Fenning & Rose, 2007).

The disproportionate incarceration rate among African-American men is also due to racial biases in police and prosecutor discretion and sentencing guidelines. African-American men face significant inequities in arrest, conviction, and incarceration rates when compared with other racial and ethnic groups (Williams, 2006). Black men are six times more likely to be held in custody as compared with their white counterparts. In addition, the incarceration rate for black men is 4,618 per 100,000 as compared with their white and Hispanic counterparts (773 per 100,000 and 1,747 per 100,000, respectively) (Sabol & Couture, 2008).

At the same time, there is evidence suggesting a connection between incarceration and health status (Graham, Treadwell, & Braithwaite, 2008; Massoglia, 2008). As noted earlier, it has been suggested that stress can lead to poor health outcomes (Baum et al., 1999). Thus, if we consider that prisons are highly stressful places, it follows that they are likely to have a negative impact on health (Massoglia, 2008). Additionally, the stressors associated with reentering society after incarceration (e.g., unemployment, inadequate access to housing and health services) may have a negative impact on the health of African-American men (Massoglia, 2008). In short, incarceration and its related stressors are other significant social determinants of health among this population.

Social Determinants of Health Behavior

As noted previously, research and programs relating to African-American men's health often focus on health behavior (Gadson, 2006). This may be due to the fact that men in general have significantly less healthy lifestyles than women. Males of all ages are more likely than females to increase their risk of morbidity, injury, and mortality by their high-risk behaviors, including the use/overuse of tobacco, alcohol, and other drugs, as well as high-risk sexual activity and violence (Courtenay, 2000). However, as pointed out earlier, explaining unhealthy behaviors simply as a matter of individual choice is problematic because it does not consider why vulnerable populations adopt these behaviors in the first place; it also leads us to blame disadvantaged populations for engaging in unhealthy coping mechanisms (Raphael et al., 2003).

As discussed in the previous section, African-American men are exposed to a whole host of social and environmental conditions that can have a negative impact on their health status. We consider that these difficult social and environmental conditions can similarly have a negative impact on *health behavior*, which can negatively impact health status. Indeed, the social environment can simultaneously *encourage the practice of unhealthy behavior* and *discourage the practice of healthy behavior* (Williams & Collins, 2001). For example, unhealthy products such as alcohol are often disproportionately marketed in the black community. LaVeist and Wallace (2000) found that liquor stores are more likely to be located in majority black census tracts than less black census tracts, and that this disparity could not be explained by census tract SES. LaVeist and Wallace's study also demonstrates significant correlations between liquor store locations and the risk of health-related problems in low-income neighborhoods.

Additionally, as indicated earlier, unfavorable social and economic conditions such as those faced by many African-American men can create psychosocial stress. This, in turn, can have a negative effect on health behavior (Xanthos, 2009). As indicated by a national survey (APA Online, 2006), Americans use unhealthy behaviors (e.g., comfort eating, smoking) as coping mechanisms for stress.

Moreover, as noted in the previous section, due to disproportionately low incomes when compared with other Americans, African-American men are often forced to reside in unfavorable neighborhood locations. High crime levels and a lack of recreational facilities in these locations can impede physical activity due to fear of being a victim of crime, and the lack of suitable places to exercise (Williams & Collins, 2001). Unfavorable neighborhood locations are also associated with reduced access to healthy foods. Many businesses (e.g., supermarkets) avoid segregated areas, which frequently results in fewer, poorer quality, and more expensive goods (e.g., food) than those available in less segregated locations. This can lead to poorer nutrition (Williams & Collins, 2001).

In short, African-American men are exposed to a whole host of social and environmental conditions (e.g., low socioeconomic status, racial discrimination, incarceration [discussed in the previous section]) that can have a negative impact on health behavior (as well as health status).

Social Determinants of Health Care

In addition to the aforementioned social determinants of health, health care has also recently started to be considered as a social determinant of health. Indeed, the barriers to accessing quality care among specific population groups plays a key role in the poor health of these populations (McGibbon, Etowa, & McPherson, 2008).

With respect to men generally, gender stereotypes can affect the quality of men's health care. For example, physicians may make the assumption that men are uninterested in psychosocial help for health problems (Bird & Rieker, 1999). African-American men, in particular, face reduced access to quality health care; health care providers who are unfamiliar with diverse populations may unconsciously be influenced by negative stereotypes of men of color (Satcher, 2003). In 2003, the groundbreaking Institute of Medicine report *Unequal Treatment* (Smedley et al., 2003) found that across a range of disease areas and clinical services, African Americans (and Hispanics) generally receive a lower of quality of health care as compared with their white counterparts. These disparities could not be explained by clinical factors (e.g., stage of disease presentation, severity of disease) or socioeconomic factors (e.g., health insurance status); furthermore, they are associated with higher mortality among these population groups. With specific reference to African-American men, Felix-Aaron et al. (2005) found that African-American men received lower quality end-stage renal disease care as compared with white men. Additionally, in a study exploring prostate cancer screening behaviors among black men, Woods, Montgomery, Belliard, Ramirez-Johnson, and Wilson (2004) found that 62.8 percent of African-American men believed that they received poor treatment because they were African-American, and 58.6 percent considered that their race/ethnicity had an effect on the quality of care provided to them. In addition, African Americans are affected by significant mental health care inequities (Braithwaite-Holden & Xanthos, 2009). To cite one example, research indicates that African Americans are more likely to be prescribed older antidepressant medications (with more serious side-effects) than whites (Melfi, Croghan, Hanna, & Robinson, 2000). (Please refer to Chapter 11 for more details on mental health care inequities affecting African-American men.)

Inequities in health care also emanate from residential factors; residence in segregated medically underserved neighborhoods particularly affects African-American men's access to quality health services. Residential segregation negatively impacts access to health care among African-American men in a number of ways, including a shortage of hospitals in African-American communities (Randall, 2006), a lack of quality physicians in poor African-American neighborhoods (Bach, Pham, Schrag, Tate, & Hargraves, 2004), as well as a lack of quality hospitals in African-American communities (Gaston, 2009). For example, research conducted by Hayanga et al. (2009) indicates that in highly segregated areas, surgical services are less readily available than in less segregated areas, and that there is a greater use of emergency services in highly segregated communities; these disparities cannot be explained by socioeconomic or health factors.

Finally, lack of access to health insurance has traditionally been a major factor in the health care inequities affecting African-American men. Indeed, in 2005, African-American men were 75 percent less likely to have health insurance when compared with their white counterparts (Office of Minority Health, 2010). Undoubtedly the health care reform legislation passed on March 23, 2010, will be an important tool in tackling these insurance-related health care inequities.

The above examples demonstrate that health care is a crucial social determinant of health among African-American men.

The Need to Apply the Social Determinants of Health Model to the Health of African-American Men

Funding bodies, researchers, program developers, and policy makers must recognize the social determinants of health inequities affecting African-American men, including the social determinants of health status, the social determinants of health behavior, and the social determinants of health care. In addition, public health research, programs, and policies for African-American men must establish a reasonable balance between focusing on health behavior and tackling the social and environmental factors that influence health behavior (Gadson, 2006). The following recommendations are not meant to be exhaustive, but rather illustrative of key issues that funding bodies, researchers, program developers, and policy makers should be concerned about when considering the health of African-American men.

Research and Programs

Funding bodies must show a greater willingness to fund research and programs that address the social determinants of health among African-American men, including the social determinants of health status, health behavior, and health care. It is imperative that researchers and program developers acknowledge the necessity of moving beyond a simple health behavior model to explore the social determinants of health behavior among this population. In short, there is a need for more research that demonstrates that health outcomes among African-American men are related to social and economic conditions, as well as interventions that address these conditions. Additionally, more diversity may be needed among health policy researchers and program developers in order to achieve a broader research and intervention agenda (Treadwell & Ro, 2003).

Social Policy

Given the impact of the social environment on the health of African-American men, policy makers must promote social policies that address these social and environmental issues. Social policies should include:

- Labor: It is necessary to strengthen systems to remove barriers to equal opportunity and adopt compensatory programs as and when necessary in employment (e.g., strengthening anti-discrimination legislation in the area of employment in relation to hiring and promotion) (Danziger, Reed, & Brown, 2004).

- Education: There is a need to strengthen systems to remove educational inequities and adopt compensatory programs as and when necessary (Danziger et al., 2004). This should include reforming the system of allocating funds to schools to address the disparities in fund allocation, and promoting race equity within schools (e.g., educational advocacy initiatives for African-American male students, increasing the numbers of African-American male teachers [Courtland, 1991], increasing the accountability of school educators with regard to exclusionary discipline practices in schools).

- Poverty and the urban environment: It is important for policy makers to strengthen systems that act as a safety net for low-income workers and individuals who are confronted with financial hardship (e.g., increasing the minimum wage, extending unemployment benefits). In addition, it is necessary to invest in revitalizing poor neighborhoods (e.g., developing walkable communities, mixed-income housing developments, crime-prevention programs) (Xanthos, 2009).

- Criminal justice: It is imperative to establish systems to tackle racial biases in the criminal justice system, including biases in police and prosecutor discretion and sentencing guidelines. In addition, it is necessary to address the various social barriers that ex-offenders face after they are released from prison (e.g., providing incentives to employers to encourage the hiring of ex-offenders) (Xanthos, 2009).

Health Policy

As argued earlier, health care is another social determinant of health. The following are examples of health policies that policy makers need to develop to address inequities in health care affecting African-American men.

- Training to promote gender-specific health services: There is a need to promote gender-specific health care within health services (Banks,

2004). For example, health service providers should receive training in gender-specific health care in order that more appropriate services for men can be provided. This would include directing health care providers away from stereotypes that disadvantage men (e.g., "men are better at coping with pain") (Banks, 2004). In addition, training should include communication, relationship building, patient education, and sensitivity to patient privacy and embarrassment (Dubé, Fuller, Rosen, Fagan, & O'Donnell, 2005). Moreover, health providers' offices should be tailored to improve men's access (e.g., services available outside working hours, availability of men's magazines in waiting rooms) (Banks, 2004).

- Training to promote race equity in health services: It is necessary to promote the provision of racially equitable health services to African-American men and other vulnerable minority populations. As argued by Xanthos (Chapter 11), health care providers should receive training to address the unconscious racial attitudes and stereotypes that negatively impact health care interactions and health care decisions. This would include developing an awareness of any biases relating to African-American men in order to improve service delivery (Cardarelli & Chiapa, 2007). This would also involve directing health care providers away from stereotypes that have a negative impact on health services (e.g., "African Americans are not likely to adhere to medical advice") (Van Ryn & Burke, 2000).

- Diverse health care workforce: It is imperative that the representation of African-American men be increased at all levels of the health care delivery system. Having health care providers who can relate to the experiences of African-American men will increase their comfort level in utilizing health services (Satcher, 2003). The authors support the recommendations of the Institute of Medicine (Smedley, Stith-Butler, & Bristow, 2004) with regard to this issue. (These recommendations are dealt with in more detail in Chapter 11.)

- Health services in underserved areas: It is crucial to improve the quality of health services in underserved African-American communities. This might include increasing federal funding for hospitals in medically underserved areas; increased funds would go towards financing high-quality medical equipment and the salaries of highly performing physicians/other medical personnel. Other initiatives might include increasing the availability of incentives to physicians to relocate to underserved areas (e.g., increase Medicaid and Medicare reimbursement rates for providers practicing in underserved communities).

Summary

In this chapter, we have argued that there are serious health inequities affecting African-American men and that these inequities are often socially determined; in other words they can often be attributed to the multitude of social and environmental factors which impact the lives of African-American men. Indeed, one would be hard pressed to find a population group that better illustrates the social determinants of health. In this chapter, we have illustrated the social determinants of health among African-American men with reference to three interrelated areas—the social determinants of health status, the social determinants of health behavior, and the social determinants of health care. Additionally we have made a number of recommendations for tackling socially determined health inequities affecting African-American men. These recommendations relate to research and programs, social policies, and health policies. Ultimately, funding bodies, researchers, program developers, and policy makers must adopt a broader framework for understanding and tackling health inequities (Gadson, 2006); they must address the underlying social determinants of health among African-American men.

Key Terms

African-American men	social determinants of health behavior
health behavior	social determinants of health care
health disparities	social determinants of health inequities
health equity	social determinants of health status
health inequities	socially determined health inequities
incarceration	underserved populations
low socioeconomic status	
racial discrimination	
social determinants of health	

Discussion Questions

1. Were you surprised to learn the extent of health status inequities affecting African-American men? Why/Why not?

2. Low socioeconomic status, racial discrimination, and incarceration were presented in this chapter as key determinants of African-American men's health. Do you agree with this assessment? Why/Why not?

3. How important are "social determinants of health status" versus "social determinants of health behavior" versus "social determinants of health care" as determinants of health among African-American men? In other words, are these three components equally important in terms of their potential to affect African-American men's health outcomes? Why/Why not?

4. Discuss the advantages and potential barriers to implementing the strategies suggested for addressing socially determined health inequities faced by African-American men. Can you think of any additional strategies?

Notes

1. This chapter draws largely from Xanthos, C., Treadwell, H., & Braithwaite-Holden, K. (2010). Social determinants of health among African-American men. *Journal of Men's Health, 7*(1): 11–19. Copyright Elsevier (2010).

References

Adler, N. E., & Snibbe, A. C. (2003). The role of psychosocial processes in explaining the gradient between socioeconomic status and health. *Current Directions in Psychological Science, 12*(4), 119–123.

American Lung Association. (2007). *State of lung disease in diverse communities: 2007.* New York, NY: American Lung Association. Available from http://www.lungusa.org/assets/documents/publications/lung-disease-data/SOLDDC_2007.pdf

APA Online. (2006). *Americans engage in unhealthy behaviors to manage stress.* Washington, DC: APA. Available from http://www.apa.org/news/press/releases/2006/01/stress-management.aspx

Bach, P. B., Pham, H. H., Schrag, D., Tate, R. C., & Hargraves, J. L. (2004). Primary care physicians who treat blacks and whites. *New England Journal of Medicine, 351,* 575–584.

Banks, I. (2004). New models for providing men with health care. *Journal of Men's Health & Gender, 1,* 155–158.

Baum, A., Garofalo, J. P., & Yali, A. M. (1999). Socioeconomic status and chronic stress: Does stress account for SES effects on health? *Annals of the New York Academy of Sciences, 896,* 131–144.

Bird, C., & Rieker, P. P. (1999). Gender matters: An integrated model for understanding men's and women's health. *Social Science and Medicine, 48*(6), 745–755.

Braithwaite-Holden K., & Xanthos, C. (2009). Disadvantages in mental health care among African Americans. *Journal of Health Care for the Poor and Underserved, 20*(2A), 17–23.

Bullard, R. D. (1990). *Dumping in Dixie: Race, class and environmental quality.* Boulder, CO: Westview Press.

Cardarelli, R., & Chiapa, A. L. (2007). Educating primary care clinicians about health disparities. *Osteopathic Medicine and Primary Care*, *1*(5).

Courtenay, W. H. (2000). Behavioral factors associated with disease, injury, and death among men: Evidence and implications for prevention. *Journal of Men's Studies*, *9*, 81–142.

Courtland, L. (1991). Empowering young black males. *ERIC Digest*, ERIC Document Reproduction Service No. ED341887.

Danziger, S., Reed, D., & Brown, T. (2004). *Poverty and prosperity: Prospects for reducing racial/ethnic economic disparities in the United States.* Geneva, Switzerland: UNRISD. Available from http://www.unrisd.org/80256B3C005BCCF9/(httpAuxPages)/ED2687548CA0C7C380256B6D0057867E/$file/danziger.pdf

Dubé, C., Fuller, B., Rosen, R., Fagan, M., & O'Donnell, J. (2005). Men's experiences of physical exams and cancer screening tests: A qualitative study. *Preventive Medicine*, *40*, 628–635.

Felix-Aaron, K., Moy, E., Kang, M., Patel, M., Chesley, F. D., & Clancy, C. (2005). Variation in quality of men's health care by race/ethnicity and social class. *Medical Care*, *43*, 172–181.

Fenning, P., & Rose, J. (2007). Overrepresentation of African American students in exclusionary discipline: The role of school policy. *Urban Education*, *42*, 536–559.

Gadson, S. L. (2006). The third world health status of black American males. *Journal of the National Medical Association*, *98*(4), 488–491.

Gaston, D. (2009). Improving African Americans access to quality healthcare, in the National Urban League (Ed.), *The state of Black America: 2009* (pp. 73–86). New York, NY: National Urban League.

Gehlert, S., Sohmer, D., Sacks, T., Mininger, C., McClintock, M., & Olopade, O. (2008). Targeting health disparities: A model linking upstream determinants to downstream interventions. *Health Affairs*, *27*(2), 339–349.

Geronimus, A. T., Hicken, M., Keene, D., & Bound, J. (2006). "Weathering" and age patterns of allostatic load scores among blacks and whites in the United States. *American Journal of Public Health*, *96*(5), 826–833.

Graham, L., Treadwell. H., & Braithwaite. K. (2008). Social policy, imperiled communities and HIV/AIDS transmission in prisons: A call for zero tolerance. *Journal of Men's Health*, *5*(4), 267–273.

Hayanga, A., Kaiser, H., Sinha, R., Berenholtz, S., Makary, M., & Chang, D. (2009). Residential segregation and access to surgical care by minority populations in US counties. *Journal of the American College of Surgeons*, *208*(6), 1017–1022.

Henry J. Kaiser Family Foundation. (2006). *Fact sheet: Young African American men in the United States.* Washington, DC: Author. Available from http://www.kff.org/minorityhealth/upload/7541.pdf

Henry J. Kaiser Family Foundation. (2007). Fact sheet. The health status of African American Men in the United States. Washington, DC: Author. Available from http://www.kff.org/minorityhealth/upload/7630.pdf

Krieger, N., & Sidney, S. (1996). Racial discrimination and blood pressure: The CARDIA study of young Black and White adults. *American Journal of Public Health*, *86*(10), 1370–1378.

LaVeist, T. A., & Wallace, Jr., J. M. (2000). Health risk and inequitable distribution of liquor stores in African American neighborhood. *Social Science & Medicine, 51*(4), 613–617.

Marmot, M. G., & Shipley, M. J. (1996). Do socioeconomic differences in mortality persist after retirement? 25-year follow up of civil servants from the first Whitehall study. *British Medical Journal, 313,* 1177–1180.

Massoglia, M. (2008). Incarceration as exposure: The prison, infectious disease, and other stress-related illnesses. *Journal of Health and Social Behavior, 49*(1), 56–71.

McGibbon, E., Etowa, J., & McPherson, C. (2008). Health care access as a social determinant of health. *Canadian Nurse, 104*(7), 22–27.

Melfi, C., Croghan, T., Hanna, M., & Robinson, R. (2000). Racial variation in antidepressant treatment in a Medicaid population. *Journal of Clinical Psychiatry, 61,* 16–21.

Monroe, C. R. (2005). Why are "bad boys" always Black? Causes of disproportionality in school discipline and recommendations for change. *Clearing House, 79*(1), 45–50.

Mullins, C. D., Blatt, L., Gbarayor, C. M., Yang, H. K., & Baquet, C. (2005). Health disparities: A barrier to high-quality care. *American Journal of Health Systems Pharmacy, 62,* 1873–1882.

National Center for Health Statistics. (2007). *Health, United States, 2007, with chartbook on trends in the health of Americans.* Hyattsville, MD: National Center for Health Statistics. Available from http://www.cdc.gov/nchs/data/hus/hus07.pdf

National Urban League. (2007). *State of Black America: Portrait of the Black male.* Silver Spring, MD: Beckham.

NIDCR. (2008). *Are you at risk for oral cancer? What African American men need to know.* Bethesda, MD: National Institute of Dental and Craniofacial Research. Available from http://www.nidcr.nih.gov/OralHealth/Topics/OralCancer/AfricanAmericanMen/oral_exam_brochure.htm

NIDCR. (2010). *Oral cancer statistics.* Bethesda, MD: National Institute of Dental and Caraniofacial Research. Available from http://www.nidcr.nih.gov/OralHealth/Topics/OralCancer/OralCancerStatistics.htm

Office of Minority Health. (2008a). *Stroke and African Americans.* Rockville, MD: U.S. Department of Health & Human Services, Office of Minority Health. Available from http://www.omhrc.gov/templates/content.aspx?lvl=2&lvlID=51&ID=3022

Office of Minority Health. (2008b). *African American profile.* Rockville, MD: U.S. Department of Health & Human Services, Office of Minority Health. Available from http://www.omhrc.gov/templates/browse.aspx?lvl=2&lvlID=51

Office of Minority Health (2010). *Men's health 101.* Available from http://minorityhealth.hhs.gov/templates/browse.aspx?lvl=3&lvlid=278

Pager, D. (2003). The mark of a criminal record. *American Journal of Sociology, 108*(5), 937–975.

Randall, V. (2006). *Dying while black.* Dayton, OH: Seven Principles Press.

Raphael, D., Anstice, S. Raine, K., McGannon, K. R., Rizvi, S. K., & Yu, V. (2003). The social determinants of the incidence and management of type 2 diabetes mellitus: Are we prepared to rethink our questions and redirect our research activities? *Leadership in Health Services, 16*(3), 10–20.

Roderick, M. (2003). What's happening to the boys? Early high school experiences and school outcomes among African American male adolescents in Chicago. *Urban Education*, *38*(5), 538–607.

Sabol, W. J., & Couture, H. (2008). *Prison inmates at midyear 2007*. NCJ 221944. Washington, DC: Bureau of Justice Statistics. Available from http://bjs.ojp.usdoj.gov/content/pub/pdf/pim07.pdf usdoj.gov/bjs/pub/pdf/pim07.pdf

Salend, S. J., Duhaney, L. M., & Montgomery, W. (2002). A comprehensive approach to identifying and addressing issues of disproportionate representation. *Remedial and Special Education*, *23*, 289–299.

Satcher, D. (2003). Overlooked and underserved: Improving the health of men of color. *American Journal of Public Health*, *93*(5), 707–709.

Schott Foundation. (2006). *Given half a chance: The Schott 50 state report on public education and Black males*. Cambridge, MA: Schott Foundation for Public Education.

Smedley, B. D., Butler, A. S., & Bristow, L. R. (2004). (Eds.). *In the nation's compelling interest: Ensuring diversity in the health-care workforce*. Washington, DC: National Academies Press.

Smedley, B. D., Stith, A. Y., & Nelson, A. R. (Eds.). (2002). *Unequal treatment: Confronting racial and ethnic disparities in health care*. Washington, DC: National Academies Press.

Taylor, T. R., Williams, C. D., Makambi, K. H., Mouton, C., Harrell, J. P., Cozier, Y., Palmer, J. R., Rosenberg, L., Adams-Campbell, L. L. (2007). Racial discrimination and breast cancer incidence in U.S. Black women: The Black Women's Health Study. *American Journal of Epidemiology*, *166*, 46–54.

Treadwell, H. M., & Ro, M. (2003). Poverty, race, and the invisible men. *American Journal of Public Health*, *93*(5), 705–707.

U.S. Department of Education. (1995). *Findings from the condition of education 1994: No 2: The educational progress of Black students*. Washington, DC: National Center for Educational Statistics, Office of Educational Research and Improvement.

USRDS. (2005). *United States renal data system*. Bethesda, MD: National Institutes of Health, National Institute of Diabetes and Digestive and Kidney Diseases. Available from http://www.usrds.org/

Van Ryn, M., & Burke, J. (2000). The effect of patient race and socio-economic status on physicians' perceptions of patients, *Social Science & Medicine*, *50*(6), 813–828.

Williams, D. R. (1999). Race, socioeconomic status, and health: the added effects of racism and discrimination. *Annals of the New York Academy of Sciences*, *896*, 173–188.

Williams, D. R., & Collins, C. (2001) Racial residential segregation: A fundamental cause of racial disparities in health. *Public Health Reports*, *116*(5), 404–416.

Williams, N. (2006). *Where are the men?: The impact of incarceration and reentry on African American Men and their children and families*. Atlanta, GA: Community Voices, Morehouse School of Medicine.

Woods, V. D., Montgomery, S., Belliard, J. C., Ramírez-Johnson, J., & Wilson, C. M. (2004). Culture, black males, and prostate cancer: What is reality? *Cancer Control*, *11*(6), 388–396.

Xanthos, C. (2008). *The secret epidemic: Exploring the mental health crisis affecting adolescent African-American males*. Atlanta, GA: Community Voices, Morehouse School of Medicine.

Xanthos, C. (2009). *Feeling the strain: The impact of stress on the health of African-American men*. Atlanta, GA: Community Voices, Morehouse School of Medicine.

Xanthos, C., Treadwell, H., & Braithwaite-Holden, K. (2010). Social determinants of health among African-American men, *Journal of Men's Health, 7*(1), 11–19.

Zerhouni, E. (2002). *Prostate cancer research plan FY 2003–FY 2008*. Bethesda, MD: NIH. Available from http://planning.cancer.gov/pdfprgreports/prostateplan.pdf

Part One

Social Determinants of Health Status

Implications of Racism for African-American Men's Cancer Risk, Morbidity, and Mortality

Derek M. Griffith
Jonetta L. Johnson

Learning Objectives

- Describe the epidemiology and patterning of African-American men's cancer morbidity and mortality.
- Explain the influence of cultural racism and cultural schemas on African-American men's cancer outcomes and lives.
- Describe how aspects of socialization influence African-American men's health behaviors and cancer health outcomes.
- Discuss how elements of African-American men's social environment affect their overall health and cancer risk.
- Describe the mechanisms by which race-based neighborhood segregation affect African-American men's cancer risk.

• • •

Although gender and racial differences in health are well documented (Dressler, Oths, & Gravlee, 2005; National Center for Health Statistics, 2008; Williams, 2003), what is less clear is how race and gender intersect to produce strikingly and consistently poor health outcomes for men of color, particularly African-American men (Griffith, Johnson, Ellis, & Schulz, 2010; Read & Gorman, 2006; Treadwell, Northridge, & Bethea, 2007). In this chapter, we explore why African-American men's cancer risk, morbidity, and mortality consistently lag behind African-American and white women, and other groups of men using a framework based on cultural and institutional racism (Griffith et al., 2010; Griffith, Neighbors, & Johnson, 2009; Griffith, Schulz, Johnson, & Herbert, 2009; Griffith, Yonas, Mason, & Havens, 2009). This framework is based on the premise that cultural and institutional racism are gendered and the intersection of racism and gender are root causes of African-American men's health, particularly cancer, outcomes.[1]

Racism may be considered a fundamental determinant of health because it is a dynamic process that endures and adapts over time, and because it influences multiple factors that ultimately affect health (Griffith, Schulz, et al., 2009; Griffith et al., 2010). Racism is both a process and an outcome that is embedded within the institutional and legal structures of U.S. society (Griffith, Childs, Eng, & Jeffries, 2007). Viewed as a process, racism is "an organized system, rooted in an ideology of inferiority that is linked to the political power to categorize, rank, and differentially allocate societal resources to human population groups" (Williams & Rucker, 2000, p. 76). As such, racism influences health over the life course by shaping access to environmental resources and stressors critical to African Americans' health behavior and health outcomes. Racial disparities in health—in this case racial disparities in cancer—can be characterized as an outcome of racism. Conceptualizing cancer risk and outcomes in terms of racism allows us to consider and incorporate links between the environment, behavior, and outcomes of African-American men diagnosed with cancer and at risk for cancer. Although this chapter primarily discusses racism as a process, the distinction between racism as a process and an outcome is useful for studying racism's contributions to racial disparities in health (Griffith, Neighbors, et al., 2009).

Racism can be perceived when individuals subjectively interpret a negative experience to be the result of racism; internalized when persons accept the ideology of racial inferiority; personally mediated when persons are discriminated against or treated differently by others because of their race; or institutionalized due to restricted access to material resources and opportunities for empowerment throughout society (Neighbors, Griffith, & Carty, 2008). Racism can also be cultural or individual and institutional expressions of racial and cultural superiority (Jones, 1997). Although the psychological experience of perceived, internalized, and personally mediated racism is important, racism also affects health through multiple environmental mechanisms and pathways.

African-American Men and Cancer

Disparities in cancer mortality rates between African Americans and whites have widened over the years for all cancers combined and for most major cancers (Powe, Jemal, Cooper, & Harmond, 2009). Men have slightly less than a 1 in 2 lifetime risk of developing cancer, a risk that increases dramatically for African-American men (American Cancer Society [ACS], 2011). For African-American men 45 and older, cancer is the first or second leading cause of death (U.S. Centers for Disease Control and Prevention [CDC], 2008; Taylor et al., 2001). African-American men have approximately a 37 percent higher death rate from cancer than white men (Powe et al., 2009). From 1975 to the early 1990s, the disparity in death rates from all cancers combined between African-American and white males widened. Though the gap narrowed during the 1990s, it remains larger than it was in 1975 (Ward et al., 2004). Of all cancers, prostate, lung, and bronchus, and colon and rectal cancers have both the highest incidence and mortality rates for African-American men. Together, these three cancers constituted 60 percent of all cancer incidence and 54 percent of all cancer mortality for African-American males (ACS, 2009). When compared to white men's rates of lung, prostate, and colon cancers, African-American men have a higher incidence and mortality rate, a lower five-year survival rate, less cancer diagnosed at early or localized stages, are less likely to undergo screening tests, and have less access to appropriate and timely cancer treatment (ACS, 2009). African-American men have the highest rate of prostate cancer in the world (twice the incidence of white men in the United States) and the lowest rate of survival (Vogt et al., 2003). African-American men's rates of developing prostate cancer also tend to be higher than African-American women's rates of developing breast cancer (34 percent versus 25 percent). These men's lifetime probability of dying from prostate cancer is higher than African-American women's probability of dying from breast cancer 4.43 (1 in 23) versus 3.22 (1 in 31) (ACS, 2009). African-American men's rates of developing and dying from colon and rectal cancer are approximately the same as African-American women's, but African-American men overall are more likely to die from cancer than African-American women and have a higher incidence and mortality rate from lung cancer.

In sum, cancer, and specifically cancer of the prostate, lung, and bronchus, and colon and rectum—have remained leading causes of cancer death for African-American men over the past three decades, while advances in public health and medicine have contributed to dramatic improvements in quality of life and life expectancy overall. The advances across the health fields have had minimal impact on persistent disparities in morbidity and mortality between racial and ethnic groups (Frohlich & Potvin, 2008; Sankar et al., 2004) and between African-American men and women (ACS, 2009). These patterns of disease suggest that race and gender play a critical role in African-American men's cancer morbidity and mortality, and that underlying social determinants of health may drive persistent racial and gender differences in health outcomes.

Cultural Racism and the Social Environment

The next section discusses how cultural and social factors affect and shape African-American men's cancer risk, morbidity, and mortality.

Cultural Racism

Culture is the medium through which race is defined and takes on meaning in society, making culture integral to any discussion of racism and racial disparities. Although some have described culture as a blueprint for living in society (Jones, 1997), micro-macro social theories explicitly recognize that social actors shape, use, and re-create culture at the same time that culture shapes and influences individuals (Carpiano & Daley, 2006; Cockerham, 2007; Ortner, 1989; Risjord, 2007). Such definitions of culture also move away from the idea of culture as a single internally consistent framework and toward the notion that culture is composed of different bits of information and schematic structures that organize that information (Dimaggio, 1997). Thus, racism is not a single fixed view of race or racism (Mullings, 2005), but a dynamic story with several subplots that incorporate power relations and historical contexts (Frederickson, 2002; Griffith et al., 2010).

In a race-conscious society, **cultural racism** reflects attitudes, values, and beliefs about races and the importance of race in society. Processes of racialization involve the emergence of cultural notions of racial and ethnic hierarchy, or cultural racism that become institutionalized in legislation or in institutional policies (Jones, 1997; Wade, 1993). To the extent that these forms of institutional racism become taken for granted as forms of practice and viewed as rational and correct, they can reinforce and accentuate cultural racism, illustrating the idea of mutual constitution (Wade, 1993). **Cultural schemas** offer one way of understanding culture and cultural racism as dynamic processes rather than static entities. Cultural schemas are plots or story lines that emerge within social groups to provide frameworks for individual actors and illustrate ways to respond to imbedded contradictions within a social system or institution (Ortner, 1989).

Cultural notions of **male gender** are similar to cultural racism. Complex and dynamic, gender intersects with cultural racism to influence the cultural schemas that shape African-American men's lives and cancer outcomes. Male gender is signified by beliefs and behaviors that are practiced in social interactions and, therefore, varies among cultures, subcultures, and individuals (Moynihan, 1998). Part of the way gender functions, however, is to hide contradictions about how men ought to behave, and what type of power and authority men should have and appear as though gender is a static fact of nature, assumed to consist of unchanging, transhistorical naturally occurring traits (Bederman, 1996). This process is based on arbitrary historical and ideological processes linking male genital anatomy, male identity, and social arrangements of authority and power, despite the fact that these factors have no intrinsic relationship. For African-American men, race, identity, and ideals of **masculinity** are often defined by white society. African-American men often become obsessed with attempts to fulfill white supremacist notions of masculinity (Gordon, 1997; hooks, 1992). For African-American males, notions of masculinity are viewed as symbols of economic standing and sexual opportunity (hooks, 1992). Notions of masculinity assigned and defined to African-American males by mainstream white society are often the cause of internal conflict and painful attempts by these men to acknowledge, fulfill, or reject such roles and identity (hooks, 1992). How men operationalize these notions and beliefs is filtered, in part, through their physical characteristics.

Physical characteristics—race, gender, height, stature—often lead to certain encounters that promote **socialization** processes (Stevenson, 1996). Although there are separate literatures on **racial socialization** (Stevenson, 1996) and **male gender socialization** (Courtenay, 2000; Nicholas, 2000; Pleck, 1981), what is less common in the literature is a description of the intersection of these processes. African-American men's lives, health, and health behaviors are shaped both by male gender socialization—the process by which men learn the gender and culturally ascribed behaviors that characterize masculinity in a particular society—and racial socialization, the process by which people's sense of racial identity is shaped by families and communities through oppressive and affirming experiences throughout the lifespan.

African-American men's sense of racial and gender identity are shaped by broader processes of cultural socialization: the broader context for understanding gender, ethnicity, sexual orientation and racial identity development (Stevenson, 1997). It is not only through interaction with people of their own race, gender, or identity group that is important, but it is how people are treated when they interact with people of other groups, and how that difference is interpreted, that influences how people see themselves and their group membership. For African-American men, this process is not one of simply race or gender, but the intersection of the two (Griffith, 2012).

African-American men, their physical bodies and images, face a complex duality in current U.S. society in which they are both worshiped and materialized as entertainers and athletes, and yet at the same time are associated with heightened notions of fear and disdain (Ferber, 2007). African-American men were characterized as criminal, sex crazed, violent and degenerate, and these characteristics were evidence of their constitutional weakness (Hutchinson, 1996). Books and articles in scholarly journals argued that African-American men were defective, hopelessly inferior, and crime- and violence-prone beings from which society had to be protected (Hutchinson, 1996). Such perceptions of African-American men in society are maintained by whites and some African Americans and work to reinforce systems of cultural racism and processes of socialization. The expectations of people outside of the African-American community, expectations of African-American women, and expectations of other African-American men shape and influence current and future health behaviors and larger social norms and expectations.

Social Environment

The **social environment** describes the cultural values, beliefs, and norms regarding diverse aspects of life (including but not limited to health), as well as the social institutions, networks, and resources in these settings. For African-American men, gender, race, and class interact in complex ways to increase the risk for various illnesses (Bowman, 1989), including cancer. Among African Americans, racism limits access to social and economic resources that may alleviate or prevent acute and chronic stress that has a direct and negative effect on health (McEwen, 1998; Schulz et al., 2009). African-American men are exposed to more psychosocial stressors than other racial and gender groups over the life course (Bowman, 1989; Watkins & Neighbors, 2007; Williams, 2003), increasing health risks.

Jackson and Knight (2006) argue that stressful social and economic living conditions, combined with restricted access to a range of potential resources to manage those conditions, may contribute to behavioral responses to stress that may adversely affect cancer outcomes. In addition to the direct and indirect influences of stressful living conditions, family members influence each others' health through socially learned and normative coping mechanisms for mediating, mitigating, and diffusing stress (Jackson & Knight, 2006). Family members provide examples of shared patterns of food preparation, eating, and other health behaviors (Semmes, 1996). Foods high in fat and carbohydrates prepared as part of holiday meals and other positive events become associated with reward, honor, and love, and eating large portions is a gendered way that African-American men can show appreciation for these expressions of love. These expressions convey and affirm common values and define collective identity (Semmes, 1996). The family provides an important social context for understanding health behavior, as it is the primary place people learn health and coping behavior; however, in some contexts these lessons can have a negative effect on health.

Coping with stress can indirectly affect health through increasing cravings and consumption of foods high in fat and carbohydrates and increasing rates of tobacco use, physical inactivity, and substance abuse (Jackson & Knight, 2006). Over time, these social and economic conditions contribute to chronic stress, increase risk for poor health outcomes, and reduce chances for social or economic success (Massey & Denton, 1988). To the extent that such **health behaviors** (e.g., unhealthy dietary practices, tobacco use, substance abuse, and physical inactivity) and health outcomes (e.g., increased cancer risk, morbidity, and mortality) become social norms, they have the potential to become parts of the social environment of African Americans. For example, opportunities to consume foods high in fats or carbohydrates, smoke tobacco, drink alcohol, and be physically inactive are disproportionately available in many predominantly African-American, poverty-dense communities and may become socially acceptable strategies for managing life stressors, increasing the risk for lung and colon cancer.

African-American men's health behavior seems to contribute to their rates of lung and colon cancer (Koh, 2009), but it is unclear how their behavior contributes to prostate cancer risk (Brawley & Wallington, 2009); thus, we briefly review behavioral risk factors for lung and colon cancer but not prostate cancer. Tobacco use, particularly smoking, is the primary risk factor for lung cancer (ACS, 2011; Koh, 2009). Despite African-American adolescents and adults smoking fewer cigarettes per day than their white counterparts, their rates of mortality from lung cancer tend to be higher (Koh, Elqura, & Short, 2009). In addition to smoking being a major risk factor for lung cancer, smokers are 30 to 40 percent more likely to die from colorectal cancer than nonsmokers, and it has been estimated that up to 12 percent of colorectal cancer deaths are due to smoking (Gatof & Ahnen, 2002). Dietary composition, physical inactivity, and alcohol use also are behavioral risk factors for colorectal cancer, as is **obesity** (Schneider, 2006). African-American men tend to have lower rates of obesity and higher levels of leisure time physical activity when compared to African-American women, but their elevated incidence and mortality from colon and prostate cancers relative to white men (ACS, 2009) suggests the continued need for diligence and improvement in health behaviors associated with cancer risk reduction.

Abuse of alcohol and illegal drugs is more common among men than women and research has demonstrated that alcohol use among various populations is associated with the presence of masculine attitudes (Hegelson, 1994). **Substance abuse** may occur as a response to stress, physiological addiction, difficult life circumstances, and other environmental factors (Brooks, 2001). African-American men may be at increased risk for substance abuse because of the daily stresses they face and the socially sanctioned nature of substance use as a coping strategy for men. Men with limited educational and employment opportunities may turn to alcohol and other drugs as an escape from their inability to live up to social expectations of men in the United States (Brooks, 2001), increasing their risk of colon cancer in particular.

Race-Based Residential Segregation and the Built Environment

U.S. cultural notions of racial inferiority and superiority become part of institutional structures and processes that organize and promote the values and standards of a race-conscious society (Jones, 1997). **Race-based residential segregation** is pervasive in the United States, structuring access to social and physical resources differentially by racial group (Schulz, Williams, Israel, & Lempert, 2002). The origins of race-based residential segregation in the United States can be traced back to efforts by white Americans to remain residentially separate from African Americans because of ideological beliefs about the inferiority of African Americans (Collins & Williams, 1999). Race-based residential segregation is a concrete example of the effects of institutional racism and represents the unequal distribution of economic, educational, and social resources and opportunities by race, not the racial distribution per se, that results in racial differences in exposure to unequal physical environments, educational systems, and economic opportunities and therefore racial disparities in health (Geronimus & Thompson, 2004). **Institutional racism** has been defined as a systematic set of patterns, procedures, practices, and policies that operate within institutions so as to consistently penalize, disadvantage, and exploit communities and individuals of color (Better, 2002). The concept describes the systematic operation of an institution and highlights the historical, social, and political aspects of systems that influence practices and policies that may not seem to be affected by race but can still produce differential outcomes (Griffith et al., 2007). Race-based residential segregation is an important aspect of institutional racism.

For African Americans, race-based residential segregation increases social isolation and limits social and economic capital and social mobility (Collins & Williams, 1999; Massey, 2004). The goal of **segregation** was to economically, politically, and socially subordinate African Americans to white Americans (Bell, 2004). In addition, allotments of money for educational facilities, infrastructure development, and economic opportunities consistently favored white Americans (Bell, 2004). Race-based residential segregation leads to poorer real estate investment return and unequal access to community resources through divestment of economic resources and reduction of services. Residential segregation, in addition to being influenced by institutional racism and its role in determining neighborhood access to economic resources, also negatively impacts African-Americans' economic independence by isolating them from key resources, such as safety, wealth, and employment opportunities (Massey & Denton, 1998; Wilson 1987).

There is a high correlation between **poverty** and residential segregation for African Americans. For example, 24 percent of African Americans live below the federal poverty threshold compared to only 8 percent of whites (ACS, 2009; DeNavas-Walt, Procter, & Smith, 2007). Opportunities for employment are more limited in poverty-dense neighborhoods, and the jobs that are available tend to be either low-paying and with few benefits, or high-skill white-collar jobs; however, due to compromised educational opportunities, many residents of poverty-dense communities are unable to compete for the white-collar positions (Darden, 1986; Farley, Danziger, & Holzer, 2000). In addition, the effect of concentrated poverty in residentially segregated African-American neighborhoods has important implications for African-Americans' ability to accumulate resources and transfer wealth to children and grandchildren (Collins & Williams, 1999).

Health insurance, which in the United States is tied to employment status, is an important health-promoting resource in African-Americans' economic environment. Greater numbers of African Americans than whites lack health insurance or are underinsured (Sandman, Simantov, & An, 2000). As discussed earlier, opportunities for employment are maldistributed as a function of race-based residential segregation and poverty (Geronimus & Thompson, 2004). Segregation and concentrated poverty also tend to be associated with low-skilled, low-paying jobs that are less likely to provide comprehensive health insurance. However, even among those who are insured, cost and access to care still can be significant factors increasing one's cancer risk. For example, African-American men are less likely than white males to undergo screening tests for colon and prostate cancers (ACS, 2009). This trend may be due to decreased access to health resources for cancer screening as a result of **low neighborhood socioeconomic status (SES)**, or decreased acquisition of personal health insurance at the levels of **individual SES**. The availability of and access to health care screening services is an important mediating factor for improving outcomes associated with colon cancer among African-American men.

Low SES at the neighborhood level influences cancer risk by minimizing and restricting access to physical activity and healthy food outlets, adult literacy resources, insurance, and participation in other behaviors and resources necessary to maintain health. African-American neighborhoods have been found to have more fast-food outlets and liquor stores, fewer supermarkets, fewer shelf choices in the stores that are available, increased exposure to tobacco products, greater distances to fitness facilities, less work-site fitness opportunities, fewer recreational facilities, and more neighborhood crime (Feighery, Schleicher, Cruz, & Unger, 2008; Schulz et al., 2005; Zenk et al., 2006a, 2006b).

Research on advertisement of tobacco products shows excess distribution of cigarette ads in stores located in minority and low socioeconomic status (SES) communities (Feighery et al., 2008; Laws, Whitman, Bowser, & Krech,

2002; Wildey et al., 1992). The sale and distribution of single cigarettes, **loosies**, is a common form of tobacco consumption that often overcomes barriers of age and price by providing a lower purchase price, easier access to cigarettes for youth smoking and may result in earlier addiction ages to tobacco (Smith et al., 2007). Research by Feighery et al. (2008) found that when controlling for income and store type, the amount of cigarette ads and the proportion of cigarette ads offering a sales promotion rose more rapidly in stores located in neighborhoods with higher proportions of African Americans. Results from a meta-analysis conducted by Primack et al. (2007) reveal that compared to majority white market areas, African-American market areas had significantly higher density and concentration of advertising materials and messages promoting tobacco use.

Research has illustrated that the availability of a grocery store in an African-American community is directly related to the consumption of fresh fruits and vegetables (Morland, Diez Roux, & Wing, 2006; Morland, Wing, & Diez Roux, 2002), making race-based residential segregation and the built environment critical factors in promoting health dietary practices. Availability of and access to physical activity outlets is another important feature of the built environment with implications for health behaviors that shape cancer incidence and mortality.

Cities and communities can have roads, schools, homes, and workplaces that are built in ways that require driving and discourage walking and bike riding (Hayne, Morgan, & Ford, 2004). Bike and walking paths, community centers, activity spaces and parks, and workplaces with usable stairwells or gyms are several features used to rate the quality of health promoting resources in an environment or neighborhood. Risk associated with colon cancer and prostate cancer may be mediated with regular physical activity (ACS, 2009; Prostate Cancer Foundation, 2009). Neighborhood level density of physical activity outlets has been found to be negatively associated with body mass index (BMI) and insulin resistance after adjusting for individual level variables such as age, sex, income, education, race/ethnicity, and family history of diabetes (Auchincloss, 2008). In addition to the quality and quantity of resources offered, residentially segregated African-American neighborhoods are often in close proximity to industrial facilities and areas such as highways and bus depots, which increase exposure to air pollution (Frumkin, 2005; Gunier, Hertz, Von Behren, & Reynold, 2003; Lopez & Hynes, 2006; Perlin, Sexton, & Wong, 1999).

Estimating cancer risk associated with ambient air toxics across several racial and ethnic groups, Morello-Frosch and Jesdale (2006) found a significant relationship between increasing levels of racial/ethnic segregation and increased cancer risk. The association between ambient air toxics and racial and ethnic segregation remained after controlling for area-level SES. In addition, the cancer risk associated with ambient air toxics for all racial groups combined was intensified with increasing levels of racial/ethnic segregation, with effects strongest in areas with the highest levels of segregation (Morello-Frosch & Jesdale, 2006). As operating within the boundaries of residential segregation, aspects of the economic environment are widespread in their patterning of access to health-enhancing forms of support and resources at levels of the built and social environments that determine and shape cancer risk, morbidity, and mortality for African-American men.

In addition to the direct availability of tobacco-related products, excess media advertising of not only tobacco, but unhealthy food and alcohol, is a common aspect of the social environment of many African-American communities. Although relatively few studies have assessed **target marketing** of unhealthy food and beverages in African-American communities (Kratz, Ponce, & Yancey, 2008), the few studies on this topic have found that more food advertisements were shown during shows targeting African-American audiences than general market shows (Grier & Kumanyika, 2008; Henderson & Kelly, 2005; Tirodkar & Jain, 2003). In addition, ads during shows targeting African-American audiences were more likely than those general market shows aired during prime time to be for unhealthy items such as fast food, candy, soda, or meats and less likely to be for cereals, grains, fruits, vegetables, and pasta (Grier & Kumanyika, 2008; Henderson & Kelly, 2005; Tirodkar & Jain, 2003). Targeted marketing of unhealthy foods and tobacco products influences the media environment encountered by African-American men and has implications for increasing their risk of lung and colon cancer.

Discussion

In this chapter, we have presented a conceptual framework for understanding how racism influences African-American men's cancer risk, morbidity, and mortality and are mediated by the social and built environments. Compared to African-American women and white men and women, African-American men have greater cancer risk, morbidity, and mortality. Interactions between gender and racism are root causes of poor health outcomes and racial disparities in cancer among African-American men. We have traced pathways by which the process of racism, as a gendered and fundamental factor, influence the environment, behavior, and health outcomes of African-American men with cancer and at risk for cancer.

Although our focus for this chapter has been on the intricate relationship between racism and cancer risk, associations between racism and health can be extended to a myriad of health outcomes and populations. Conceptually linking gender, racism, and the environments in which they interact are important steps necessary to uncover fundamental causes of health disparities and develop substantive ways in which they can be eliminated. We suggest that without recognition of the direct and indirect influence of racism as a fundamental and gendered factor shaping environments, health behaviors, and health outcomes, evidence-based and theoretical research is incomplete and has the potential to propose unfounded and risky conclusions for considering African-American men's increased cancer risk, morbidity, and mortality.

Policy Implications and Recommendations

The utility of policy efforts to aid the elimination of cancer disparities facing African-American men are particularly applicable to the discussion of the interaction of racism, gender, and health. Although research on social determinants of health has illustrated the importance of considering race-based residential segregation, poverty, and other environmental factors, less attention has been paid to the role that cultural beliefs, norms, and stereotypes play in shaping health policies and outcomes over time. Although structural and institutional factors resulting from explicit policies and practices are critical, efforts to construct a robust theory of racial inequities in health based solely on these factors is conceptually incomplete. A more fully specified frame for analysis of racial inequality requires examination of the intricate interplay between culture and social structure in forming, shaping, and perpetuating a range of policies and practices that contribute to the persistence of cancer disparities.

It is not enough to examine health policies that affect African Americans; there is an explicit need to consider how policies are differentially affecting people by gender. Health policies that limit and impose restrictions on the content of media advertising of cigarettes, and unhealthy food outlets and liquor stores in racially segregated minority neighborhoods must be examined through a gendered lens to have greater potential to reduce African-American men's cancer risk. Researchers and policy makers should consider how racism is gendered, and how using a gendered lens to examine cancer risk, morbidity, and mortality may help to highlight cultural schemas that underlie formal policies and informal practices that affect African-American men's health.

Summary

In this chapter, we focused on multiple sites of cancer (i.e., lung and bronchus, colon and rectum, and prostate) to illustrate the ways in which gendered aspects of racism are fundamental determinants of African-American men's cancer risk. Specifically, we argue that fundamental factors structured around race and gender influence the intermediate social and physical environments within which individuals live and act, and that African-American men disproportionately live and act in social environments and physical environments that expose them to higher levels of risk associated with the development of cancer, and reduced access to the resources that might help them reduce the negative effects of cancer (Griffith, Schulz et al., 2009). The definition of a fundamental factor—which in this case we argue is racism—is that it operates through multiple pathways to influence health outcomes. Above, we have traced multiple aspects of the social environment (e.g., local policies associated with advertising, effectiveness of policing in maintaining public order) and the physical environment (e.g., presence, location, and quality of food stores, safety of neighborhoods, and conduciveness of physical activity) that place African-American men—particularly those residing in predominantly African-American neighborhoods with high rates of poverty—at heightened risk of developing cancer, and once cancer has developed, offers fewer resources with which to effectively manage this chronic disease.

Key Terms

cultural racism

cultural schemas

culture

diet

disparities

health behavior

health insurance

individual SES

institutional racism

loosies

low neighborhood SES

male gender socialization

male gender

masculinity

obesity

physical activity

poverty

race-based residential segregation

racial socialization

racism

segregation

smokers

social environment

socialization

substance abuse

target marketing

tobacco use

Discussion Questions

1. How do African-American men's patterns of cancer morbidity and mortality compare with African-American women and white men?

2. How does racism affect African-American men's cancer morbidity and mortality?

3. How do socialization processes influence African-American men's health behaviors and cancer health outcomes?

4. How do elements of African-American men's social environment affect their overall health and cancer risk?

5. What are the mechanisms by which race-based neighborhood segregation affects African-American men's cancer risk?

Note

1. This chapter was supported in part by grants from the American Cancer Society (grant number MRSGT-07-167-01-CPPB), the Michigan Center for Urban African American Aging Research, and the University of Michigan Comprehensive Cancer Center, and by two centers at the University of Michigan School of Public Health: the Center on Men's Health Disparities and the Center for Research on Ethnicity, Culture and Health. Its contents are solely the responsibility of the authors and do not necessarily represent the official views of the American Cancer Society or the University of Michigan.

References

American Cancer Society. (2009). *Cancer facts & figures for African Americans 2009–2010*. Atlanta, GA: Author.

American Cancer Society. (2011). *Cancer facts & figures for African Americans 2011–2012*. Atlanta, GA: Author.

Auchincloss, A. H., Diez Roux, A. V., Brown, D. G., Erdmann, C. A., & Bertoni, A. G. (2008). Neighborhood resources for physical activity and healthy foods and their association with insulin resistance. *Epidemiology, 19*(1), 146–157.

Bederman, G. (1996). *Manliness & civilization: A cultural history of gender and race in the United States, 1880–1917*. London, UK: University of Chicago Press.

Bell, D. (2004). *Silent covenants: Brown v. Board of Education and the unfulfilled hopes for racial reform*. New York, NY: Oxford University Press.

Better, S. (2002). *Institutional racism: A primer on theory and strategies for social change*. Chicago, IL: Burnham.

Bowman, P. J. (1989). Research perspectives on black men: Role strain and adaptation across the adult life cycle. In R. L. Jones (Ed.), *Black adult development and aging* (pp. 117–150). Berkeley, CA: Cobb & Henry.

Brooks, G. (2001). Masculinity and men's mental health. *Journal of American College Health, 49*(6), 285.

Brawley, O.W., & Wallington, S. F. (2009). Disparities in prostate. In H. K. Koh (Ed.), *Toward the elimination of cancer disparities* (pp. 179–202). New York, NY: Springer.

Carpiano, R. M., & Daley, D. M. (2006). A guide and glossary on postpositivist theory building for population health. *Journal of Epidemiology and Community Health, 60*, 564–570.

Cockerham, W. C. (2007). *Social causes of health and disease*. Malden, MA: Polity Press.

Collins, C. A., & Williams, D. R. (1999). Segregation and mortality: The deadly effects of racism? *Sociological Forum, 14*, 495–523.

Courtenay, W. H. (2000). Constructions of masculinity and their influence on men's well-being: A theory of gender and health. *Social Science Medicine*, *50*, 1385–1401.

Darden, J. T. (1986). The residential segregation of blacks in Detroit, 1960–1970. *International Journal of Comparative Sociology*, *17*(1–2), 84–91.

DeNavas-Walt C., Proctor, B. D., & Smith, J. (2007). *Income, poverty, and health insurance coverage in the United States: 2006*. Washington, DC: U.S. Census Bureau, Current Population Reports, P60–233.

Dimaggio, P. (1997). Culture and cognition. *Annual Review of Sociology*, *23*, 263–288.

Dressler, W. W., Oths, K.S. & Gravlee, C.C. (2005). Race and ethnicity in public health research: models to explain health disparities. *Annual Review of Anthropology*, *34*, 231–252.

Farley, R., Danzinger, S., & Holzer, H. J. (2000). *Detroit divided*. New York, NY: Russell Sage Foundation.

Feighery, E. C., Schleicher, N. C., Cruz, T. B., & Unger, J. B. (2008). An examination of trends in amount and type of cigarette advertising and sales promotions in California stores, 2002–2005. *Tobacco Control*, *17*(2), 93.

Ferber, A. L. (2007). The construction of black masculinity: White supremacy now and then. *Journal of Sport and Social Issues*, *31*(1), 11–24.

Frederickson, G. M. (2002). *Racism: A short history*. Princeton, NJ: Princeton University Press.

Frohlich, K. L., & Potvin, L. (2008). The inequality paradox: the population approach to vulnerable populations. *American Journal of Public Health*, *98*(2), 216–221.

Frumkin, H. (2005). Health, equity, and the built environment. *Environmental Health Perspectives*, *113*: A290–291.

Gatof, D., & Ahnen, D. (2002). Primary prevention of colorectal cancer: diet and drugs. *Gastroenterology Clinics of North America*, *31*(2), xi, 587–623.

Geronimus, A.T., & Thompson, J. P. (2004). To denigrate, ignore, or disrupt: Racial inequality in health and impact of a policy-induced breakdown of African-American communities. *Du Bois Review: Social Science Research on Race*, *1*(2), 247–279.

Gordon, E. T. (1997). Cultural politics of black masculinity. *Transforming Anthropology*, *6*(1&2), 36–53.

Grier, S. A., & Kumanyika, S. K. (2008). The context for choice: Health implications of targeted food and beverage marketing to African Americans. *American Journal of Public Health*, *98*(9), 1616–1629.

Griffith, D. M. (2012). An intersectional approach to men's health. *Journal of Men's Health*, *9*(2), 106–112.

Griffith, D. M., Childs, E. L., Eng, E., & Jeffries, V. (2007). Racism in organizations: The case of a county public health department. *Journal of Community Psychology*, *35*(3), 291–306.

Griffith, D. M., Johnson, J., Ellis, K., & Schulz, A. J. (2010). Cultural context and a critical approach to eliminating health disparities. *Ethnicity and Disease*, *20*, 71–76.

Griffith, D. M., Neighbors, H. W., & Johnson, J. (2009). Using national data sets to improve the health and mental health of Black Americans: Challenges and opportunities. *Cultural Diversity and Ethnic Minority Psychology*, *15*(1), 86–95.

Griffith, D. M., Schulz, A. J., Johnson, J., & Herbert, K. (2009). Implications of racism for black Americans' diabetes management and outcomes. In L. Jack (Ed.), *Diabetes in black America: Public health and clinical solutions to a national crisis.* Munster, IN: Hilton.

Griffith, D. M., Yonas, M., Mason, M., & Havens, B. (2009). Considering organizational factors in addressing healthcare disparities: Two case examples. *Health Promotion Practice*, e-pub ahead of print April 3, 2009.

Gunier, R. B., Hertz, A., Von Behren, J., & Reynold, P. (2003). Traffic density in California: Socioeconomic and ethnic differences among potentially exposed children. *Journal of Exposure Analysis & Environmental Epidemiology, 13*, 240–246.

Henderson, V. R., & Kelly, B. (2005). Food advertising in the age of obesity: Content analysis of food advertising on general market and African American television. *Journal of Nutrition Education and Behavior, 37*, 191–196.

hooks, b. (1992). Reconstructing black masculinity. In *Black looks: Race and representation* (pp. 87–113). Boston, MA: South End Press.

Hutchinson, E. O. (1996). *The assassination of the black male image.* New York, NY: Simon & Schuster.

Jackson, J. S., & Knight, K. M. (2006). Race and self-regulatory health behaviors: The role of the stress response and the HPA axis in physical and mental health disparities. In K. W. Schair & L. L. Carstensen (Eds.), *Social structures, aging, and self regulation in the elderly* (pp. 189–214), New York, NY: Springer.

Jones, J. M. (1997). *Prejudice and racism* (2nd ed.). New York, NY: McGraw-Hill.

Koh, H. K. (2009). *Toward the elimination of cancer disparities.* New York, NY: Springer.

Koh, H. K., Elqura, L., & Short, S. M. (2009). Disparities in tobacco use and lung cancer. In H. K. Koh (Ed.), *Toward the elimination of cancer disparities* (pp. 109–136). New York, NY: Springer.

Kratz, R. E., Ponce, N. A., & Yancey, A. K. (2008). Process evaluation of the Los Angeles Unified School District. *Preventing Chronic Disease, 5*(2), 1–9.

Laws, M. B., Whitman, J., Bowser, D. M., & Krech, L. (2002). Tobacco availability and point of sale marketing in demographically contrasting districts of Massachusetts. *Tobacco Control, 11*(suppl 2), ii71–ii73.

Lopez, R. P., & Hynes, H. P. (2006). Obesity, physical activity, and the urban environment: Public health research needs. *Environmental Health, 5*, 25–35.

Massey, D. S. (2004). Segregation and stratification: A biosocial perspective. *Du Bois Review, 1*(1), 7–25.

Massey, D. S., & Denton, N. A. (1988). *American apartheid: Segregation and the making of the underclass.* Cambridge, MA: Harvard University Press.

McEwen, B. S. (1998). Stress, adaptation, and disease: Allostasis and allostatic load. *Annals of the New York Academy of Sciences, 840*, 33–34.

Morello-Frosch, R., & Jesdale, B. M. (2006). Separate and unequal: Residential segregation and estimated cancer risks associated with ambient air toxics in U. S. metropolitan areas. *Environmental Health Perspectives, 114*(3), 386–393.

Morland, K., Diez Roux, A. V., & Wing, S. (2006). Supermarkets, other food stores, and obesity: the atherosclerosis risk in communities study. *American Journal of Preventative Medicine, 30*(4), 333–339.

Moynihan, C. (1998). Theories in health care and research: Theories of masculinity. *British Medical Journal, 317*, 1072–1075.

Mullings, L. (2005). Interrogating racism: Toward an antiracist anthropology. *Annual Review of Anthropology*, *34*, 667–693.

Neighbors, H. W., Griffith, D. M., & Carty, D. (2008). Racism. *Encyclopedia of the life course and human development*. Farmington Hills, MI: Gale Cengage.

Nicholas, D. R. (2000). Men, masculinity, and cancer: risk-factor behaviors, early detection, and psychosocial adaptation. *American Journal of College Health*, *49*(1), 27–33.

Nyberg, F., Gustavsson, P., Jarup, L., Bellander, T., Berglind, N., Jakobsson, R., & Pershagen, G. (2000). Urban air pollution and lung cancer in Stockholm. *Epidemiology*, *11*(5), 487–495.

Perlin, S. A., Sexton, K., & Wong, D. W. (1999). An examination of race and poverty for populations living near industrial sources of air pollution. *Journal of Exposure Analysis & Environmental Epidemiology*, *9*, 29–48.

Pleck, J. H. (1981). *The myth of masculinity*. Cambridge, MA: MIT Press.

Powe, B. D., Jemal, A., Cooper, D., & Harmond, L. (2009). Cancer disparities: Data systems, sources and interpretation. In H. K. Koh (Ed.), *Toward the elimination of cancer disparities* (pp. 29–48). New York, NY: Springer.

Prostate Cancer Foundation. (2009). *Nutrition, exercise and prostate cancer*. Santa Monica, CA: Prostate Cancer Foundation.

Read, J. G., & Gorman, B. K. (2006). Gender inequalities in US adult health: the interplay of race and ethnicity. *Social Science and Medicine*, *62*(5), 1045–1065.

Risjord, M. (2007). Ethnography and culture. In S. P. Turner & M. W. Pisjord (Eds.), *Philosophy of anthropology and sociology* (pp. 399–428). Amsterdam, The Netherlands: Elsevier.

Sandman, D., Simantov, E., & An, C. (2000). *Out of touch: American men and the health care system*. New York, NY: Commonwealth Fund.

Sankar, P., Cho, M. K., Condit, C. M., Hunt, L. M., Koenig, B., Marshall, P., . . . Spicer, P. (2004). Genetic research and health disparities. *Journal of the American Medical Association*, *291*(24), 2985–2989.

Schneider, E. C. (2009). Disparities and colorectal cancer. In H. K. Koh (Ed.), *Toward the elimination of cancer disparities* (pp. 161–178). New York, NY: Springer.

Schulz, A. J., Israel, B. A., Zenk, S. N., Parker, E. A., Lichtenstien, R., Shellman-Weir, S. & Klem, A. B. (2006). Psychosocial stress and social support as mediators of relationships between income, length of residence and depressive symptoms among African American women on Detroit's eastside. *Social Science & Medicine*, *62*(2), 510–522.

Schulz, A. J., Williams, D. R., Israel, B. A., & Lempert, L. B. (2002). Racial and spatial relations as fundamental determinants of health in Detroit. *Milbank Quarterly*, *80*(4), 677–707.

Schulz, A. J., Zenk, S., Odoms-Young, A., Hollis-Neely, T., Nwankwo, R., Lockett, M., . . . Kannan, S. (2005). Healthy eating and exercising to reduce diabetes: Exploring the potential of social determinants of health frameworks within the context of community-based participatory diabetes prevention. *American Journal of Public Health*, *95*(4), 645–651.

Semmes, C. E. (1996). Emancipation and the roots of health. In C. E. Semmes (Ed.), *Racism, health, and post-industrialism* (pp. 1–16). Westport, CT: Praeger.

Smith, K., Stillman, F., Bone, L., Yancey, N., Price, E., Belin, P., & Kromm, E. (2007). Buying and selling "loosies" in Baltimore: The informal exchange of cigarettes in the community context. *Journal of Urban Health, 84*(4), 494–507.

Stevenson, H. C. (1996). Development of the scale of racial socialization for African American adolescents. In R. L. Jones (Ed.), *Handbook of tests and measurements for black populations* (Vol. 1, pp. 309–326) Hampton, VA: Cobb & Henry.

Stevenson, H. C. (1997). Managing anger: Protective, proactive or adaptive racial socialization identity profiles and African-American manhood development. In R. J. Watts & R. J. Jagers (Eds), *Manhood development in urban African-American communities* (pp. 35–61). Boca Raton, FL: Hawthorne Press.

Taylor, K. L., Turner, R. O., Davis, J. L. 3rd, Johnson, L., Schwartz, M. D., Kerner, J., & Leak, C. (2001). Improving knowledge of the prostate cancer screening dilemma among African American men: An academic-community partnership in Washington, DC. *Public Health Reports, 116*(6), 590–598.

Tirodkar, M. A., & Jain, A. (2003). Food messages on African American television shows. *American Journal of Public Health, 93*(3), 439–441.

Treadwell, H. M., Northridge, M. E., & Bethea, T. N. (2007). Confronting racism and sexism to improve men's health. *American Journal of Men's Health, 1*(1), 81–86.

Vogt, T. M., Ziegler, R. G., Graubard, B. I., Swanson, C. A., Greenberg, R. S., Schoenberg, J. B., . . . Mayne, S. T. (2003). Serum selenium and risk of prostate cancer in U.S. blacks and whites. *International Journal of Cancer, 103*(5), 664–670.

Wade, J. C. (1993). Institutional racism: An analysis of the mental health system. *American Journal of Orthopsychiatry, 63*(4), 536–544.

Ward, E., Jemal, A., Cokkinides, V., Singh, G., Cardinez, C., Ghafoor, A. & Thun, M. (2004). Cancer disparities by race/ethnicity and socioeconomic status. *CA: A Cancer Journal for Clinicians, 54*, 78–93.

Watkins, D. C., & Neighbors, H. W. (2007). An initial exploration of what mental health means to young black men. *The Journal of Men's Health & Gender, 4*(3), 271–282.

Wildey, M. B., Young, R. L., Elder, J. P., de Moor, C., Wolf, K. R., Fiske, K. E., & Sharp, E. (1992). Cigarette point-of-sale advertising in ethnic neighborhoods in San Diego, California. *Health Values: The Journal of Health Behavior, Education & Promotion, 16*(1), 23–28.

Williams, D. R. (2003). The health of men: Structured inequalities and opportunities. *American Journal of Public Health, 93*, 724–731.

Williams, D. R., & Rucker, T. D. (2000). Understanding and addressing racial disparities in health care. *Health Care Financing Review, 21*(4), 75–90.

Wilson, W. J. (1987). *The truly disadvantaged.* Chicago, IL: University of Chicago Press.

Zenk, S. N., Schulz, A. J., Israel, B. A., James, S. A., Bao, S., & Wilson, M. L. (2006a). Neighborhood racial composition, neighborhood poverty, and the spatial accessibility of supermarkets in metropolitan Detroit. *American Journal of Public Health, 95*(4), 660–667.

Zenk, S. N., Schulz, A. J., Israel, B. A., James, S. A., Bao, S., & Wilson, M. L. (2006b). Fruit and vegetable access differs by community racial composition and socioeconomic position in Detroit, Michigan. *Ethnicity & Disease, 16*(1), 275–280.

Chapter 3

Social Determinants of Depression and the Black Male Experience

Daphne C. Watkins
Harold W. Neighbors

Learning Objectives

- Introduce depression as a mental health disorder in black men.
- Present the social determinants that contribute to depression in black men.
- Discuss the methodological challenges that influence the clinical and epidemiologic assessment of depression in black men.
- Explore the policy implications for depression diagnoses and treatment in black men.
- Examine the lessons learned from previous work on black men and depression and provide recommendations for future pursuits.

• • •

Innumerable characteristics are unique to black men and have implications for their mental health. A report by the Kaiser Family Foundation suggested that the experiences of black men differ from those of men from other racial and ethnic groups. For example, fewer than 8 percent of black men have graduated from college compared to 17 percent of white men and 35 percent of Asian men (Kaiser, 2006). The unemployment rate for black men is more than twice the rate for white, Hispanic, and Asian men. Likewise, fewer black men between the ages of 16 and 29 are in the labor force compared to white, Hispanic, and Asian men in the same age group (Kaiser, 2006). More than 20 percent of black men live in poverty, compared to 18 percent of Hispanic, 12 percent of Asian, and 10 percent of white men. The percentage of black men in prison is nearly three times that of Hispanic men and nearly seven times that of white men. Black men also represent more than 40 percent of the prison population, although they represent only 14 percent of men in the United States (Harrison & Beck, 2005). The percentage of uninsured black men, though higher than that of whites, is lower than that of Hispanics, American Indian, and Native Hawaiian men (Kaiser, 2006). The above social determinants may not influence the lives of all black men; however, these determinants are precursors for **depression** in many black men. In this chapter, we provide an in-depth examination of the social determinants of depression for black men. There is notable variance in the terms used to describe men of African descent in mental health research. For the most part, the studies reviewed here have used either "black" or "African American." In this chapter, we use the more inclusive term *black* to describe men who self-identify as men of African descent.

We begin with an overview of depression in black men. Next, we discuss the recent and relevant literature on depression as well as some of the key social determinants of mental health for black men, including employment and socioeconomic status, kinship and social support, masculinities, stress (as described via racial discrimination, violence, and gender), and incarceration. Then we present methodological issues that arise with assessment and diagnosis of depression in black men and review the importance of social policies and programs that address the social determinants of depression for black men. Finally, we discuss the lessons learned and provide recommendations for closing the disparity gap and improving the mental health and overall well-being of black men.

Depression in Black Men

Rarely has depression in black men been explored as a centralized topic. Instead of depression, most studies have chronicled the broad mental health status of black men. Specifically, the majority of studies have focused on psychosocial coping (Gaines, 2007; Watkins, Green, Rivers, & Rowell, 2006), invisibility (Franklin, 1999); economic status/income (Broman, 1997; Watkins et al., 2006; Williams, 2003); failure to live up to the expectations placed on their gender (Bowman, 1989); and chronic exposures to racism (Broman, 1997; Fernando, 1984; Pearson, 1994; Pierre & Mahalik, 2005; Sellers, Bonham, Neighbors, & Amell, 2006; Utsey & Payne, 2000; Watkins et al., 2006; Williams, 2003). Findings from these studies usually suggest an inverse relationship between mental health and psychosocial coping, economic status, and racism/discrimination for black men of various educational and socioeconomic backgrounds (Watkins et al., 2006; Watkins, Walker, & Griffith, 2010; Williams, 2003).

Certain groups have a greater susceptibility to depression than others, such as individuals who are homeless or incarcerated, children in foster care and the child welfare system, and people who are exposed to violence. Since more than one in four black men experience some form of a mental health or substance abuse disorder (U.S. Department of Health and Human Services [USDHHS], 2001) and 7 percent of all black men will develop clinical levels of depression during their lifetime, being a black man has considerable implications for mental health. The *Supplement to Mental Health: A Report of the Surgeon General* identified risk factors that are common to depression on an individual, family, and community level (see USDHHS, 2001, for a review of these factors). Unless acted on by protective factors, these risk factors can influence the prevalence of depression in black men. Despite the increasing number of studies on depression, there remains a meager effort toward research on depression in black men and how social factors, symptoms, diagnosis, and treatment manifest across subgroups (e.g., incarcerated, college students, middle class) of black men. Results from large, epidemiologic community surveys imply that the prevalence of depression symptoms is lower in black men compared to white men and black women (Breslau, Su, Kendler, Aguilar-Gaxiola, & Kessler, 2005; Brown, Ahmed, Gary, & Milburn, 1995). These findings suggest that the impact of social stress on the mental health of black men may not be as harmful as it is for white men and black women. Other research underscores the misconstrued picture that depression findings present for blacks because the course and persistence of mood disorders may be more chronic for blacks than for whites (Williams et al., 2007). These studies also reported high prevalence rates for lifetime mood disorders for blacks compared to whites, which could lead to tragic occurrences such as suicide.

Studies that explore gender differences for suicide attempts among blacks are rare in the literature. Early studies on suicide and black men from the Epidemiologic Catchment Area (ECA) study reported a 2.3 percent lifetime estimate of attempted suicide while later studies found that the rates of suicide in black men made significant increases since the mid-1980s (Garlow, Purselle, & Heninger, 2005; Joe & Kaplan, 2001). A number of studies have reported that black men ages 15 to 24 are among the highest at risk for attempted suicide (Garlow, 2002). In the study by Joe and colleagues (2006), African-American women reported attempting suicide more than African-American men (5.0 percent versus 2.74 percent, respectively), but the men were more likely to die by suicide than the women. Black men and women who were at higher risk for suicide attempts were those in younger birth cohorts, less educated, residents in the Midwest region of the United States, and who had one or more disorders from the *Diagnostic and Statistical Manual of Mental Disorders, Fourth Edition (DSM-IV-TR)* (American Psychiatric Association, 2000). Some studies propose that increases in suicide are the result of younger blacks having increased access to lethal methods (Hawton, 2001), more psychiatric disorders, and more acceptable attitudes toward suicide (Joe, 2003). Others believe that institutional racism and the criminal justice system (Gaines, 2007) play more of an instrumental role in the suicide ideation for blacks than previously reported. Although there are a few studies on gender differences in suicide among blacks, there are too few studies addressing this important topic. More should be done to clarify precisely why black men are less prone to suicide attempts but much more likely than black women to die from a suicide attempt.

Social Determinants of Depression for Black Men

The World Health Organization (WHO) defines **social determinants** as the conditions in which people are born, grow, live, work, and age. These conditions include the health system and are shaped by the distribution of money, power, and resources at global, national, and local levels, which are themselves influenced by policy. Social determinants are primarily responsible for gender disparities that exist with regard to depression in blacks. Later, we discuss some of the social determinants that influence depression in black men; namely, employment and socioeconomic status, kinship and social support, masculinities, stress (in the context of racism and discrimination, violence, and gendered stress), and incarceration. We begin by framing our discussion within the sociocultural context of employment and socioeconomic status.

Employment and Socioeconomic Status

Socioeconomic status (SES) is the most robust and consistent factor affecting health outcomes whether measured by income, education, or occupation; or measured during childhood, adolescence, or adulthood (Geronimus, 2000; LaVeist, 2005). Twenty-seven percent of black families earn wages that are below the federal poverty level, compared to 10 percent of non-Hispanic white families (Staveteig & Wigton, 2000). According to economic studies, not only do blacks have a comparatively higher unemployment rate than whites, but blacks also average only 66 percent of the income of whites ($30,439 versus $45,904, respectively; McKinnon, 2003). Resource, opportunity, and environmental differences by race have important mental health consequences (Williams & Williams-Morris, 2000). For example, a recent analysis of national data on African Americans found that home value and parental education predicted higher depression but conversely, household income and years of education predicted lower rates of depression. However, the inverse association between education, income, and depression was only observed once the effects of home values were included (Hudson, 2009). On average, the unemployment rate for black men is two times greater than that of white men and black men earn 62 cents for every dollar earned by white men (Oliver, 2006). Some studies have reported that access to educational and employment opportunities are obstructed for black men due to the adverse effects of the restructuring of the economy and the historical and contemporary patterns of racial discrimination (Wilson, 1996).

Education correlates highly with measures of occupational and employment status. For many black men, idleness, often resulting from imprisonment, unemployment, or underemployment, is a major contributing factor to their availability for and participation in street-related activities (Oliver, 2006). In terms of within-group differences, black men with fewer education and financial resources may have different concerns (i.e., drug infestation, economic barriers, crime, lack of affordable health insurance, perceived discrimination in health care settings) than black men with more formal education and financial resources (i.e., managed care, chronic diseases; Watkins et al., 2010). Education level is a determining factor for job type, so educational attainment is often predictive of the type of employment (entry- versus managerial-level) black men will obtain. Lower educational attainment is associated with entry-level positions, which are known for rapid turnovers and lack of job security.

Lower levels of education may lead to increased risks for depression; the literature, though, is conflicting on this. For example, the social and environmental context associated with higher SES and more educational success for black men may buffer some of the adverse effects of depression. On the contrary, SES is inversely related to stress for black women and positively related to stress for black men. Black men face environments that are often impoverished and where few economic opportunities exist because of social inequalities and racism (Utsey, 1997). Even when middle-class black men earn similar incomes as their white male counterparts, doing so does not translate into more desirable housing and neighborhood conditions, economic stability, equivalent levels of wealth, or income levels that reflect their level of education (Braboy-Jackson & Williams, 2006; Williams, 2003). Due to such challenges, black men have often struggled to achieve success in highly valued social roles, such as being a good provider, spouse/partner, father, or employee. Consequently, success in any one of these areas is a taxing priority that often supersedes mental health for black men (Bowman,

1989; Courtenay, 2000). Just as studies have found a relationship between social roles and mental health for blacks (Barrett, 2003), studies have also presented a picture of the role of kinship and social support in the lives of black men.

Kinship and Social Support

White (2004) suggested that a large network of kinship and family support (i.e., uncles, aunts, preachers, significant others) are involved in the functioning of a black home. In terms of social support, research comparing blacks to whites found that high levels of critical and intrusive behaviors by family members predicted better mental health outcomes for blacks (Rosenbarb, Bellack, & Aziz, 2006). According to the authors, the cultural beliefs of black families hold that confrontation is an expression of concern. Existing research on the social support networks of black men generally focuses on the relationships of socially marginalized men, such as those entrenched in gang activity (Mac An Ghaill, 1994), the criminal justice system (Gaines, 2007), homeless men (Littrell & Beck, 2001), and low-income nonresidential fathers (Anderson, Kohler, & Letiecq, 2005). Despite these shortcomings in the literature, kinship and support are found to be especially important in terms of maintaining a sense of community and support for issues surrounding the health of black men. For example, Plowden and Young (2003) identified the influence of significant others as a critical social factor in motivating their sample of urban black men to seek health care and participate in health-related activities. A 2006 study by Plowden and colleagues (Plowden, John, Vasquez, & Kimani, 2006) also identified the influence of "trusted and respected individuals," described as family members, political officials, and members of the media. Although race was not discussed as a dominating factor with regard to outreach for black men, informants discussed men with whom they shared common characteristics—such as economic status and age—as individuals whom they considered helpful in reaching black men and connecting them with their health needs. A robust literature on the influence of significant others suggests that marriage is more psychologically beneficial for black men than black women (e.g., James, Tucker, & Kernan, 1996) such that separated and divorced black males and females have higher rates of depression than their married counterparts. Relative rates of psychiatric disorder are higher in separated/divorced and never-married black men compared to nonmarried black women and their peers (Williams, Takeuchi, & Adair, 1992). Equally important as black men's roles in partnerships are their gender identities as they pertain to how they define manhood.

Masculinities

Masculinities affect the pressing concerns of men as well as their potential resources to address problems (Levant, 1995). In this chapter, we refer to the various ideologies of masculinity as *masculinities*, because a number of scholars have acknowledged that there are more than one masculine ideology by which men identify. Addis and Cohane (2005) have acknowledged the importance of understanding the multiple ways that masculinities can be conceptualized beyond a sole focus on sex differences between men and women. For example, there are advantages and disadvantages for men who engage in traditional gender roles. In this context, **traditional gender norms** refer to the idea that a man should be confident, dominant, and not exude feminine characteristics (Courtenay, 2000). Men who are young, have lower educational levels, lower family incomes, and who identify as black tend to endorse more traditional, dominant norms of masculinity. The endorsement of traditional gender norms by black men compared to non-black men is consistent across studies (Courtenay, 2000; Levant, Majors, & Kelley, 1998) and the endorsement of traditional norms of masculinity changes depending on the age and professional or nonprofessional status of the men.

With regard to engagement, *conformity* to masculine gender norms may result in benefits including acceptance by social groups, and social and financial rewards. Conformity to masculine gender norms could also result in the man being described by others as "emotionally distant" or "interpersonally dominant" in his relationships. On the other hand, *nonconformity* to masculine norms is associated with a reduction in some of the psychological distress connected to traditional masculine gender roles (e.g., the breadwinner, man of the house; Good et al., 1995; Hayes & Mahalik, 2000; Mahalik, Good, & Englar-Carson, 2003). Likewise, nonconforming men tend to avoid problems such as violence, high-risk behaviors, and absent fathering—all problems associated with the negative outcomes of men who identify with more traditional masculine norms (Brooks & Silverstein, 1995). Nonconforming males may be able to avoid some of the negative mental health consequences associated with conformity to masculine norms. However, social and gender norms research also suggests that nonconformers are more likely to experience group rejection than conformers (Cialdini & Trost, 1998), and that individuals are evaluated more negatively when they contravene traditional gender roles, with men evaluated more negatively compared with women (Sirin, McCreary, & Mahalik, 2004).

Phenomena associated with the concept of black male masculinities strongly influence the mental health of black men. For instance, Majors and Billson (1992) have discussed the mental health implications of using "**cool pose**" (or, behaviors by black males that deliver a message of strength and control) to conceal feelings of self-doubt and insecurity. Clyde Franklin (1986) presents black masculinities in the contexts of such characteristics as stoicism, self-concealment, and the ability to maintain three role expectations: a "societal male sex role" (which includes competitiveness, aggression, independence, and work ethic); a "black" American role (which includes cooperation, survival of the group, and promotion of the group); and a "black male group" role (which tends to be defined by individual black male circles, but may include hypersexuality, violence, and intraracism). Franklin suggests that the black American role is in direct opposition to the societal male sex role and that a successful black man can only dwell partially in both in order to achieve societal success and cultural acceptance. A meta-study of black male mental health and well-being found that black men are more likely to experience poor mental health, at least in part from adhering to traditional masculine norms that promote the avoidance of medical care (Watkins et al., 2010). Often the behavioral norms associated with masculine identity evoke various stressors in the lives of black men.

Stress

Here we discuss stress in the context of four phenomena often experienced by black men: racial discrimination, violence, gendered stress, and incarceration.

Racial Discrimination

Combined with the innumerable stressors that influence their daily lives, black men experience challenges associated with the effects of racial discrimination on their mental health (Pierre & Mahalik, 2005; Utsey & Payne, 2000; Watkins et al., 2006). The cultural context of racism plays a particularly important role in understanding the stress and mental health status of black men. For example, Rich and Grey (2005) reported that the black men in their study expressed a lack of faith in the police and the judicial system due to being victimized and racially profiled. The victims of violent crimes from the Rich and Grey study discussed the desire to protect themselves because the police were more a part of the problem than the solution. Similarly, participants from the Kendrick, Anderson, and Moore (2006) study reported that their rights as Americans were constantly violated by the police; for instance, never being told why they were pulled over by a patrol officer.

Black men contend with numerous stressors related to overt and covert racial discrimination manifested in many forms, including racial residential segregation, diminished returns for investments in social and cultural capital, and limited advancement in occupational settings due to racialized glass ceilings (Cole & Omari, 2003; Williams, 2003). Previous studies on psychological distress and black men have documented that experiencing racism and discrimination lowers their psychological health (Pieterse & Carter, 2007; Utsey, 1997). One interpretation of this is that over the life course for black men, they are more likely to encounter racial discrimination or experience noxious encounters in their social environments (i.e., school and the workplace), thus threatening their mental health. Perhaps the mental health effects of social incongruence coupled with exposure to racial discrimination remain consistent for black men beginning in their youth and continuing well into adulthood.

Violence

Black men are more likely to participate in violence, rather than demonstrate dominance through professional and economic achievement (Pearson, 1994; Whaley, 1998). However, a small number of studies have emphasized the role that racial profiling has in black men's likelihood to be involved in violent acts. Violence and homicide are leading causes of death for black men (Hammond & Yung, 1993). Likewise, black-on-black crime is a virulent malaise often prevalent in inner city and urban African-American communities (Baffour, 2007; Beverly, 1998). For some black males, participation in life on "the streets" (Oliver, 2006) is helpful in establishing their ability to convey symbolic and overt displays of masculinities and can resort to violence as a means to resolving disputes (Majors & Billson, 1992). In this context, "the streets" is a socialized institution that is composed of the network of public and semi-public social settings (e.g., street corners, bars, after-hours locations, drug houses, vacant lots) that serve as important influences on the psychosocial development and life course trajectories and transitions of black men (Oliver, 2006). Paxton and colleagues have demonstrated a noteworthy relationship between exposure to violence and psychological distress in adolescent black males (Paxton, Robinson, Shah, & Schoeny, 2004). Likewise, chronic exposure to violence has been associated with depression, anxiety, and suicidal ideation.

Gendered Stress

Gendered stress emerges at the intersection of a series of interwoven social formations that include historic, economic, political, linguistic, interpersonal, and psychological threads. Certainly, the behaviors of some black men, particularly of those affiliated with street-oriented lifestyles, may result in psychosocial stressors associated with perceived gender norms in the context of their environments. These men may also render less desirable partners that lead to relationship disruption resulting in high divorce rates, female-headed families, out-of-wedlock births, less commitment of men to relationships, and negative perceptions of black men on the part of the black women (Tucker & Mitchell-Kernan, 1995). Under this type of gender-induced stress, many black men are limited in their ability to serve as responsible father figures, which may include providing love, social, and financial support for their children (Oliver, 2006). Active participation in street life that derives from conforming to certain street-related gender norms can diminish a black man's role in the household and limit his abilities to fulfill the responsibilities associated with fatherhood, specifically (Wilson, 1996), and manhood, generally.

The black family unit is most often affected by the social responsibilities of black men and can experience direct repercussions when black men are indisposed. For example, when a man is ill or away from the household, fulfilling his expected obligations to his family and others in his social network may be more difficult to perform. Sickness, injuries, or imprisonment can have multiple effects on the black family unit and ultimately lead to other stressful events such as marital discord and changes in personal habits and social activities (Bowman, 1989; Neighbors, Jackson, Bowman, & Gurin, 1983). In the first cross-sectional study on a national probability sample of black adults, Neighbors and colleagues found that the majority of the interpersonal problems among black men were the result of family difficulties, including marital discord and economic disadvantage. Black men from the study reported difficulty fulfilling their roles as providers and protectors of their families—logically, a factor that often contributes to their reluctance to seek strong relationships and social support (Neighbors et al. 1983).

Incarceration

Black men remain the most disproportionately incarcerated group, constituting about 45 percent of the prison population, or more than 818,000 men (Harrison & Karberg, 2004). Some have estimated that black men have a 32 percent chance of going to prison at some time in their lives, compared to just 6 percent for white men (Bonczar, 2003). Black men are also about seven times more likely than white men to have a prison record (Pettit & Western, 2004). Between the 1980s and 1990s, class inequalities increased and the frequency of imprisonment overshadowed that of military service and college graduation for birth cohorts of black males (Pettit & Western, 2004). Endemic incarceration leaves few black male role models in the community. Likewise, Pettit and Western (2004) have posited that incarceration represents a significant reordering of the life course that can have lifelong effects, particularly for black men. The high risk of imprisonment for black men is a significant social ordering of the distinctive life course and is said to distinguish the young adulthood of black men from the life course of others more than military enlistment, marriage, or college graduation (Pettit & Western, 2004). In fact, one could even argue that the mass imprisonment of noncollege black men should be included in the discussion of the influence of social contexts we use to describe the key institutional influences on U.S. social inequality (Pettit & Western, 2004).

A study by the National Institute of Justice estimated that 16 percent of individuals in jail and prison had a mental illness (Ditton, 1999). Individuals who are substance users, are unemployed, have lower incomes, and have fewer years of education are also at greater risk of incarceration (Draine, Salzer, Culhane, & Hadley, 2002). Many of these incarcerated individuals are black men who suffer from mental disorders and could benefit from interventions that treat them as both criminal offenders and recipients of mental health services. Unfortunately, the experience of incarceration for black men has come to be an aspect of their rite of passage into manhood, particularly for black males who reside in underserved neighborhoods (Whitehead, 2000). The involvement of black men and boys in so-called *street life* (Oliver, 2006) is also associated with their high rates of incarceration. Often the result of men rejoining society from prison means that they lack the skills needed to secure employment, lack occupational skills, and/or have fewer skills to seek jobs or confront potential employers who may be hesitant to hire an ex-offender (Finn, 1999).

Methodological Challenges to the Clinical and Epidemiologic Assessment of Black Men

Largely, studies that examine the mental health of blacks have included an overrepresentation of women, thereby limiting the ability to draw conclusions about black men. Past approaches to studying depression in blacks have been limited due to challenges with identifying the variables that best explain their mental health (Mizell, 1999). Few epidemiologic studies on the incidence and prevalence of major depressive disorder, for example, have included samples of black men that were representative of the population (Bennett, Merritt, Edwards, & Sollers, 2004; Paxton, Robinson, Shah, & Schoeny, 2004; Utsey & Payne, 2000). Furthermore, as black adults tend to conceal mental health problems (Baker, 2001) it becomes more difficult to assess the incidence and prevalence of depression for black men. Although positive associations between self-concealment and depression have been uncovered, generally (Cramer & Barry, 1999), measurement issues have presented barriers for the diagnosis of depression in black men, specifically. The methodological limitations that contribute to low diagnostic reliability raise questions about the validity of the procedures used to apply the *Diagnostic and Statistical Manual of Mental Disorders (DSM-IV-TR)* criteria to black men (Love & Love, 2006; Watkins et al., 2010).

Findings like those reported for gender differences in major depressive disorder point to important methodological challenges of measuring gender differences in mental disorders. In an interesting reversal of the feminist critique popular in the early 1980s (Kaplan, 1983), some scholars argue that currently there is gender bias in the *DSM* that works to the detriment of men rather than women (Cochran & Rabinowitz, 2003). For example, instead of overpathologizing women, it is now argued that clinicians using the *DSM* underdiagnose depression in men. Consequently, men are at increased risk for adverse outcomes, including underrecognition of depression that leads to the underutilization of services, inadequate treatment, and potentially increased risk for suicide. Although it is not yet clear why men with depression may go undetected, a number of explanations have been proposed. For example, it has been suggested that the underdiagnosis of men with depression occurs because men express symptoms of depression in ways that are inconsistent with the *DSM* major depression symptom criteria, and that because the criteria are biased toward the manner in which women tend to express depression, clinicians tend to miss depressive symptoms expressed by men.

Many have written extensively about the problems of making a psychiatric diagnosis within the context of race (Bell, Williamson, & Chien, 2008). Fewer have addressed these challenges while considering the **intersectionality** of race and gender (Head, 2004; Metzl, 2010). Black men in particular are overdiagnosed with psychosis and underdiagnosed with depression (USDHHS, 1999). As a function of racial and gender bias, black men experience "double jeopardy" in terms of risk for the underdiagnosis of depression. Labeling a symptom as pathological is a subtle and difficult process, especially when clinicians are influenced by the subtle gender stereotypes (e.g., the "angry black men") that can influence clinical judgment. This view underscores the importance of expert clinical opinion in the process of applying *DSM* criteria to black men. We want to emphasize that the valid diagnosis of mental disorders like depression in black men is a function of the diagnostic criteria *as well as* the method and procedures employed to apply those criteria to a particular black man. Thus, in pursing an initial, provisional diagnosis, it is crucial that every effort is made by clinicians to ascertain the historical, structural, and situational contexts that provide the surrounding context by which black men are required to function. The broader cultural experiences of black men play a role in the attitudes of mistrust, as one example, they bring to the clinical assessment (Whaley, 1998). The potential for misinterpreting symptoms of psychopathology has profound implications for our understanding of depression in black men and should be considered during clinical evaluations and observations with depressed black men.

How psychiatric epidemiology should address the problem of gender bias is less obvious because epidemiologic interviewing procedures rely so heavily on highly structured survey instruments and as a result, diminish the role of clinical judgment in case-designation. These highly standardized procedures make it difficult for present epidemiologic methods to address the argument that *DSM* criteria are gender-biased. Clinical expertise is one source of the information needed to identify the signs and symptoms of psychopathology within the cultural contexts of black men. Clinicians, by virtue of their specialized training, are in a better position to learn and incorporate gender-specific vocabularies of distress (e.g., slang) used by black men. Consequently, the extent to which gender bias is a problem in epidemiologic community surveys is not well understood (Shin, Martin, & Howren, 2009). In order to achieve an accurate assessment of mental disorders within the social and cultural context of the lives of black men, future research must develop and apply the necessary procedural modifications to the diagnostic criteria and to the instruments used to assess disorders such as depression.

Policy Implications

Public policies aimed at closing the gap in social conditions between blacks and whites will reduce disparities in mental health status (Alegria, Perez, & Williams, 2003). The development of public policies and social programs that address the social determinants of depression in black men will be important for reducing disparities. Although there is concurrence about the importance of social determinants for mental health, there remains conflict surrounding the mechanisms operating in favor of changing social conditions as a strategy to improve mental health, particularly for black men. Identifying the structural relationship between social conditions and mental health status is influenced by the varying mechanisms by which social factors are acknowledged and acted upon. For example, more than 20 percent of black men live in poverty (U.S. Census Bureau, 2005) and the connection between poverty and poor mental health suggests any policy that purports to reduce poverty will have a positive effect on the mental health of black men (Albee & Ryan, 1998). For social policies to benefit black men, policies must first be effective at changing social and economic conditions for black men.

Next, mental health education has a strong influence on mental health; however, if social conditions to cope with adversity and maintain control are fragmented, chances of receptivity to mental health education by black men are decreased. Rich (2000) noted that the future of health for black men is contingent on improving their access to health care that addresses health behaviors in their social context while also providing access to primary care. One way that public and social policies can play a more active role in these efforts is to increase education and awareness about the mental health care system within the black community, with respect to social determinants. Furthermore, reducing stigma and the social conditions that discourage black men from seeking mental health care may increase utilization of mental health services by black men and their families.

Finally, using the context by which current research and practice on black men are examined will expand the range of activities needed to improve mental health. This approach involves innovations in policy, including those that are not necessarily linked to the conventional roles of mental health professionals. These roles include, but are not limited to, "community-level interventions, social welfare programs, conventional and alternative law-enforcement programs, and the development of greater infrastructure for supporting self-help and mutual-aid associations among persons whose lives are affected by mental illness" (Draine et al., 2002, p. 571). In terms of more broad-based policy, those that reduce the risk of pertinent social problems for black men should be considered (e.g., unemployment, crime, poverty, incarceration, education, insurance); as well as social policies that reduce the prevalence of risk factors in black men with depression.

Lessons Learned

Existing evidence on the social determinants of mental health for black men propose best practices to be considered by the next generation of researchers and practitioners. Here, we will discuss three. First, **social and cultural context** plays an important role in understanding the mental health of black men (Watkins et al., 2010). Although services and programs have been implemented for black men with depression, these efforts have meagerly included elements from the lived experiences of black men. In other words, the experiences of black men with depression are often contextualized in disadvantaged social settings (Draine et al., 2002). Yet, only recently have these social settings been acknowledged and considered in the development and delivery of interventions and treatment. For instance, understanding the positive and negative aspects of factors such as social support and mental health literacy is a critical piece to depression diagnosis and treatment for black men (Watkins & Neighbors, 2007). In addition, prior studies have implied that racial factors are a major marker for mental health, but the health behaviors, attitudes, and beliefs of black men may be similar to that of other men. We cannot attribute black men's mental health outcomes to them being black because being male also plays an important part. Furthermore, as blacks tend to conceal emotional health status (Baker, 2001), researchers have reported positive associations between self-concealment and indications of compromised mental health, such as depression, poor self-esteem, and lower levels of perceived social support (Cramer & Barry, 1999). Quantitative studies on race and gender suggest that race plays an essential role in mental health outcomes for blacks (Williams & Williams-Morris, 2000). However, what prior research does not do is identify which aspects of being black and being male influences these outcomes.

Second, ***targeted interventions*** are a driving force in addressing mental health problems. Studies have documented successful interventions that reduced the severity of depression in both minority and nonminority groups. For example, low-income minority adults at risk for depression participated in a program on cognitive-behavioral methods tailored to their culture to control their moods. At the end of the one-year follow-up, the adults in the study showed fewer symptoms of depression than did the control group (Munoz et al., 1995). Similar efforts are promising for black men across different life stages. For example, targeted interventions for black men could focus on prevention and intervention efforts that address racism, both individually and collectively. The development and implementation of programs that focus on self-esteem and mastery of their environment will also benefit the mental health of black men. A sequence of negative life events and pressing economic hardships may mean that older black men, for example, require targeted interventions that differ from those of their younger counterparts. Positive mental health for older black men requires integrity and the ability to cope effectively with despair based on successes and failures from earlier in their lives (Bowman, 1989). Black men in late adulthood may benefit most from targeted interventions that focus on health care and social services, including income and retirement services and those that enhance self-esteem.

Lastly, research and practice efforts that consider the social construction of ***manhood and masculinities*** empower black men to care for their health (Rich, 2000; Watkins et al., 2010). Such practices may be more effective than those that focus solely on enhancing self-esteem. For example, Cochran and Rabinowitz (2003) have outlined masculine-specific assessment approaches to detecting depression in men that integrate the idiosyncratic manner in which many men cope with depressed mood with traditional diagnostic criteria for depression used by most clinicians. Sociocultural constructions of masculinity contribute to gender-related health concepts as well as to subjective experiences and the presentation of depressive symptoms. Depression in men is associated with rigid adherence to traditional masculine gender roles (Levant et al., 2003), masculine gender role conflict (Good & Wood, 1995), work, concentration, and performance-related difficulties, and increased interpersonal conflict. Using traditional diagnostic criteria only will result in some black men slipping under the radar and not undergoing an accurate depression diagnosis. Masculine gender role conflict themes (i.e., irritability, anger, and violence), externalizing defenses, and work-related concerns should also supplement future work with black men.

Recommendations for Addressing Depression in Black Men

Often the dream of an education, a decent job, a house, and a family become impossible to attain for black men. Not only are social barriers in place to limit the progress of black men, but so are barriers that restrict them from living long, healthy lives. According to the World Health Organization (WHO, 2009), disparities in social determinants of health can be reduced if researchers and practitioners make an effort to: improve daily living conditions; tackle the inequitable distribution of power, money, and resources; and understand the problem and assess the impact of action. These efforts, tailored to subgroups of black men and coupled with the following three recommendations, will help to address depression in black men.

1. *Increase collaborations among researchers, practitioners, black men, and other stakeholders who are interested in depression among black men.* Engaging in collaborative efforts with stakeholders and other interested associates will result in the design of culturally sensitive and gender-appropriate programs that achieve optimal mental health for black men. By increasing the collaborations among researchers, community practitioners, black men, and other stakeholders, depression in black men can be addressed in the context of their lived experiences and efforts tailored to their individual and community needs can be achieved. Not only should each component of the team increase their knowledge about depression, but they should also become more familiar with the mental health needs of black communities in general. Collaborators can work with black men and their families amid the intrapersonal and environmental adversities that affect them, predispose them to depression, and limit their ability to make use of the resources and services provided.

2. *Incorporate a life course perspective in the study of depression in black men.* A life course perspective on black men and depression may be important when considering strategies for targeting mental health promotion and prevention efforts. Therefore, increased knowledge of the risk and protective factors influencing depression in black men at different age-linked life

stages is needed to inform research and practice. There is a need for a focus on prevention at early adult life stages and intervention at all adult developmental stages for black men. If early prevention and successful intervention efforts to improving and maintaining the mental health and well-being of black men are implemented, threatening social determinants could potentially have less of an impact on their mental health over the life course. Empirical examinations of the buffering effects of potentially damaging factors are needed and could be highly informative to clinicians working with black men. One strategy may be for mental health service providers to assess the needs of black men at different life stages and tailor mental health promotion and disorder prevention programs specifically to these needs.

3. *Adopt an intersectional approach to the study of depression in black men.* Future research and practice should consider an intersectional approach to understanding black men's depression and overall mental health (Weber & Parra-Medina, 2003). An intersectional approach calls for simultaneously addressing the intersection of multiple aspects of socially constructed identity, including race, ethnicity, gender, class, SES, and context. Inclusion of biological, sociocultural, psychological, and environmental factors and how these factors are manifested through individual identities (e.g., racial, cultural, gender) will help to develop a comprehensive understanding of depression in black men. Future inquiries should continue to examine the impact of black men's lived experiences and incorporate intrinsically important social and psychosocial factors that influence their lives such as SES, successful life transitions, and gender role socialization. Logical next steps include proposing other factors that lead to depression in black men and exerting greater effort toward understanding within and between group differences. Strategies to improve black men's psychological resilience to risk factors are needed, and more focused research can help inform efforts to promote their positive transitions and mental health trajectories.

Summary

This chapter examines the social determinants of depression in black men because no other race-by-gender population group has been stigmatized as much as black men. Black men are often thought to be detached, unintelligent, lazy, irresponsible, sexually promiscuous, angry, and violent. As a result, black men in the United States live under a microscope that questions their manhood and at times, their humanity. Unique culturally grounded coping styles such as Majors' (1992) "cool pose" and Anderson's (1999) "code of the street" have been developed by black men as a means of deflecting these negative images. This chapter has shown that a number of underlying factors contribute to the misperception that there is something wrong with black men. However, one must also ask what is wrong with a society that so effectively uses race and gender to differentiate those who are afforded the opportunities to attain positions of prestige and power and those who are not. This will involve confronting the racism and sexism ingrained in the very institutions (e.g., education, employment, and housing) into which black men aspire to integrate. The reality for many black men is that the quest for the "American Dream" is a chronic stressor that reminds them of their inability to achieve desired life goals. This state of affairs most certainly has deleterious effects on mental health. The mental health problems of black men should be addressed by developing services and interventions that are accessible, empowering, culturally sensitive, age-specific, and gender-appropriate. However, the concept of mental health is more than the treatment of mental disorders. It involves ensuring that black men have every opportunity to reach their full potential.

Key Terms

conformity	nonconformity
cool pose	social and cultural context
depression	social determinants
gendered stress	socioeconomic status
intersectionality	targeted interventions
masculinities	traditional gender norms

Discussion Questions

1. How do masculinities that are shaped over a life course influence depression in black men?

2. How can researchers and practitioners work together to develop targeted efforts that raise awareness, educate, and reduce the prevalence and incidence of depression in black men?

3. Can the harmful aspects of "traditional" masculinities be modified for black men while maintaining the more adaptive aspects (e.g., strength, self-determination, sacrifice, caretaker, and breadwinner) that contribute to the masculine identities embraced by black men? Why or why not?

4. Does the success of Barack Obama challenge the view that the existence of racial discrimination requires black men to place realistic limits on the heights to which they can aspire? Why or why not?

5. Are the positive efforts of some black men strong enough to change the historical and institutional undertones of racism in society? Why or why not?

References

Addis, M. E., & Cohane, G. H. (2005). Social scientific paradigms of masculinity and their implications for research and practice in men's mental health. *Journal of Clinical Psychology*, *61*, 1–15.

Albee, G. W., & Ryan, K. (1998). An overview of primary prevention. *Journal of Mental Health*, *7*, 439–447.

Alegria, M., Perez, D., & Williams, D. R. (2003). The role of public policies in reducing mental health status disparities for people of color, *Health Affairs*, *22*(5), 51–64.

American Psychiatric Association. (2000). *Diagnostic and statistical manual of mental disorders* (4th ed., text rev., p. 341). Washington, DC: Author.

Anderson, E. (1999). *Code of the street: Decency, violence and the moral life of the inner city*. New York, NY: Norton.

Anderson, E. A., Kohler, J. K., & Letiecq, B. L. (2005). Predictors of depression among low-income, nonresidential fathers. *Journal of Family Issues*, *26*, 547–567.

Baffour, T. D. (2007). Prevalence and incidence of black-on-black crime among youth. In L. A. See (Ed.), *Human behavior in the social environment from an African-American perspective* (2nd ed., pp. 293–308). New York, NY: Hawthorne Press.

Baker, F. M. (2001). Diagnosing depression in African Americans. *Community Mental Health Journal*, *37*(1), 31–38.

Barrett, A. E. (2003). Race differences in the mental health effects of divorce: a reexamination incorporating temporal dimensions of the dissolution process. *Journal of Family Issues*, *24*(8), 995–1019.

Bell, C. C., Williamson, J. L., & Chien, P. (2008). Cultural, racial, and ethnic competence in psychiatric diagnosis. *Ethnicity and Inequalities in Health and Social Care*, *1*(1), 34–41.

Bennett, G. G., Merritt, M. M., Edwards, C. L., & Sollers, J. T. (2004). Perceived racism and affective responses to ambiguous interpersonal interactions among African American men. *American Behavioral Scientist*, *47*(7), 963–976.

Beverly, C. C. (1998). Black on black crime: Compensation for idiomatic purposelessness. *Journal of Human Behavior in the Social Environment*, *1*(2–3), 183–201.

Bonczar, Thomas P. (2003). *Prevalence of imprisonment in the U.S. population, 1974–2001*. Bureau of Justice Statistics Special Report, NCJ 197976.

Bowman, P. J. (1989). Research perspectives on black men: Role strain and adaptation across the adult life cycle. In R. L. Jones (Ed.), *Black adult development and aging* (pp. 117–150). Berkeley, CA: Cobb & Henry.

Braboy-Jackson, P., & Williams, D. (2006). Culture, race/ethnicity, and depression. In C. L. M. Keyes & S. H. Goodman (Eds.), *Women and depression: A handbook for the social, behavioral, and biomedical sciences* (pp. 328–359). New York, NY: Cambridge University Press.

Breslau, J., Su, M., Kendler, K., Aguilar-Gaxiola, S., & Kessler, R. C. (2005). Lifetime risk and persistence of psychiatric disorders across groups in the United States. *Psychological Medicine*, *35*, 317–327.

Broman, C. L. (1997). Race-related factors and life satisfaction among African-Americans. *Journal of Black Psychology*, *23*, 36–49.

Brooks, G. (2001). Masculinity and men's mental health. *Journal of American College Health*, *49*, 285–297.

Brooks, G. R., & Silverstein, L. B. (1995). The dark side of masculinity. In R. F. Levant & W. S. Pollack (Eds.), *A new psychology of men* (pp. 280–305). New York, NY: Basic Books.

Brown, D. R., Ahmed, F., Gary, L. E., & Milburn, N. G. (1995). Major depression in a community sample of African Americans. *American Journal of Psychiatry*, *152*(3), 373–378.

Bureau of Justice Statistics. (2009). *Criminal offenders statistics*. Available from http://www.ojp.usdoj.gov/bjs/crimoff.htm#lifetime

Cialdini, R. B., & Trost, M. R. (1998). Social influence: Social norms, conformity, and compliance. In D. Gilbert, S. Fiske, & G. Lindzey (Eds.), *The handbook of social psychology* (pp. 151–192). New York, NY: McGraw-Hill.

Cochran, S. V., & Rabinowitz, F. E. (2003). Gender-sensitive recommendations for assessment and treatment of depression in men. *Professional Psychology*, *34*, 132–140.

Cole, E. R., & Omari, S. R. (2003). Race, class, and the dilemma of upward mobility for African Americans. *Journal of Social Issues*, *59*, 785–802.

Courtenay, W. H. (2000). Constructions of masculinity and their influence on men's well-being: A theory of gender and health. *Social Science Medicine*, *50*(10), 1385–1401.

Cramer, K. M., & Barry, J. E. (1999). Conceptualizations and measures of loneliness: A comparison of subscales. *Personality and Individual Differences*, *27*, 491–502.

Ditton, P. (1999). *Mental health and treatment for inmates and probationers*. Washington, DC: Bureau of Justice Statistics.

Draine, J., Salzer, M. S., Culhane, D. P., & Hadley, T. R. (2002). Role of social disadvantage in crime, joblessness, and homelessness among persons with serious mental illness. *Psychiatric Services*, *53*, 565–573.

Fernando, S. (1984). Racism as a cause of depression. *International Journal of Social Psychiatry*, *30*, 41–49.

Finn, P. (1999). Job placement for offenders: A promising approach to reducing recidivism and correctional costs. *National Institute of Justice Journal*, 2–11.

Franklin, A. J. (1999). Invisibility syndrome and racial identity development in psychotherapy and counseling African American men. *Counseling Psychologist*, *27*, 761–793.

Franklin, C. W. (1986). Conceptual and logical issues in theory and research related to black masculinity. *Western Journal of Black Studies*, *10*(4), 161–166.

Gaines, J. S. (2007). Social correlates of psychological distress among adult African American males. *Journal of Black Studies*, *37*, 827–858.

Garlow, S. J. (2002). Age, gender, and ethnicity differences in patters of cocaine and ethanol use preceding suicide. *American Journal of Psychiatry*, *159*, 615–619.

Garlow, S. J., Purselle, D., & Heninger, M. (2005). Ethnic differences in patterns of suicide across the life cycle. *American Journal of Psychiatry*, *162*, 319–323.

Geronimus, A. T. (2000). To mitigate, resist, or undo: Addressing structural influences on the health of urban populations. *American Journal of Public Health*, *90*, 867–872.

Good, G. E., Robertson, J. M., O'Neil, J. M., Fitzgerald, L. F., Stevens, M., Debord, K. A., & Bartels, K. M. (1995). Male gender role conflict: Psychometric issues and relations to psychological distress. *Journal of Counseling Psychology*, *42*, 3–10.

Good, G. E., & Wood, P. K. (1995). Male gender role conflict, depression, and help seeking: Do college men face double jeopardy? *Journal of Counseling and Development*, *74*, 70–75.

Hammond, W. R., & Yung, B. (1993). Psychology's role in the public health response to assaultive violence among young African-American men. *American Psychologist*, *48*(2), 142–154.

Harris, I., Torres, J. B., & Allender, D. (1994). The responses of African American men to dominant norms of masculinity within the United States. *Sex Roles*, *31*, 703–719.

Harrison, P. M., & Beck, A. J. (October, 2005). *Prisoners in 2004*. Bureau of Justice Statistics Bulletin.

Harrison, P., & Karberg, J. (2004). *Prison and jail inmates at mid-year 2003* (NCJ 203947). Washington, DC: U.S. Department of Justice, Bureau of Justice Statistics.

Hayes, J. A., & Mahalik, J. R. (2000). Gender role conflict and psychopathology in a clinical population. *Psychology of Men and Masculinity*, *1*, 116–125.

Hawton, K. (2001). Studying survivors of nearly lethal suicide attempts: An important strategy in suicide research. *Suicide and Life-Threatening Behavior*, *32*(Suppl.), 76–84.

Head, J. (2004). *Black men and depression: Saving our lives, healing our families and friends*. New York, NY: Broadway Books.

Henry J. Kaiser Family Foundation. (July, 2006). *Race, ethnicity, and health fact sheet: Young African American men in the United States*. Available from http://www.kff .org/minorityhealth/upload/7541.pdf

Hudson, D. L. (2009). *Race, socioeconomic position and depression: The mental health costs of upward mobility*. University of Michigan Dissertations and Theses. Available from http://hdl.handle.net/2027.42/64820

James, A., Tucker, B., & Mitchell-Kernan, C. (1996). Marital attitudes, perceived mate availability, and subjective well-being among partnered African American men and women. *Journal of Black Psychology*, *22*(1), 20–36.

Joe, S., & Kaplan, M. S. (2001). Suicide among African American men. *Suicide and life-threatening behavior*, *31*(1), 106–121.

Joe, S. (2003). Implications of focusing on black youth self-destructive behaviors instead of suicide when designing preventative interventions (pp. 325–332). In D. Romer (Ed.), *Reducing adolescent risk: Toward an integrated approach*. Thousand Oaks, CA: Sage.

Joe, S., Baser, R. E., Breeden, G., Neighbors, H. W., & Jackson, J. S. (2006). Prevalence of and risk factors for lifetime suicide attempts among blacks in the United States. *Journal of the American Medical Association*, *296*, 2112–2123.

Kaplan, E. A. (1983). *Women and film: Both sides of the camera*. New York, NY and London, UK: Methuen.

Kendrick, L., Anderson, N. L., & Moore, B. (2006). Perceptions of depression among young African American men. *Family & Community Health*, *30*(1), 63–73.

King, G., & Williams, D. R. (1995). Race and health: A multidimensional approach to African American health. In B. C. Amick, S. Levine, A. R. Tarlov, & D. C. Walsh (Eds.), *Society & health* (pp. 93–130). Oxford, UK: Oxford University Press.

LaVeist, T. A. (2005). Disentangling race and socioeconomic status: A key to understanding health inequalities. *Journal of Urban Health*, *82*(2 Suppl. 3), iii, 26–34.

Levant, R. F. (1995). *Masculinity reconstructed: Changing the rules of manhood at work, in relationships and in family life*. New York, NY: Penguin.

Levant, R. F., Majors, R. G., & Kelley, M. L. (1998). Masculinity ideology among young African American and European American women and men in different regions of the United States. *Cultural Diversity and Ethnic Minority Psychology*, *4*(3), 227–236.

Levant, R. F., Richmond, K., Majors, R. G., Inclan, J. E., Rossello, J. M., Heesacker, M., . . . Sellers, A. (2003). A multicultural investigation of masculinity ideology and alexithymia. *Psychology of Men & Masculinity*, *4*, 91–99.

Littrell, J., & Beck, E. (2001). Predictors of depression in a sample of African-American homeless men: Identifying effective coping strategies given varying levels of daily stressors. *Community Mental Health Journal*, *37*, 15–29.

Love, A. S., & Love, R. J. (2006). Measurement suitability of the Center for Epidemiological Studies: Depression scale among older urban black men. *International Journal of Men's Health*, *5*(2), 173–189.

Mac An Ghaill, M. (1994). *The making of men: Masculinities, sexualities and schooling*. Buckingham, UK: Open University Press.

Mahalik, J. R., Good, G. E., & Englar-Carson, M. E. (2003). Masculinity scripts, presenting concerns and help seeking: Implications for practice and training. *Professional Psychology: Research and Practice*, *34*, 123–131.

Majors, R., & Billson, J. (1992). *Cool pose: The dilemmas of black manhood in America*. New York, NY: Lexington Books.

McKinnon, J. (2003). *The black population in the United States: March 2002*. Washington, DC: U.S. Census Bureau, Current Population Reports, Series P20–541.

Metzl, J. M. (2010). *The protest psychosis: How schizophrenia became a black disease*. Boston, MA: Beacon Press.

Mizell, A. C. (1999). Life course influences on African American men's depression: Adolescent parental composition, self-concept and adult earnings. *Journal of Black Studies*, *29*(4), 467–490.

Munoz, R. F., Ying, Y. W., Bernal, G., Perez-Stable, E. J., Sorensen, J. L., Hargreaves, W. A., . . . Miller, L. S. (1995). Prevention of depression with primary care patients: A randomized controlled trial. *American Journal of Community Psychology*, *23*, 199–222.

Neighbors, H., Jackson, J., Bowman, P., & Gurin, G. (1983). *Stress, coping, and black mental health: Preliminary findings from a national study*. Newbury Park, CA: Sage.

Neighbors, H. W., & Williams, D. R. (2001). *The epidemiology of mental disorder 1985 to 2000*. In R. L. Braithwaite & S. E. Taylor (Eds.), *Health issues in the black community*. San Francisco, CA: Jossey-Bass.

Oliver, W. (2006). "The streets": An alternative black male socialization institution. *Journal of Black Studies, 36*(6), 918–937.

Paxton, K., Robinson, W. L., Shah, S., & Schoeny, M. (2004). Psychological distress for African-American adolescent males: Exposure to community violence and social support as factors. *Child Psychiatry and Human Development, 34*(4), 281–295.

Pearson, D. F. (1994). The black man: Health issues and implications for clinical practice. *Journal Black Studies, 25*, 81–98.

Pettit, B., & Western, B. (2004). Mass imprisonment and the life course: Race and class inequality in U.S. incarceration. *American Sociological Review, 69*, 151–169.

Pierre, M. R., & Mahalik, J. R. (2005). Examining African self-consciousness and black racial identity as predictors of black men's psychological well-being. *Cultural Diversity and Ethnic Minority Psychology, 11*, 28–40.

Pieterse, A. L., & Carter, R. T. (2007). An examination of the relationship between general life stress, racism-related stress and psychological health among black men. *Journal of Counseling Psychology, 54*, 102–109.

Plowden, K., & Young, A. (2003). Socio-structural factors influencing health behaviors of urban African-American men. *Journal of National Black Nurses' Association, 14*(1), 45–51.

Plowden, K. O., John, W., Vasquez, E., & Kimani, J. (2006). Reaching African American men: A qualitative analysis. *Journal of Community Health Nursing, 23*, 147–158.

Rich, J. (2000). The health of African American men. *Annals of the American Academy of Political and Social Science, 569*, 149–159.

Rich, J. A., & Grey, C. M. (2005). Pathways to recurrent trauma among young black men: Traumatic stress, substance use, and the "code of the street." *American Journal of Public Health, 95*, 816–824.

Sellers, S. L., Bonham, V., Neighbors, H. W., & Amell, J. W. (2006). Effects of racial discrimination and health behaviors on mental and physical health of middle-class African American men. *Health Education and Behavior, 3*(6), 1.

Shin, J. Y., Martin, R., & Howren, M. B. (2009). Influence of assessment methods on reports of gender differences in AMI symptoms. *Western Journal of Nursing Research, 31*(5), 552–568.

Sirin, S. R., McCreary, D. R., & Mahalik, J. (2004). Differential reactions to men's and women's gender role transgressions: Perceptions of social status, sexual orientation, and value dissimilarity. *Journal of Men's Studies, 12*(2), 119–132.

Staveteig, S., & Wigton, A. (2000). *Key findings by race and ethnicity*. 1999 snapshots of America's families II: A view of the nation and 13 states from the National Survey of America's Families. Washington, DC: Urban Institute Press.

Tucker, M. B., & Mitchell-Kernan, C. (1995). African American marital trends in context: Towards a synthesis. In M. B. Tucker & C. Mitchell-Kernan (Eds.), *The decline in marriage among African Americans: Causes, consequences and policy implications*. New York, NY: RussellSage Foundation.

U.S. Census Bureau Current Population Survey, Annual Social and Economic Supplement, 2005. Available from http://www.census.gov/hhes/www/cpstc/cps_table_creator.html

U.S. Department of Health and Human Services, USDHHS. (1999). *Mental health: A report of the Surgeon General.* Rockville, MD: U.S. Department of Health and Human Services, Substance Abuse and Mental Health Services Administration, Center for Mental Health Services, National Institutes of Health, National Institute of Mental Health.

U.S. Department of Health and Human Services. (2001). *Mental health: Culture, race, and ethnicity—A supplement to Mental health: A report of the Surgeon General.* Rockville, MD: U.S. Department of Health and Human Services, Public Health Service, Office of the Surgeon General.

Utsey, S. O. (1997). Racism and the psychological well-being of African American men. *Journal of African American Men*, *3*, 69–87.

Utsey, S. O., & Payne, Y. A. (2000). Differential psychological and emotional impacts of race related stress. *Journal of African American Men*, *5*, 56–72.

Watkins, D. C., Green, B. L., Rivers, B. M., & Rowell, K. L. (2006). Depression in black men: Implications for future research. *Journal of Men's Health and Gender*, *3*, 227–235.

Watkins, D. C., & Neighbors, H. W. (2007). An initial exploration of what "mental health" means to young black men. *Journal of Men's Health and Gender*, *4*, 271–282.

Watkins, D. C., Walker, R. L., & Griffith, D. M. (2010). A meta-study of black male mental health and well-being. *Journal of Black Psychology*, *36*(3), 303–330.

Weber, L., & Parra-Medina, D. (2003). Intersectionality and women's health: Charting a path to eliminating health disparities. *Advances in Gender Research*, *7*, 181–230

Whaley, A. L. (1998). Black psychiatric patients' reactions to the cultural mistrust inventory. *Journal National Medical Association*, *90*(12), 776–778.

White, J. (2004). Toward a black psychology. In R. Jones (Ed.), *Black psychology* (4th ed., pp. 5–16.) Hampton, VA: Cobb & Henry.

Whitehead, T. L. (2000). The "epidemic" and "cultural legends" of black male incarceration: The socialization of African American children to a life of incarceration. In J. P. May (Ed.), *Building violence: How America's rush to incarcerate creates more violence.* Thousand Oaks, CA: Sage.

Williams, D., Takeuchi, D., & Adair, R. (1992). Marital status and psychiatric disorders among blacks and whites. *Journal of Health and Social Behavior*, *33*, 140–157.

Williams, D. R. (2003). The health of men: Structured inequalities and opportunities. *American Journal of Public Health*, *93*, 724–731.

Williams, D. R., Gonzalez, H. M., Neighbors, H., Nesse, R., Abelson, J. M., Sweetman, J., & Jackson, J. S. (2007). Prevalence and distribution of major depressive disorder in African Americans, Caribbean blacks, and non-Hispanic whites. *Archives of General Psychiatry*, *64*, 305–315.

Williams, D. R., & Williams-Morris, R. (2000). Racism and mental health: The African American experience. *Ethnicity & Health*, *5*(3–4), 243–268.

Wilson, W. J. (1996). *When work disappears: The new world of the urban poor.* New York, NY: Knopf.

World Health Organization. (2009). Social determinants of health. Available from http://www.who.int/social_determinants/en/

Chapter 4

Psychosocial Health of Black Sexually Marginalized Men

Louis F. Graham

Learning Objectives

- Gain awareness of major themes related to the social determinants of black sexually marginalized men's psychosocial health.
- Identify factors related to mental disorder acquisition by black sexually marginalized men.
- Understand the relationships between mental health and attitudes and beliefs, relationship functionality, identity development, and violence discrimination and harassment.

• • •

I could not bear the burden of living as a gay man of color in a world grown cold and hateful towards those of us who live and love differently than the so-called mainstream.

—*Joseph Jefferson, 26*

Joseph Jefferson	Tyler Clementi
Raymond Chase	Zach Harrington
Terrel Williams	Billy Lucas
Austin Aaberg	Seth Walsh
Asher Brown	

These are the names of some of the young gay, same-gender-loving, and bisexual men who committed suicide in 2010. This chapter is dedicated to their lives and memory.

The dead offer no answer. We must question the living.

–Marvin K. White, Poet

There is a paucity of research on the psychosocial health of black sexually marginalized men. The little research that exists suggests that black sexually marginalized men (BSMM) are disproportionately burdened by mental health problems and disorders, the most severe of which are depression, anxiety, and **suicidality** (i.e., suicidal ideation, suicide attempts, and completed suicides). A number of theoretical models have been conceptualized to explain health outcomes among both ethnic and sexual minorities, the most comprehensive of which include three primary pathways: internalization of negative attitudes, beliefs, and stigma; structural inequalities; and perceived discrimination and harassment (Clark, Anderson, Clark, & Williams, 1999; Jones, 2000; Krieger, 2001; Link & Phelan, 2001). The **minority stress model**, which has been used with ethnic and racial minorities as well as lesbian, gay, and bisexual communities (LGBs) (Crocker & Major, 1989; Jones et al., 1984; Mirowsky & Ross, 1980, 1989; Pearlin, 1982), posits that minorities who face oppression from a dominant group are likely to experience stress due to this oppression and consequently suffer greater morbidity (Hamilton & Mahlik, 2009).

Meyer (2003) carried out a meta-analytic study that documented the high prevalence of psychiatric morbidity among LGBs and conceptualized a minority stress model to explain the somatic and mental health concerns among gay men, which proposes that gay communities, similar to other marginalized groups, experience stress as a result of oppression and stigmatization (Meyer, 1995). The model casts discrimination and harassment as key elements of harsh social environments that contribute to internalized homophobia, being closeted, expectations of rejection, and experience of prejudice, which then results in compromised mental health (Battle & Crum, 2007). Although evidence supporting constructs and relationships between them delineated in the minority stress model for predominately heterosexual samples of ethnic minorities or predominately white samples of sexual minorities are not readily generalizable to BSMM, there is undoubtedly overlap and some empirical evidence substantiates similarities. Nevertheless, models are needed that address the particular sociocultural context of BSMM's lives in order to better understand how and why minority stress model factors and others contribute to mental disorder occurrence among this specific subpopulation.

Based on the literature broadly, key empirical evidence, and drawing from minority stress models, discrimination effects models, and social interaction and norms theory, a model to understand mental health outcomes among

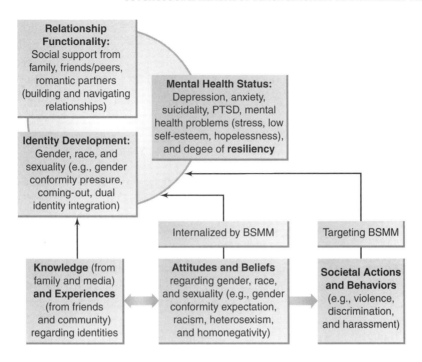

Figure 4.1. Black Sexually Marginalized Men's Psychosocial Health Model

BSMM is expanded in Figure 4.1. A number of constructs across domains of the **socioecologic framework** have been identified as key factors influencing outcomes among this subpopulation. The limited research conducted with BSMM and sexually marginalized and black men in general indicates that ethnic, sexual, and gender **identity development** (intrapersonal); **relationship functionality** (interpersonal); exposure to violence, discrimination, and harassment (institutional/structural); and resilience may play particularly important roles (Graham, Aronson, Nichols, Stephens, & Rhodes, 2011; Graham, Braithwaite, Spikes, Stephens, & Edu, 2009). Researchers have pointed to societal negative attitudes and beliefs regarding gender, race, and sexuality; and policies and practices of community institutions, as forces underlying these factors.

Knowledge produced and shared in families and learned through popular media and experiences with friends and institutions shape the gendered, racial, and sexual terrains community members must navigate, including BSMM. Often this identity landscape and the experience of its inhabitants are imbued with gender conformity pressure, racism, **homonegativity**, and mental illness stigma, among other "isms" and stigma. The effects of these negative attitudes and beliefs regarding gender, race, and sexuality, if internalized by BSMM or if acted on by others in the form of violence, discrimination, or harassment

(VDH) perpetuated against BSMM, can lead to poor mental health outcomes among this subpopulation both directly and by impacting identity development of BSMM and the degree to which they are successful in building and maintaining healthy relationships with family, friends, and romantic partners. The degree of resilience within BSMM communities may moderate these relationships.

Mental Health Outcomes

Major depressive disorder is the leading cause of disability in the United States and Canada among those between the ages of 15 and 44 (WHO, 2008). Although there are no available sample statistics of mental disorder prevalence among BSMM in the United States that can accurately estimate population parameters due, in part, to methodological challenges in obtaining random samples, measurement issues related to accuracy and precision of tools (Perreira, Deeb-Sossa, Harris, & Bollen, 2005), and small sample sizes; research suggests that the prevalence of depression may be as high as 32 percent, anxiety as high as 33 percent, and that BSMM may be 1.2 times more likely than white gay men to attempt suicide (Cochran & Mays, 1994; Graham, Aronson et al., 2011; Meyer, Dietrich, & Schwartz, 2008). Epidemiological research shows that sexual minorities are at significantly greater risk for psychiatric morbidity across a wide range of outcomes, including depression, anxiety, and suicidality, throughout the life course (Cochran & Mays, 2000a, 2000b; Cochran, Sullivan, & Mays, 2003; Fergusson, Horwood, Ridder, & Beautrais, 2005; Gilman, Cochran, Mays, Ostrow, & Kessler, 2001; Sandfort, de Graaf, Bijl, & Schnabel, 2001). In fact, the aforementioned meta-analysis (Meyer, 2003) indicated that sexual minorities are twice as likely as heterosexuals to have a lifetime mood disorder and nearly three times as likely to have a current mood disorder.

A study by Cochran, Sullivan, and Mays (2003) found a 31 percent one-year prevalence of major depression and 17.9 percent one-year prevalence of panic disorder among gay and bisexual men in a U.S. population-based random sample using the Composite International Diagnostic Interview Short Form (CIDI) from the MacArthur Foundation National Survey of Midlife Development. This represents a prevalence 3.57 and 5.09 times ($p < .05$) more than that of heterosexual men in the study (10.2 percent, 3.8 percent, respectively). Additionally, the investigators found higher levels of current and past psychological concerns among men who have sex with men (MSM) compared to heterosexual men in the study; 17.8 and 20.4 percent of MSM self-rated their own mental health as "fair" or "poor" at age 16 and at present age, respectively. These percentages were 3.10 ($p < .05$) and 3.47 ($p < .05$) times greater than that of heterosexual men. This study is consistent with other previous studies, concluding that MSM suffer greater lifetime prevalence rates of major depression and suicide symptoms than men reporting only female partners.

Though mainly based on convenience samples, research indicates that LGBs have higher rates of suicidality than do heterosexuals (Paul et al., 2002). Among adult gay men and lesbians, lifetime suicidal ideation prevalence rates have been reported ranging from 24 to 41 percent, with lifetime suicide attempts prevalence rates ranging from 7 to 20 percent (Bell & Weinberg, 1978; Jay & Young, 1979; Saghir & Robins, 1973). In 2002, suicide was the third leading cause of death among males ages 10 to 24, and males are four times more likely to commit suicide than females (National Alliance on Mental Illness [NAMI], 2007). More than 90 percent of those who die by suicide have a diagnosable mental disorder (National Institute of Mental Health [NIMH], 2005). Oppressive attitudes and beliefs contribute to these rates both directly and indirectly.

Oppressive Attitudes and Beliefs: Racism and Homonegativity

Ethnic minority youth, including sexually marginalized youth, are already confronting racist attitudes, beliefs, discriminatory policies, and practices regularly by the time they reach adolescence and become teenagers (Parks, 2001). Ethnic minority families often intentionally and proactively try to teach their children how to deal with blatant and covert racism experienced in predominately white heterosexual spaces (Jones, 1997), through, for example, imparting race-conscious ethnic relations perspectives that offer children language of critique and views that help insulate them from the harmful effects of racism (Graham, Brown-Jeffy, Aronson, & Stephens, 2011). BSMM also encounter racism and cultural orientation incongruence (Graham, Brown-Jeffy et al., 2011) in sexually marginalized communities. Racism and cultural orientation incongruence in gay communities are present in political and service organizations, social spaces, and in the sexual stereotyping of black men (Parks, 2001) ranging from sexual predator to pornographic object. Racism in sexually marginalized communities is expressed in many ways, including: differential treatment and regard (DeMarco, 1983; Icard, 1986), invisibility, lack of acknowledgement, tokenism (Jackson & Brown, 1996), European derived standards of beauty (Loiacano, 1989), and sexual objectification or perceptions of exoticism (Burstin, 1999; Diaz, Ayala, Bein, Henne, & Marin, 2001). This reality can negatively affect the social relations within community institutions; and, racism is not the only oppressive force BSMM face. Throughout the next three sections, we draw heavily from Battle and Crum's (2007) theorizing and insights on homophobia, parental social support, and identity development.

Homonegativity pervades our society, including black communities. A number of issues have been identified as likely contributing to homonegativity in black communities, including Christian doctrine and beliefs that often view homosexuality as sinful, the legacy of slavery, and gender conformity expectations that center heterosexuality as an ideal construct of black masculinities, among other issues. Although homonegativity exists in black communities, this is not to say that there is more or a greater degree of homonegativity in black communities compared to white communities or society generally. How it is experienced, what it means, and the impact it has on black sexual minorities may, however, be different.

Homonegativity may hurt more or may be felt more severely when it comes from community members and institutions that are regarded as places of refuge from racism, networks of support, and groups with which black sexual minorities may strongly identify. Loiacan (1989) uncovered through in-depth interviews that black gay men who viewed black communities as "extremely homophobic" did not view them as any more homophobic than white communities. Also, black gay and bisexual men rated their experiences with black heterosexuals in black straight organizations significantly more positively than their experiences with white LGBs in white gay organizations, but agreed more with the statement that "homophobia is a problem within the black community" than with the statement that "racism is a problem for GLBT blacks dealing with the GLBT community" (Battle, Cohen, Warren, Fergerson, & Audam, 2002). In this study, although participants' experiences alluded to racism in gay communities as a more pervasive problem, homonegativity in black communities was deemed more problematic (Battle & Crum, 2007).

Additionally, Herek and Capitanio (1995) found no significant differences between African-Americans and Euro-Americans in heterosexist attitudes toward gay men. Battle comments that homonegativity in black communities is problematic "not because of its magnitude but because of its relevance" (Battle & Crum, 2007, p. 339) in the eyes of black sexual minorities. BSMM cannot afford to lose the social support of black communities because of their role in helping community members contend with racism and discrimination in society writ large. BSMM have, to some degree, been equipped to deal with racism and its consequences, but the same is not true for homonegativity.

BSMM have been taught approaches for managing stress related to racial and ethnic discrimination and violence, albeit not specifically in gay communities. They are not as equipped, though, to be resilient against the alienation and hostility of homonegativity in black communities. Even less is known about how internalized isms may play out in BSMM communities. And controlling and negotiating degrees of being "out" or "closeted" in particular spaces and to particular people contributes to stress and poor mental health outcomes. BSMM may endure high levels of stress because of the aggregate effects of institutionalized racism and cultural orientation incongruence in institutions, homonegativity, and heterosexism.

Relationship Functionality

Mental health outcomes among BSMM are influenced by the degree to which BSMM's interpersonal relationships are supportive, functional, and beneficial. Low levels of social support have been shown to predict depression and slowed recovery from major depressive episodes (Kessler, Price, & Wortman, 1985; McLeod, Kessler, & Landis, 1992). Research with sexual minorities has established the importance of both familial and peer/friendship support in promoting and protecting mental health (M. Goldfried & Goldfried, 2001; Radkowsky & Siegel, 1997). Research has shown that sexual minorities report less social support than heterosexuals and that this difference partially explains mental health disparities, including depressive symptoms (Eisenberg & Renick, 2006; Safren & Heimberg, 1999).

Graham and colleagues (2009) found that among BSMM, relationships of support sometimes became relationships of shunning and ostracism. This study defined relationship functionality as the degree to which individuals were able to build, grow, and maintain healthy relationships with family, friends, and romantic partners. Some BSMM in this study reported developing and sustaining unhealthy relationships that contributed to their depression and anxiety. LGB identities often are viewed by ethnic minority families as being in conflict with "traditional" family structures, value systems, and religious beliefs (Morales, 1990).

Some ethnic minority families may discuss issues of sexuality frankly, whereas others may have a hard time overcoming taboos, adjusting their attitudes and beliefs positively, or regarding the marginalized identities of family members in healthy ways. In response to a family member's **coming-out**, the negative views of families can vary from considering this a threat to the existing family unit, an unwanted and unworthy distraction from other more urgent problems and stressors they are facing, to unnecessary increased exposure to HIV. BSMM often fear rejection and expulsion from their family when coming-out. Pilkington and D'Augelli (1995) revealed that 10 percent of ethnic minority LGB youth reported verbal abuse from fathers, 11 percent from brothers, and 7 percent from sisters. Twenty percent characterized the possibility of coming-out to their family as "extremely troubling." Twenty-two percent considered their mothers' reactions to their sexual orientation as "rejecting," 25 percent judged their fathers' reactions as "rejecting," and 8 percent assessed their sisters' reactions as "rejecting."

Identity development commences early and Caldwell and colleagues' study (2002) suggests that families play a purposeful and primary role in instilling positive self-concepts in their children to help buffer the effects of negative external views regarding race, which may partially explain elevated levels of self-esteem found among black adolescents (Jordan, 2004). It is doubtful that families of BSMM intentionally attempt to impart tactics that protect against the effects of negative external views related to their child's sexuality that do not also harm their identity (Battle & Crum, 2007). In fact, it is more likely that heterosexual families do not recognize, acknowledge, or envision the possibility that their children will grow and develop as anything other than heterosexual, until well after same-sex orientation becomes discernible in desire, action, and/or identity. Given this case, it is largely unavoidable for BSMM to internalize some of their families' and communities' homonegative and heterosexist attitudes and beliefs, whereas black families may work to shield their children from internalizing the larger society's racist attitudes and beliefs; and this is to say nothing of the unique experience and nonadditive considerations of being positioned at intersecting identities. Consequently, budding realization and development of an orientation other than heterosexual is more likely to be initially accompanied at best by confusion, fear, and uncertainty, and at worst by shame and self-hatred, rather than pride; thus all but guaranteeing a difficult and vulnerable adolescence for BSMM (Cochran, 2001). BSMM likely do not possess parallel assets vis-à-vis identity development that facilitate ethnic minorities' well-being (Ryff, Keyes, & Hughes, 2003).

Identity Development

Mental health outcomes among BSMM are influenced by the degree to which they are able to achieve positive integrated ethnic, sexual, and gender identities. Generally, identities, being simultaneously culturally bound and porous, aid in social grouping, a sense of life satisfaction, and self-definition (Howard, 2000; Lewin, 1948; Tajfel & Turner, 1979). Strong, positive, and integrated identities are particularly important for marginalized communities as a core factor in how political, social, and psychological resources for protecting against stressors associated with marginalized status are garnered, developed, distributed, and accessed (Cass, 1979; Cross, Parham, & Helms, 1998; Icard, 1996; Lemert, 1997; Sellers, Smith, Shelton, Rowley, & Chavous, 1998; Troiden, 1989). Our self-concept is in part composed of a reflection of how others view, treat, and regard us (Cooley, 1956; Mead, 1934). Consequently, the attitudes and beliefs of communities about BSMM and societal actions targeting BSMM (e.g., VDH) affect their identity development and by extension their mental health. Identity development includes a number of components (e.g., racial, ethnic, gender, sexual) and they have been operationalized in a number of ways by researchers. We begin this discussion by highlighting the effects of internalized homonegativity and identity achievement and integration on the mental health of BSMM, followed by a discussion of racial and sexual identity development models generally, coming-out, and unique features of identity development among BSMM in particular.

In the survey study by Graham and colleagues (2011), internalized homonegativity (measured using the Internalized Homonegativity Inventory revised for use among BSMM) explained 13 percent of the variance in depression (CESD) and 46 percent of the variance in anxiety (STAI) among BSMM. Also, the study by Crawford, Allison, Zamboni, and Soto (2002) among African-American gay and bisexual men found that BSMM with less-developed racial and sexual identities were significantly more likely to have mental distress and less likely to have greater life satisfaction and self-esteem than BSMM with strong dual identities. Additionally, Graham, Braithwaite, Spikes, Stephens, and Edu (2009) conducted focus groups to shed light on the potential factors influencing mental health outcomes among BSMM. They found that BSMM were challenged in developing a healthy overarching identity. Authors concluded that struggles related to the unique experience of being BSMM, such as negative attitudes and beliefs concerning race, sexuality, and gender conformity expectations, contributed to the burden of depression and anxiety.

Cross's Nigrescence Model and Troiden's Sexual Identity Development Model

Although racial and sexual identity development models have been theorized separately, no models have been theorized that consider the simultaneous development of racial and sexual identities. **Cross's Nigrescence model** was one of the first racial identity models conceptualized. In accordance with this model, individuals begin with low race salience. Next, consequent to a race-related "encounter," individuals recognize the oppressed nature of their race and begin to contemplate their racial identity. Following this, in the immersion/emersion phase, there is a heightened awareness and sensitivity to racial identity, and assessments of the dominant external or white communities are inclined to be negative. The last phase, called *internalization/commitment*, is marked by a positive complete identity wherein race is seamlessly integrated with other identities, such as gender, age, and religious affiliation (Cross, 2001).

Troiden (1993) proposed the most well-received model of sexual identity development, which suggests that the healthiest stage of functioning is the **Committed state**. The Committed state exemplifies embracing an identity that matches sexual desire and emotional feelings, perceiving a "nontraditional" or "alternative" identity as legitimate and not inferior to a heterosexual orientation and straight identity, thus commencing and sustaining same-sex romantic relationships—divulging this identity to the general public. This process, commonly known as coming-out, is especially difficult for BSMM and often contributes to psychological distress until successful and complete sexual identity is achieved (Troiden, 1979). Grov, Bimbi, Nanin, and Parsons (2006) found that only 61.8 percent of African-American MSM in their sample were "out" to their parents, compared to 76.8 percent of white MSM (p < .001). Given findings in the Meyer study on the relationship between being closeted and suicidality, evidence suggests that BSMM may be at increased risk. Additionally, a study by Mills et al. (2004) found that nonqueer (i.e., no sexual identity indicated or straight identified) sexually identified MSM in their sample had a 39 percent depression prevalence rate (CES-D > 15) that was statistically significantly different from queer sexually identified MSM who had a 28 percent depression prevalence rate (p < .001). These results are suggestive in that those MSM who have not reached the committed state may be at increased risk for depression. However, the developmental trajectories of BSMM, with respect to coming-out processes, may vary considerably from the Euro-centric standard.

Coming-Out and Unique Features of Identity Development among BSMM

Most models of the coming-out process in the LGB identity literature are Euro-centric. Limited investigation of the coming-out process among black sexual minorities suggests that BSMM's experiences differ from that of white sexually marginalized men. A study by Dube and Savin-Williams (1999), for example, showed that older BSMM came to recognize and self-identify as gay much later than current models suggest. Socially, psychologically, and politically BSMM cannot afford exclusion from or rejection of homonegative heterosexist communities that is frequently theorized as a stage or phase in LGB identity development, because homophile communities often do not provide parallel sociopolitical or psychological resources for them as they do white sexually marginalized community members (Eliason, 1996). This may also partially shed light on the rejection of gay identity among many BSMM (Icard, 1996), choosing instead to identify as Same Gender Loving.

A few have suggested that BSMM may be challenged in simultaneously developing a healthy sexual identity while preventing damage to their ethnic identity (Akerlund & Cheung, 2000). Akerlund and Cheung (2000) found, in reviewing literature on sexual minority issues from 1989 to 1998, that oppression, discrimination, rejection, assimilation, and lack of social support were major factors contributing to the challenge of healthy identity development. In spite of the acknowledged homonegativity in African-American and other communities, BSMM maintain a strong connection with their ethnic cultural heritage and to their communities, and often cite their ethnic identity as primary (Acosta, 1979; Mays, Cochran, & Rhue, 1993). Even so, BSMM allude to feelings of conflicting loyalties between African-American communities and gay communities, when challenged by homophobia in African-American communities or racism in gay communities (Greene, 1994). There are realistic concerns about rejection by both communities (Dyne, 1980; Icard, 1986; Mays & Cochran, 1988), and consequently, there is the potential for negative effects on the health and psychosocial well-being of gay men who are members of ethnic minority groups.

Loiacano (1989) conducted a qualitative study in which black gay men were interviewed about their sexual identities. One of the salient themes delineated was an expressed need to integrate better multiple identities, namely ethnic and sexual identities. The author describes this as a strong desire to acquire simultaneous and inclusive validation and support for black gay men's diverse identities. Most people have multiple components of a collective identity, each of which can assume lesser or greater importance or prominence in disparate circumstances. When two or more of those identities are marginalized, one could become the target of multiple prejudices in majority group contexts (e.g., as black, gay, low socioeconomic status) but could also experience prejudice in minority community environments (e.g., racial prejudice from white gay men, sexual prejudice from black heterosexuals) (Herek & Garnets, 2007). Possessing multiple minority identities raises an individual's likelihood of experiencing marginalization and subjugation (Diaz et al., 2001; Greene, 1994), which could lead to mental disorders like depression and anxiety.

Violence, Discrimination, and Harassment

Black sexually marginalized men face unique challenges in managing a double minority status (i.e., facing racism and heterosexism), putting them at risk for negative life events (e.g., loss of employment, home, or custody of children) and chronic daily hassles due to discrimination. Perceived unfair treatment or discrimination contributes to psychiatric morbidity among BSMM. Both qualitative and quantitative studies have found significant relationships between racial and sexual discrimination, violence, and perceived racist events, and the life satisfaction, anxiety, depression, and general mental health status of BSMM. The most recent was an observational, cross-sectional study that examined the relationships between depression and anxiety; ethnic and sexual identity development; violence, discrimination, and harassment; and coping skills (Graham, Aronson et al., 2011). In this study, 95 percent of BSMM reported experiencing violence, discrimination, and harassment (VDH) in the past year at least once; and of those experiencing any VDH in the past year, 40 percent indicated their race as being primarily involved, and 32 percent indicated both race and sexuality as being primarily involved. Fifty-two percent of participants reported experiencing VDH in public places, 43 percent in retail, customer services, or other business settings, and 35 percent in the criminal justice system. VDH accounted for 52 percent of the variance in depression and 7 percent of the variance in anxiety among respondents.

In regard to the prevalence of hate crimes in African-American communities targeting ethnic minority LGB youth because of their racial or sexual identities, Pilkington and D'Augelli (1995) found that 48 percent of ethnic sexually marginalized youth reported experiencing one form of victimization, and 33 percent experienced two or more forms of victimization. These same authors documented that 56 percent of sexually marginalized youth experienced more than one occurrence of verbal assault, 26 percent of sexually marginalized youth were threatened once, and 10 percent were threatened three or more times. In this same study, 8 percent of LGB ethnic minority youth had objects thrown at them, 7 percent were physically assaulted twice or more, and 5 percent had been a victim of assault with a weapon. LGB adolescents are more likely than their heterosexual peers to be victims of peer violence. Physical and verbal abuse are related to suicide, school problems, and substance abuse among LGB youth.

Sexually Marginalized Men

Research on minority stress among gay men has shown that discrimination and experiences of negative treatment in society are associated with more mental health problems. Meyer (1995) found that gay-related discrimination corresponded with a threefold increase in risk for severe mental distress. Similarly, Huebner, Rebchook, and Kegeles (2004) found that among young MSM those who experienced discrimination within the past six months were 2.13 times more likely to have suicidal ideation within the past two months ($p < .001$) than those who had not experienced discrimination. Likewise, those who were victims of physical violence within the past six months were also 2.06 times more likely to have suicidal ideation in the past two months than those who had not. Hate crimes are common among this population.

In a national probability sample of sexual minorities, Herek (2009) found that nearly 25 percent of participants reported a person or a property crime, and more than 50 percent had been verbally harassed; and Badgett, Lau, Sear, and Ho (2007) found that gay men earn 10 to 32 percent less than equally qualified heterosexual men with the same job. Mays and Cochran (2001) found that a nationally representative sample (Midlife Development in the United States—MIDUS) of MSM were 4.30 times more likely to be fired from a job and 1.82 times more likely to experience any type of discrimination than heterosexuals ($p < .05$). Authors also reported that 42 percent of MSM attributed lifetime discrimination to their sexual orientation, in whole or part, and 76 percent reported any personal experience of discrimination. In comparison, 98 percent of heterosexuals attributed lifetime discrimination to factors other than sexual orientation, and 65 percent indicated that they had ever experienced discrimination.

Black Men

A 2000 review of the literature on racial/ethnic discrimination and mental health not bound by sexuality criteria identified 13 studies (Williams & Williams-Morris, 2000). Four investigations (Brown et al., 2000; Karlsen & Nazroo, 2002; Kessler, Mickelson, & Williams, 1999; Siefert, Bowman, Helfin, Danzinger, & Williams, 2000) explored the relationship between a diagnosis of major depression and perceived discrimination, and three showed a positive association. None of the investigations revealed a negative association. One investigation (Kessler et al., 1999) explored the relationship between generalized anxiety disorder and perceived discrimination, which showed a positive association.

Another study conducted by Jackson and colleagues (1996) reported a relationship between a negative perception of whites' intentions and mental health distress among a national sample of black Americans, while Landrine and Klonoff (1996) reported a relationship between perceived racism and mental distress among black university sub-populations. Additionally, Sellers, Caldwell, Schmeelk-Cone, and Zimmerman (2003) reported direct and indirect longitudinal associations between perceived discrimination and mental distress among black youth. Generally, racial discrimination is associated with poor mental health outcomes; however, we do not yet understand the degree to which exposure to perceived discrimination contributes to increased risk of illness, disorder, or problems, the circumstances in which this may happen, or the processes and mechanisms that may be implicated. Study of ethnic discrimination and mental health in this regard is still in a formative phase.

Summary

BSMM appear to learn and become aware of what it means to exemplify manliness, blackness, and gayness from their families, friends, through popular media, and in community institutions. This knowledge and experience are often infused with oppressive attitudes and beliefs surrounding identity designations, which may include racism, homonegativity, heterosexism, and hegemonic gender conformity expectations that may be both internalized by BSMM and lead to societal actions and behaviors perpetuated against BSMM, such as violence, discrimination, and harassment. These constructs: knowledge/experiences, attitudes/beliefs, and societal actions/behaviors, can influence and affect BSMM's core sense of self, ability to sustain healthy relationships, and their mental health status. Additionally, there may exist bidirectional relationships between these constructs: identity development, relationship functionality, and mental health status. Resilience may moderate these factors' influence on mental health outcomes.

The unique standpoint and experience of BSMM adds a layer of complexity, problematizes current conceptions and presents disparate challenges and opportunities for expanding theoretical frameworks to better understand pathways to mental health problems and disorders among this subpopulation and others. From a standpoint theory perspective, BSMM are of particular interest because they are positioned at the intersection of multiple marginalized identities. We stand to learn the most from those most marginalized among us. Theoretical suppositions and recent research findings have been drawn on to expand a model that highlights social factors likely playing important roles in mental health outcomes among BSMM.

Key Terms

coming-out

committed state

Cross's Nigrescence model

homonegativity

identity development

minority stress model

relationship functionality

socioecologic framework

suicidality

Discussion Questions

1. What institutional policies and practices contribute to the violence, discrimination, and harassment that black sexually marginalized men experience?

2. How might the concept of intersectionality influence how mental health disorders are diagnosed and measured among black sexually marginalized men?

References

Acosta, E. (1979, October 11). Affinity for black heritage: Seeking life-style within a community. *Washington Blade*, A–1, A–25.

Akerlund, M., & Cheung, M. (2000). Teaching beyond the deficit model: Gay and lesbian issues among African Americans, Latino, and Asian Americans. *Journal of Social Work Education*, 36, 279–293.

Badgett, M. L., Lau, H., Sear, B., & Ho, D. (2007). *Bias in the workplace: Consistent evidence of sexual orientation and gender identity discrimination*. Williams Institute. http://www.law.ucla.edu/williamsinstitute/publications/Bias%20in%20the%20Workplace.pdf

Battle, J., Cohen, C., Warren, D., Gergerson, G., & Audam, S. (2002). *Say it loud: I'm black and I'm proud: Black pride survey 2000*. Policy Institute of the National Gay and Lesbian Task Force, New York.

Battle, J., & Crum, M. (2007). Black LGB health and well-being. In I. H. Meyer, & M. E. Northridge (Eds.), *The health of sexual minorities: Public health perspectives on lesbian, gay, bisexual, and transgender populations* (pp. 320–352). New York, NY: Springer.

Bell, A., & Weinberg, M. (1978). *Homosexualities: A study of human diversity among men and women*. New York, NY: Simon & Schuster.

Brown, T. N., Williams, D. R., Jackson, J. S., Neighbors, H. W., Torres, M., Sellers, S. L., & Brown, K. T. (2000). Being black and feeling blue: The mental health consequences of racial discrimination. *Race and Society*, *2*(2), 117–131.

Burstin, H. E. (1999). Looking out, looking in: Anti-Semitism and racism in lesbian communities. *Journal of Homosexuality*, *36*, 143–157.

Caldwell, C., Zimmerman, M., Bernat, D., Sellers, R., & Notaro, P. (2002). Racial identity, maternal support and psychological distress among African American adolescents. *Child Development*, *73*, 1322–1336.

Cass, V. C. (1979). Homosexual identity formation: A theoretical model. *Journal of Homosexuality*, *4*, 219–235.

Clark, R., Anderson, N. B., Clark, V. R., & Williams, D. R. (1999). Racism as a stressor for African Americans: A biopsychosocial model. *American Psychologist*, *54*, 805–816.

Cochran, S. D. (2001). Emerging issues in research on lesbians and gay men's mental health: Does sexual orientation really matter? *American Psychology*, *56*, 931–947.

Cochran, S. D., & Mays, V. M. (1994). Depressive distress among homosexually active African American men and women. *American Journal of Psychiatry*, *151*, 524–529.

Cochran, S. D., & Mays, V. M. (2000a). Lifetime prevalence of suicide symptoms and affective disorders among men reporting same-sex sexual partners: Results from NHANES III. *American Journal of Public Health*, *90*, 573–578.

Cochran, S. D., & Mays, V. M. (2000b). Relation between psychiatric syndromes and behaviorally defined sexual orientation in a sample of the US population. *American Journal of Epidemiology*, *151*, 516–523.

Cochran, S. D., Sullivan, J. G., & Mays, V. M. (2003). Prevalence of mental disorders, psychological distress, and mental health services use among lesbian, gay, and bisexual adults in the United States. *Journal of Consulting and Clinical Psychology*, *71*, 53–61.

Cooley, C. H. (1956). *Human nature and the social order*. New York, NY: Free Press.

Crawford, I., Allison, K. W., Zamboni, B. D., & Soto, T. (2002). The influence of dual-identity development on the psychosocial functioning of African-American gay and bisexual men. *Journal of Sex Research*, *39*(3), 179–189.

Crocker, J., & Major, B. (1989). Social stigma and self-esteem: The self-protective properties of stigma. *Psychological Review*, *96*, 608–630.

Cross, W. E. (2001). The psychology of nigrescence. In J. G. Ponterotte, J. M. Casas, L.A. Suzuki, & C. M. Alexander (Eds.), *Handbook of multicultural counseling* (pp. 93–122). London, UK: Sage.

Cross, W. E., Parham, T. A., & Helms, J. E. (1991). The stages of black identity development: Nigrescence models. In R. Jones (Ed.), *Black psychology* (pp. 319–338). Oakland, CA: Cobb & Henry.

DeMarco, J. (1983). Gay racism. In M. J. Smith (Ed), *Black men/white men: A gay anthology* (pp. 109–118). San Francisco, CA: Gay Sunshine Press.

Diaz, R. M., Ayala, G., Bein, E., Henne, J., & Marin, B. V. (2001). The impact of homophobia, poverty, and racism on the mental health of gay and bisexual Latino men: Findings from 3 US cities. *American Journal of Public Health, 91*(6), 927–932.

Dube, E. M., & Savin-Williams, R. C. (1999). Sexual identity development among ethnic sexual-minority male youths. *Developmental Psychology, 35*, 1389–1398.

Dyne, L. (1980, September). Is D.C. becoming the gay capitol of America? *Washingtonian*, 96–101, 133–141.

Eisenberg, M. E., & Resnick M. D. (2006). Suicidality among gay, lesbian, and bisexual youth: The role of protective factors. *Journal of Adolescent Health, 39*, 662–668.

Eliason, M. J. (1996). Identity formation for lesbian, bisexual and gay persons: Beyond a "minoritizing" view. *Journal of Homosexuality, 30*, 31–58.

Fergusson, D. M., Horwood, L. J., Ridder, E. M., & Beautrais, A. L. (2005). Sexual orientation and mental health in birth cohort of young adults. *Psychological Medicine, 35*, 971–981.

Gilman, S. E., Cochran, S. D., Mays, V. M., Hughes, M., Ostrow, D., & Kessler, R. C. (2001). Risk of psychiatric disorders among individuals reporting same-sex sexual partners in the National Comorbidity Survey. *American Journal of Public Health, 91*, 933–939.

Goldfried, M. R., & Goldfried, A. P. (2001). The importance of parental support in the lives of gay, lesbian, and bisexual individuals. *Journal of Clinical Psychology, 57*, 681–693.

Graham, L. F., Aronson, R. E., Nichols, T., Stephens, C. F., & Rhodes, S. (2011). Factors influencing depression and anxiety among black sexual minority men. *Depression Research and Treatment*, 2011, 587984. doi: 10.1155/2011/587984

Graham, L. F., Braithwaite, K., Spikes, P., Stephens, C. F., & Edu, U. F. (2009). Exploring the mental health of lack men who have sex with men. *Community Mental Health Journal, 45*, 272–284.

Graham, L. F., Brown-Jeffy, S., Aronson, R. E., & Stephens, C. F. (2011). Critical race theory as theoretical framework and analysis tool for population health research. *Critical Public Health Journal, 21*(1), 81–93.

Greene, B. (1994). Lesbian women of color. In L. Comas-Diaz & B. Greene (Eds.), *Women of color: Integrating ethnic and gender identities in psychotherapy*. New York, NY: Guilford Press.

Grov, C., Bimbi, D., Nanin, J., & Parsons, J. (2006). Race, ethnicity, gender, and generational factors associated with the coming-out process among gay, lesbian, and bisexual individuals. *Journal of Sex Research, 43*(2), 115–121.

Hamilton, C. J., & Mahalik, J. R. (2009). Minority stress, masculinity, and social norms predicting gay men's health risk behaviors. *Journal of Counseling Psychology, 56*, 132–141.

Herek, G. M. (2009). Hate crimes and stigma-related experiences among sexually marginalized adults in the United States: Prevalence estimates from a national probability sample. *Journal of Interpersonal Violence*, *24*, 54–74.

Herek, G. M., & Capitanio, J. (1995). Black heterosexuals' attitudes towards lesbians and gay men in the United States. *Journal of Sex Research*, *32*, 95–105.

Herek, G. M., & Garnets, L. D. (2007). Sexual orientation and mental health. *Annual Reviews of Clinical Psychology*, *3*, 353–375.

Howard, J. A., (2000). Social psychology of identities. *Annual Review of Sociology*, *26*, 267–393.

Huebner, D., Rebchook, G., & Kegeles, S. (2004). Experiences of harassment, discrimination, and physical violence among young gay and bisexual men. *American Journal of Public Health*, *94*, 1200–1203.

Icard, L. (1986). Black gay men and conflicting social identities: Sexual orientation versus racial identity. *Journal of Social Work and Human Sexuality*, *4*, 83–93.

Icard, L. (1996). Assessing the psychosocial well being of African American gays: A multidimensional perspective. *Journal of Gay & Lesbian Social Services*, *5*, 25–49.

Jackson, J. S., Brown, T. N., Williams, D. R., Torres, M., Sellers, R. L., & Brown, K. (1996). Racism and the physical and mental health status of African Americans: A thirteen year national panel study. *Ethnicity and Disease*, *6*, 132–147.

Jackson, K., & Brown, L. (1996). Lesbians of African heritage: Coming out in the straight community. *Journal of Gay & Lesbian Social Services*, *5*, 53–61.

Jay, K., & Young, A. (1979). *The gay report: Lesbian and gay men speak out about sexual experiences and lifestyles*. New York, NY: Summit Books.

Jones, C. P. (2000). Levels of racism: A theoretic framework and a gardener's tale. *American Journal of Public Health*, *90*, 1212–1215.

Jones, E. E., Farina, A., Hestrof, A. H., Markus, H., Miller, D. T., & Scott, R. A. (1984). *Social stigma: The psychology of marked relationships*. New York, NY: Freeman.

Jones, J. M. (1997). *Prejudice and racism* (2nd ed.). New York, NY: McGraw-Hill.

Jordan, M. (2004, June 18). Ethnic diversity doesn't blend in kids' lives. *Wall Street Journal*, Marketplace.

Karlsen, S., & Nazroo, J. Y. (2002). Relation between racial discrimination, social class, and health among ethnic minority groups. *American Journal of Public Health*, *92*, 624–631.

Kessler, R. C., Mickelson, K. D., & Williams, D. R. (1999). The prevalence, distribution, and mental health correlates of perceived discrimination in the United States. *Journal of Health and Social Behavior*, *40*, 208–230.

Kessler, R. C., Price, R. H., & Wartman, C. B. (1985). Social factors in psychopathology: Stress, social support, and coping processes. *Annual Review of Psychology*, *36*, 531–572.

Krieger, N. (2001). Theories for social epidemiology in the 21st century: An ecosocial perspective. *International Journal of Epidemiology*, *30*, 155–163.

Landrine, H., & Klonoff, E. A. (1996). The schedule of racist events: A measure of racial discrimination and a study of its negative physical and mental health consequences. *Journal of Black Psychology*, *22*, 144–168.

Lemert, C. (1997). *Postmodernism is not what you think*. Malden, MA: Blackwell.

Lewin, K. (1948). *Resolving social conflicts*. New York, NY: Harper.

Link, B. G., & Phelan, J. C. (2001). Conceptualizing stigma. *Annual Review of Sociology*, *27*, 363–385.

Loiacano, D. K. (1989). Gay identity issues among black Americans: Racism, homophobia, and the need for validation. *Journal of Counseling & Development*, *68*, 21–25.

Mays, V. M., & Cochran, S. (1988). The black women's relationship project: A national survey of black lesbians. In M. Shernoff & W. Scott (Eds.), *The sourcebook on lesbian/gay health care* (2nd ed., pp. 54–62). Washington, DC: National Lesbian and Gay Health Foundation.

Mays, V. M., & Cochran, S. D. (2001). Mental health correlates of perceived discrimination among lesbian, gay, and bisexual adults in the United States. *American Journal of Public Health*, *91*, 1869–1876.

Mays, V. M., Cochran, S. D., & Rhue, S. (1993). The impact of perceived discrimination on the intimate relationships of black lesbians. *Journal of Homosexuality*, *25*(4), 1–14.

McLeod, J. D., Kessler, R. C., & Landis, K. R. (1992). Speed of recovery from major depressive episodes in a community sample of married men and women. *Journal of Abnormal Psychology*, *101*, 277–286.

Mead, G. H. (1934). *Mind, self and society*. Chicago, IL: University of Chicago Press.

Meyer, I. H. (1995). Minority stress and mental health in gay men. *Journal of Health and Social Behavior*, *36*, 38–56.

Meyer, I. H. (2003). Prejudice, social stress, and mental health in lesbian, gay, and bisexual populations: Conceptual issues and research evidence. *Psychological Bulletin*, *129*, 674–697.

Meyer, I. H., Dietrich, J., & Schwarts, S. (2008). Lifetime prevalence of mental disorders and suicide attempts in diverse lesbian, gay, and bisexual populations. *American Journal of Public Health*, *98*(6), 1001–1006.

Mills, T. C., Paul, J., Stall, R., Pollack, L., Canchola, J., Chang, Y. J., . . . Catania, J. A. (2004). Distress and depression in men who have sex with men: The urban men's health study. *American Journal of Psychiatry*, *161*, 278–285.

Mirowsky, J., & Ross, C. E. (1980). Minority stress, ethnic culture, and distress: A comparison of blacks, whites, Mexicans, and Mexican Americans. *American Journal of Sociology*, *86*, 479–495.

Mirowsky, J., & Ross, C. E. (1989). *Social causes of psychological distress*. Hawthorne, NY: Aldine de Gruyter.

Morales, E. (1990). Ethnic minority families and minority gays and lesbians. In F. W. Bozett & M. B. Sussman (Eds.), *Homosexuality and family relations* (pp. 217–239). Binghamton, NY: Harrington Park Press.

National Alliance on Mental Illness. (2007). *Mental illness: Facts and numbers*. www.nami.org

National Institute of Mental Health. (2005). *Suicide in the U.S.: Statistics and prevention*. Available at http://www.nimh.nih.gov/publicat/harmsway.cfm

Parks, C. W. (2001). African-American same-gender–loving youths and families in urban schools. *Journal of Gay & Lesbian Social Services*, *13*, 41–56.

Paul, J. P., Catania, J., Pollack, L., Moskowitz, J., Canchola, M. S., Mills, T. . . . Stall, R. (2002). Suicide attempts among gay and bisexual men: Lifetime prevalence and antecedents. *American Journal of Public Health*, *92*, 1338–1345.

Pearlin, L. I. (1982). The social context of stress. In L. Goldberger & S. Breznitz (Eds.), *Handbook of stress: Theoretical and clinical aspects* (pp. 367–379). New York, NY: Academic Press.

Perreira, K. M., Deeb-Sossa, N., Harris, K. M., & Bollen, K. (2005). What are we measuring? An evaluation of the CES-D across race/ethnicity and immigrant generation. *Social Forces, 83*(4), 1567–1602.

Pilkington, N. W., & D'Augelli, A. R. (1995). Victimization of lesbian, gay, and bisexual youths in community settings. *Journal of Community Psychology, 23,* 34–56.

Radkowsky, M., & Siegel, L. J. (1997). The gay adolescent: Stressors, adaptations, and psychosocial interventions. *Clinical Psychology Review, 17,* 191–216.

Ryff, C. D., Keyes, C. M., & Hughes, D. L. (2003). Status inequalities, perceived discrimination, and eudaimonic well-being: Do the challenges of minority life hone purpose and growth? *Journal of Health and Social Behavior, 44,* 275–291.

Safren, S. A., & Heimberg, R. G. (1999). Depression, hopelessness, suicidality, and related factors in sexually marginalized and heterosexual adolescents. *Journal of Consulting and Clinical Psychology, 67,* 859–866.

Saghir, M. T., & Robins, E. (1973). *Male and female homosexuality: A comprehensive investigation.* Baltimore, MD: Williams & Wilkins.

Sandfort, T. G., de Graaf, R., Bijl, R. V., & Schnabel, P. (2001). Same-sex sexual behavior and psychiatric disorders: Findings from the Netherlands Mental Health Survey and Incidence Study (NEMESIS). *Archives of General Psychiatry, 58,* 85–91.

Sellers, R. M., Caldwell, C. H., Schmeelk-Cone, K., & Zimmerman, M. A. (2003). Racial identity, racial discrimination, perceived stress, and psychological distress among African American young adults. *Journal of Health and Social Behavior, 44,* 302–317.

Sellers, R. M., Smith, M. A., Shelton, J. N., Rowley, S. J., & Chavous, T. M. (1998). Multidimensional Model of Racial Identity: A reconceptualization of African American racial identity. *Personality and Social Psychology Review, 2*(1), 18–39.

Siefert, K., Bowman, P. J., Helfin, C. M., Danzinger, S., & Williams, D. R. (2000). Social and environmental predictors of maternal depression in current and recent welfare recipients. *American Journal of Orthopsychiatry, 70,* 510–522.

Tajfel, H., & Turner, J. (1979). An integrative theory of intergroup conflict. In W. G. Austin & S. Worchel (Eds.), *The social psychology of intergroup relations* (pp. 33–47). Monterey, CA: Brooks/Cole.

Troiden, R. R. (1979). Becoming homosexual: A model of gay identity acquisition. *Psychiatry, 42,* 362–373.

Troiden, R. R. (1989). The formation of homosexual identities. *Journal of Homosexuality, 17,* 43–73.

Troiden, R. R. (1993). The formation of homosexual identities. In L. Garnets & D. Kimmel (Eds.), *Psychological perspectives on lesbian and gay male experiences* (pp. 191–217). New York, NY: Columbia University Press.

Williams, D. R., & Williams-Morris, R. (2000). Racism and mental health: The African American experience. *Ethnicity & Health, 29,* 243–268.

World Health Organization (WHO). (2008). *Depression.* http://www.who.int/mental_health/management/depression/definition/en/

Parental Incarceration as a Social Determinant of Male African-American Adolescents' Mental Health

Susan D. Phillips
Qiana R. Cryer-Coupet

Learning Objectives

- Understand ways in which high rates of incarceration adversely affect African-American *communities* and the mental health and developmental outcomes of African-American adolescent males.
- Understand ways in which parental incarceration adversely affects African-American *families* and indirectly affects the mental health and developmental outcomes of African-American adolescent males.
- Understand ways in which parental incarceration directly affects the mental health of African-American adolescent males.
- Understand how high incarceration rates within one generation of African Americans increase the risk that members of the next generation will be incarcerated.

• • •

Although mental health is recognized as an important component of overall health, African Americans are disproportionately exposed to social conditions that can impinge on mental well-being (U.S. Department of Health and

Human Services [DHHS], 2001). Among these are racial discrimination, chronic poverty, and unemployment. These same social conditions are also linked to the increased risk of being sent to jail or prison (Chaiken, 2000; Pratt, 2001; Sampson, 1985; Sampson & Groves, 1989), an experience that is epidemic within some low-income, urban, African-American communities. Studies in Baltimore and D.C. neighborhoods, for example, find that as many as one in four African-American males in their twenties are under the supervision of criminal justice authorities (Mauer, 2004). Moreover, statisticians estimate that at recent rates of incarceration, one in three African-American boys born in 2001 will spend time in prison at some point in their lives (Bonczar & Beck, 1997).

In this chapter, we examine the complex ways in which high rates of incarceration in general, and the incarceration of parents in particular, negatively affect the mental health and developmental outcomes of African-American adolescent males. More specifically, this chapter describes how adolescents' outcomes are influenced indirectly by changes brought about by incarceration in communities and families as well as more direct links between incarcerating African-American parents and their adolescent sons' mental well-being. Additionally, this chapter describes how the mental health consequences of parental incarceration, coupled with **disparities** (*the lack of equality*) in access to mental health care and the proliferation of the criminal justice system, combine to create a pathway linking the incarceration of one generation of African Americans to the increased potential for incarceration among members of the next.

How Incarceration Adversely Affects Adolescents' Communities

African-American adults are more likely to experience incarceration than are adults in general. Point prevalence estimates show that out of all the adults in the United States, 1 in 134 is in jail or prison. In contrast, the incarceration rate among African-American adults is nearly 1 in 20 (Wildeman, 2009). Incarceration is not equally distributed among African Americans. Instead, it is concentrated among members of a relatively small number of communities and, moreover, often within a relatively small number of blocks within those communities (Brooks, Solomon, Keegan, Kohl, & Lahue, 2005; Visher & Farrell, 2005). High levels of incarceration within communities adversely affect the outcomes of community youth—even youth who do not personally have a parent who has been to prison. This is because, paradoxically, high rates of incarceration feed many of the same neighborhood social problems that contribute to crime.

Crime rates are persistently highest in communities with high rates of poverty, single-parent households, and population mobility. Because of longstanding **structural racism** (*a system of social structures that produces durable, race-based inequalities*) in areas such as education, employment, and housing, African Americans and members of other minority groups disproportionately occupy neighborhoods with these characteristics. Incarceration contributes to the social problems associated with crime by perpetuating poverty and destabilizing families and communities (Clear, 1996). For example, incarceration perpetuates poverty because people who have been to prison face numerous barriers obtaining employment when they are released (Grogger, 1995; Needels, 1996). Incarceration also changes the structure of families, sometimes turning two-parent households into single-parent households (Glaze & Maruschak, 2008). The flux of community residents constantly leaving the community to go to prison and then returning adds to mobility and instability within communities (Clear, Rose, Warring, & Scully, 2005).

In addition to perpetuating social problems associated with crime, high community levels of incarceration also play a role in adolescent African-American males' identity formation and their perceptions of what their futures hold. One can readily imagine that African-American teens in neighborhoods with high rates of incarceration may have dim hopes for their futures when as many as one in four young adult males around them are under the supervision of the criminal justice system. In turn, African-American adolescent boys who lack confidence in their futures experience higher levels of depressive symptoms (Hawkins, Hawkins, Sabatino, & Ley, 1998).

How Incarceration Adversely Affects Adolescents' Families

Approximately one in seven African-American children has a parent in state or federal prison on any given day. In terms of lifetime prevalence, one in four African-American children born in 1990 experienced the incarceration of at least one parent by age 14. Among African-American children whose fathers dropped out of high school, the rate is one out of two (Wildeman, 2009).

Many parents in prison have problems that may adversely affect adolescents' family circumstances and adolescents' mental health and developmental outcomes. For example, approximately 20 percent of parents in prison report a history of physical or sexual abuse, 57 percent have mental health problems, and 67 percent have substance abuse problems (Glaze & Maruschak, 2008). A substantial body of research links these parent problems to family problems of household poverty, single-parent households, and multiple disruptions in children's living arrangements or caregivers. These family problems are associated with a plethora of adverse mental health and development outcomes in children and adolescents, including higher rates of emotional and behavioral problems, school failure, teen pregnancy, delinquency, and so on (Ammerman, Kolko, Kirisci, Blackson, & Dawes, 1999; Chaffin, Kelleher, & Hollenberg, 1996;

Giancola, 2000; Kumpfer, 1987; Loukas, Fitzgerald, Zucker, & von Eye, 2001; Stanger, Higgins, & Bickel, 1999).

Sending parents to prison can contribute to their children's adverse outcomes in two ways. First, the criminal justice system rarely acts on the opportunity it has to improve children's outcomes by helping parents while parents are in custody. These missed opportunities are tantamount to **acts of omission** (*the legal concept that damages can ensue not only from someone's action, but also from someone's inaction*). Second, incarcerating parents contributes to adversity in children's families, such as poverty and family disruption, increasing the likelihood of adverse mental health and developmental outcomes.

Acts of Omission

Although it was not their intent, when policy makers enacted criminal justice policies that sent a historically unprecedented number of parents to prison, they effectively made the criminal justice system a *de facto* partner with other child- and family-serving systems in addressing adolescent mental health (Phillips & Dettlaff, 2007). Youth could potentially benefit from this unintentional partnership if, during the period parents are incarcerated, parents received interventions and rehabilitation services that addressed problems that interfere with their abilities to function in their roles as parents. However, fewer than half (42 percent) of the people who are sent to prison who have substance abuse problems receive treatment while incarcerated. The picture is even bleaker for people with mental health problems—only 31 percent receive treatment (Glaze & Maruschak, 2008).

We err, however, if we only consider the shortcomings of the criminal justice system. One of the most consistent findings in studies of children who experience parental incarceration is that they are more likely than their peers to live in households with a greater number of co-occurring problems (Murray, Janson, & Farrington, 2007; Phillips, Burns, Wagner, & Barth, 2004; Phillips, Burns, Wagner, Kramer, & Robbins, 2002; Phillips, Leathers, & Erkanli, 2009). These include parental substance abuse, mental illness, inadequate education, family violence, housing instability, and extreme poverty. Research shows that the risk for adverse outcomes increases exponentially as the number of risk factors youth experience increases (Biederman et al., 1995; Bry, McKeon, & Pandina, 1982; Johnson & Waldfogel, 2002; McCrae & Barth, 2007). This means that the adolescents who experience parental incarceration are at greatest risk for developing problems in those families with the most complex needs.

High incarceration rates are in some ways a symptom of the failure of multiple systems (e.g., health care, mental health, substance abuse, workforce development, welfare, education) to adequately prevent or address parents' problems that have negative consequences for families and children and which also place parents at risk for arrest and incarceration. That failure is attributable, in part, to the fragmented nature of existing services: one system addresses parents' substance abuse problems; another, their mental health problems; another, poverty, and so forth. The problem is compounded by the fact that services for parents often overlook their children's needs for intervention. At the same time, child and adolescent services often treat parents' problems only as a peripheral concern, if they acknowledge those problems at all.

The Role of Parental Incarceration in Family Adversity

The problem is not only that the criminal justice and other public systems are failing to act on opportunities to improve adolescents' outcomes by helping their parents, but incarcerating parents denigrates teens' family circumstances. Research shows, for example, that beyond any adverse effects parents' substance abuse, mental illness, or lack of education may have on families, incarceration acts independently to increase family poverty and disruption (Phillips, Erkanli, Keeler, Costello, & Angold, 2006).

Poverty

Studies of children in the general population, mental health settings, and the child welfare system repeatedly show that children whose parents have been incarcerated are more likely than are their peers to live in households with annual incomes below $10,000 (Phillips et al., 2004; Phillips et al., 2002; Phillips, Erkanli, Costello, & Angold, 2007). The extreme economic hardship these children and their families face is partly a result of their parents' incarceration. Approximately 50 percent of parents in prison were the primary source of financial support for their children before they were sent to prison (Glaze & Maruschak, 2008). The incarceration of parents, therefore, means a loss of support in the short term.

Incarceration, however, also has an enduring effect on an individual's employability and earnings (Freeman, 1992; Sampson & Laub, 1993). A number of laws have been passed that preclude people with criminal records from obtaining employment in a variety of occupations. Even in the absence of legal barriers, employers often hesitate to hire someone with a criminal record. This may be particularly damaging to people re-entering the community after being in prison, as programs that people often depend on as a safety net are not accessible to individuals who have been convicted of felonies. Among these are Temporary Assistance to Needy Families, food stamps, subsidized housing, and student loans (Allard, 2002; Hirsch et al., 2002). The combined effects of these policies make it difficult for parents who are sent to prison to support themselves and provide for the instrumental needs of their children.

The resulting economic strain can lead to children's caregivers experiencing emotional distress, particularly if they are raising children alone, are socially isolated, or have few financial resources to begin with (McLoyd, 1990). Perhaps more importantly, the economic problems associated with having a prison record may contribute to children being **persistently poor** (*living in extreme poverty for extended periods of their childhoods*). Youth who experience persistent poverty are at greater risk for developing emotional and behavioral problems than are those who are never poor or only transiently poor. Moreover, researchers have found that youth who experience poverty for a number of years during childhood not only have higher levels of depression and antisocial behaviors, but their symptoms endure beyond the period of childhood poverty (McLeod & Shanahan, 1996). Consistent with this, researchers in England have found that children who are separated from their parents because their parents were incarcerated are more likely than children separated from their parents for other reasons to have persistent internalizing problems and antisocial behaviors (Murray & Farrington, 2005, 2008).

Family Disruption

Nearly half of the parents in prison (44 percent) lived with their children immediately prior to beginning their current sentence (Glaze & Maruschak, 2008). Approximately 18 percent of these parents lived with their children in two-parent households, and a similar proportion lived with their children in single-parent households. Incarcerating parents from two-parent households creates new single-parent households. Incarcerating those from single-parent households necessitates someone other than a parent assuming responsibility for the parent's children; this is often a grandparent. In addition to separation from their parents, studies indicate that 20 to 30 percent of children whose mothers go to prison are separated from their siblings (Harm & Thompson, 1995; Koban, 1983; Stanton, 1980; Zalba, 1964) and that approximately 1 in 10 youth change households multiple times (Zalba, 1964).

Disruptive family experiences are a concern because of their potential adverse effects on children's ability to form secure attachments (Johnson & Waldfogel, 2002; Poehlmann, 2005). Secure attachments influence children's mental representations of themselves and others that provide the lens for their interpretation of future interpersonal interactions. As such, attachments influence children's developmental trajectories leading toward interpersonal competence or incompetence (Poehlmann, 2005, p. 679). Research indicates that the more changes in residences or caregivers children with incarcerated parents experienced, the more likely they were to have disruptive behaviors (Johnston, 1995).

How Parental Incarceration Directly Affects Adolescents

Thus far, we have described ways in which incarceration indirectly affects adolescents' mental health and developmental outcomes by adversely affecting their communities or their family lives. Sending parents to prison, however, can also directly affect adolescents' well-being and development.

Posttraumatic Stress

Individuals working with children whose parents are in jails and prisons have long contended that witnessing a parent's arrest traumatizes children (e.g., Bernstein, 2005; Puddefoot & Foster, 2007). Research on this issue is extremely limited, but available studies suggest that this claim has merit (Bocknek, Sanderson, & Britner, 2008; Stanton, 1980). The most rigorous study to date is based on a nationally representative sample of youth who were subjects of reports of maltreatment (Phillips & Zhao, 2010), a sample that may not be typical of all youth whose parents are imprisoned. Nonetheless, this study found that children who witnessed the arrest of someone in their household (not exclusively their parent) were more likely than were other children to witness someone in their home dealing drugs or stealing. They were also more likely to witness and be the victims of a greater number of acts of violence in their homes, including being threatened with knives and guns. These findings are not particularly surprising as these types of events potentially explain why arrests occurred. It was also not surprising that exposure to these types of events was associated with symptoms of **posttraumatic stress** (*a severe anxiety disorder that can develop in response to an event such as the threat of death to oneself or to someone else and which includes symptoms such as nightmares, avoidance, anger, sleep disturbances, and hypervigilance*). What *was* surprising is that witnessing the arrest of a household member was a risk factor for posttraumatic stress symptoms in its own right, after accounting for multiple other experiences that might explain children's symptoms of posttraumatic stress.

Ambiguous Loss

Parental imprisonment is thought to be a particularly harmful form of parent–child separation because it is often unexpected, children may not be told or understand what happened to their parents, and they have limited contact with their parents in the wake of the loss (Murray, 2008). The loss of a parent due to incarceration has been described as an ambiguous loss (Bocknek et al., 2008)—the type of loss people experience when a family member is kidnapped and his or her fate is unknown, or when a person is missing in action in a war. Research shows that the loss of a parent, combined with possible traumatic circumstances surrounding that loss, increases the likelihood of children developing emotional and behavioral problems (Dowdney, 2005). Rather than extending the same support and concern we offer children who lose parents for other reasons, children separated from their parents because of imprisonment are left to struggle with their loss alone.

Stigmatization

Stigmatization (*treating people in a discriminatory manner because they are different in some way*) is often mentioned as one of the adverse unintended consequences of parental imprisonment (Arditti, Lambert-Shute, & Joest, 2003; Hagan & Dinovitzer 1999; Murray, 2007; Sack, Seidler, & Thomas, 1976). Although there has been little research on the stigmatization associated with parental incarceration, studies of other stigmatized conditions have found that, in the short run, children worry about how they and their parents will be viewed by others after learning their parent has a stigmatized condition. In the case of children whose parents are arrested and incarcerated, there is speculation that children's concerns about being stigmatized at school may contribute to school phobias and nonattendance, particularly in the first few weeks following a parent's arrest.

In the end, to protect themselves from stigmatizing treatment, children may try to keep their parent's incarceration a secret from others or withdraw from social situations and activities in which their status might be discovered (Hagan & Myers, 2003; Nesmith & Ruhland, 2008; Sack et al., 1976). Even if children do not personally encounter stigmatizing treatment, they are aware of negative societal attitudes about stigmatized groups. The anticipation of rejection and discriminatory treatment can also lead to the avoidance of interactions with others. Consistent with these findings, researchers in Canada who interviewed children with incarcerated fathers concluded that the fear of stigma had a much more debilitating effect on families than did the way in which they were actually treated (Benaquisto & Coulthard, 2008).

More insidious still is the fact that membership in a stigmatized group does not protect children from adopting negative societal attitudes about their group, or accepting those views as true of themselves personally. Studies of various groups of stigmatized children have found that children who internalize negative societal attitudes about a group to which they belong are more likely to subsequently have lower self-esteem, a reduced sense of self-efficacy, and higher rates of various mental and physical health problems (Bos & Van

Blen, 2008; Gershon, Tschann, & Jemerin, 1999; Kidd, 2007). The belief that negative stereotypes about one's group (e.g., "the apple doesn't fall far from the tree") are personally true about oneself can also result in behaviors that are consistent with the stereotypes.

Parental Incarceration, Adolescents' Mental Health, and Pathways of Intergenerational Incarceration

As we have shown, high rates of incarceration in general, and the incarceration of parents in particular, can adversely affect male African-American adolescents' mental health. In doing so, the incarceration of African-American parents creates a pathway that increases the chances of their son's becoming involved with the criminal justice system.

Professionals working in the mental health field need to be aware that the emotional and behavioral problems of adolescent African-American males may be associated with issues of parental incarceration such as witnessing arrests, the ambiguous loss of a parent who is in prison, or stigmatization. They also need to recognize the role that incarceration plays in family disruption and the despair youth may feel when they see so many others around them involved with the criminal justice system. Considering these factors could help mental health professionals shape interventions to alleviate some of the distress youth experience because of parental incarceration.

At the same time, youth cannot benefit from **incarceration-sensitive mental health interventions** (interventions that take into consideration children's emotional, social, and psychological response to a parent going to jail or prison) if they cannot access mental health services. One of the recalcitrant problems with child and adolescent mental health services is that many African-American youth who might benefit from mental health services never receive them. Disparities in accessing mental health services may, indirectly, contribute to African-American males becoming involved with criminal authorities and to intergenerational incarceration because many of the behavioral problems that might arise from the incarceration of parents or other community members place youth in jeopardy of becoming involved in the juvenile justice system.

Although African-American youth experience barriers to adequate and appropriate mental health care (DHHS, 2001), they have high exposure to law enforcement officers in their schools and communities. Once involved in the justice system, African-American youth receive harsher sanctions and punishments for behaviors in comparison to white youth with similar charges. Consequently, the adverse consequences incarceration has on the mental health of adolescent African-American males, when coupled with barriers to receiving mental health services and the greater likelihood of contact with the criminal justice system, create a pathway linking the incarceration of one generation of African Americans to the incarceration of members of the next.

Summary

The high rate of incarceration within some African-American communities in the United States is increasingly being regarded as a public health issue. It is an especially important issue given that African-American children are eight times more likely than their white peers to have at least one parent who is incarcerated (Mumola, 2000). This chapter highlighted ways in which experiences of parental incarceration can negatively impact the social, emotional, and behavioral outcomes of African-American adolescent males. Understanding that adolescence is an important developmental and transitional period in a young man's life, it is important for mental health researchers and practitioners to find ways of helping young people cope effectively with parental incarceration, while at the same time joining forces with other professionals (e.g., public health, social work, economic development) and members of affected communities to tackle the deeply seated social and systemic problems that contribute to high incarceration rates.

Key Terms

acts of omission

ambiguous loss

disparities

incarceration-sensitive mental
   health interventions

persistently poor

posttraumatic stress

stigmatization

structural racism

Discussion Questions

1. How might the stigma associated with a parent going to prison affect African-American males' mental health across their life span?

2. What do you believe needs to happen to address the direct and indirect impacts of parental incarceration on the mental health outcomes of adolescent African-American males?

3. Given the fragmented nature of social services in the United States, how might policy makers better address the needs of African-American families impacted by incarceration?

4. Do you believe it is completely accidental that policies for addressing the problem of crime in low-income African-American communities actually contribute to the problem of poverty in those neighborhoods?

References

Allard, P. (2002). *Life Sentences: Denying welfare benefits to women convicted of drug offenses* (Report). Washington, DC: Sentencing Project.

Ammerman, R. T., Kolko, D. J., Kirisci, L., Blackson, T. C., & Dawes, M. A. (1999). Child abuse potential in parents with histories of substance use disorder. *Child Abuse & Neglect*, *23*, 1225–1238.

Arditti, J. A., Lambert-Shute, J., & Joest, K. (2003). Saturday morning at the jail: Implications of incarceration for families and children. *Family Relations*, *52*, 195–204.

Benaquisto, L., & Coulthard, J. (2008). *Children of incarcerated offenders: The impact of secrecy due to fear of shame and stigma.* Paper presented at the annual meeting of the American Society of Criminology Annual Meeting. St. Louis, Missouri.

Bernstein, N. (2005). *All alone in the world: Children of the incarcerated.* New York, NY: New Press.

Biederman, J., Milberger, S., Faraone, S. V., Kiely, K., Gutie, J., Mick, E., . . . Reed, E. (1995). Family-environment risk factors for attention-deficit hyperactivity disorder: A test of Rutter's indicators of adversity. *Archive of General Psychiatry*, *52*, 464–470.

Bocknek, E. L., Sanderson, J., & Britner, P. A. (2008). Ambiguous loss and posttraumatic stress in school-age children of prisoners. *Journal of Child and Family Studies*, *18*, 323–333.

Bonczar, T. P., & Beck, A. J. (1997). *Lifetime likelihood of going to state or federal prison* (NCJ 160092). Washington, DC: Bureau of Justice Statistics.

Bos, H. M. W., & Van Balen, F. (2008). Children in planned lesbian families: Stigmatization, psychological adjustment and protective factors. *Health & Sexuality*, *10*, 221–236.

Brooks, L. D., Solomon, A. L., Keegan, S., Kohl, R., & Lahue, L. (2005). *Prisoner re-entry in Massachusetts.* Washington, DC: Urban Institute Policy Justice Center.

Bry, B. H., McKeon, P., & Pandina, R. (1982). Extent of drug use as a function of number of risk factors. *Journal of Abnormal Psychology*, *91*, 273–279.

Chaffin, M., Kelleher, K., & Hollenberg, J. (1996). Onset of physical abuse and neglect: Psychiatric, substance abuse, and social risk factors from prospective community data. *Child Abuse & Neglect*, *20*, 193–203.

Chaiken, J. M. (2000). Crunching numbers: Crime and incarceration at the end of the millennium. *Nation Institute of Justice Journal*, 10–17.

Clear, T. R. (1996). *When incarceration increases crime.* New York, NY: Vera Institute of Justice.

Clear, T. R., Rose, D. R., Warring, E., & Scully, C. (2005). Coercive mobility and crime: A preliminary examination of concentrated incarceration and social disorganization. *Justice Quarterly*, *20*, 33–64.

Dowdney, L. (2005). Children bereaved by parent or sibling death. *Psychiatry*, *4*, 118–132.

Freeman, R. (Ed.). (1992). *Crime and the economic status of disadvantaged young men.* Washington, DC: Urban Institute.

Gershon, T. D., Tschann, J. M., & Jemerin, J. M. (1999). Stigmatization, self-esteem, and coping among the adolescent children of lesbian mothers. *Journal of Adolescent Health*, *24*, 437–445.

Giancola, P. R. (2000). Temperament and antisocial behavior in preadolescent boys with or without a family history of a substance use disorder. *Psychology of Addictive Behaviors, 14*, 56–68.

Glaze, L. E., & Maruschak, L. M. (2008). *Parents in prison and their minor children* (NCJ 222984). Washington, DC: Bureau of Justice Statistics. Available from http://www .ojp.usdoj.gov/bjs/pub/pdf/pptmc.pdf

Grogger, J. (1995). The effects of arrest on the employment and earnings of young men. *Quarterly Journal of Economics, 110*, 51–72.

Hagan, J., & Dinovitzer, R. (1999). Collateral consequences of imprisonment for children, communities, and prisoners. *Crime and Justice, 26*, 121–162.

Hagan, K. A., & Myers, M. J. (2003). The effect of secrecy and social support on behavioral problems in children of incarcerated women. *Journal of Child and Family Studies, 12*, 229–242.

Harm, N. J., & Thompson, P. J. (1995). *Needs assessment: Children of incarcerated women and their caregivers*. Little Rock, AR: Centers for Youth & Families.

Hawkins, W. E., Hawkins, M. J., Sabatino, C., & Ley, S. (1998). Relationship of perceived future opportunity to depressive symptomatology of inner-city African American adolescents. *Children and Youth Services Review, 20*, 757–764.

Hirsch, A. E., Dietrich, S. M., Landau, R., Schneider, P. D., Ackelsberg, I., Bernstein-Baker, J., & Hohenstein, J. (2002). *Every door closed: Barriers facing parents with criminal records*. Joint publication of the Center for Law and Social Policy, Washington, DC, and Community Legal Services, Philadelphia, PA.

Johnson, E. I., & Waldfogel, J. (2002). *Children of incarcerated parents: Cumulative risk and children's living arrangement* (Report). New York, NY: Columbia University.

Johnston, D. (1995). Effects of parental incarceration. In K. Gabel & D. Johnston (Eds.), *Children of incarcerated parents* (pp. 59–88). New York, NY: Lexington Books.

Kidd, S. A. (2007). Youth homelessness and social stigma. *Journal of Youth and Adolescence, 36*, 291–299.

Koban, L. A. (1983). Parents in prison: A comparative analysis of the effects of incarceration on the families of men and women. *Research in Law, Deviance and Social Control, 5*, 171–183.

Kumpfer, K. L. (1987). Special populations etiology with and prevention of vulnerability to chemical dependency in children of substance abusers. In B. S. Brown & A. R. Ifills (Eds.), *Youth at high risk for substance abuse* (pp. 1–72). Washington, DC: National Institute on Drug Abuse.

Loukas, A., Fitzgerald, H. E., Zucker, R. A., & von Eye, A. (2001). Parental alcoholism and co-occurring antisocial behavior: Prospective relationships to externalizing behavior problems in their young sons. *Journal of Abnormal Child Psychology, 29*, 91–106.

Mauer, M. (2004, May/June). Disenfranchising felons hurts entire communities. *Focus*, 5–6.

McCrae, J. S., & Barth, R. P. (2007). Using cumulative risk to screen for mental health problems in child welfare. *Research on Social Work Practice, 18*, 144–159.

McLeod, J. D., & Shanahan, M. J. (1996). Trajectories of poverty and children's mental health. *Journal of Health and Social Behavior, 37*, 207–220.

McLoyd, V. C. (1990). The impact of economic hardship on black families and children: Psychological distress, parenting, and socioemotional development. *Child Development*, *61*, 311–146.

Mumola, C. (2000). *Incarcerated parents and their children*. Washington, DC: U.S. Department of Justice, Bureau of Justice Statistics.

Murray, J. (2007). The cycle of punishment: Social exclusion of prisoners and their children. *Journal of Criminology and Criminal Justice*, *7*, 55–81.

Murray, J. (2008). The effects of imprisonment on families and children. In A. Liebling & S. Maruna (Eds.), *The effects of imprisonment* (pp. 442–462). Cullompton, UK: Willan.

Murray, J., & Farrington, D. P. (2005). Parental imprisonment: Effects on boys' antisocial behaviour and delinquency through the life course. *Journal of Child Psychology and Psychiatry*, *46*, 1269–1278.

Murray, J., & Farrington, D. P. (2008). Parental imprisonment: Long-lasting effects on boys' internalizing problems through the life course. *Development and Psychopathology*, *20*, 279–290.

Murray, J., Janson, C., & Farrington, D. P. (2007). Crime in adult offspring of prisoners: A cross-national comparison of two longitudinal samples. *Criminal Justice and Behavior*, *34*, 133–149.

Needels, K. E. (1996). Go directly to jail and do not collect? A long-term study of recidivism, employment, and earnings patterns among prison releasees. *Journal of Research in Crime and Delinquency*, *33*, 471–496.

Nesmith, A., & Ruhland, E. (2008). Children of incarcerated parents: Challenges and resiliency, in their own words. *Children and Youth Services Review*, *30*, 1119–1130.

Phillips, S. D., Burns, B. J., Wagner, H. R., & Barth, R. P. (2004). Parental arrest and children in child welfare services agencies. *American Journal of Orthopsychiatry*, *2*, 174–186.

Phillips, S. D., Burns, B. J., Wagner, H. R., Kramer, T. L., & Robbins, J. R. (2002). Parental incarceration among youth receiving mental health services. *Journal of Child and Family Studies*, *11*(4), 385–399.

Phillips, S. D., & Dettlaff, A. J. (2007). More than parents in prison: The broader overlap between the criminal justice and child welfare systems. *Journal of Public Child Welfare*, *3*, 3–13.

Phillips, S. D., Erkanli, A., Costello, E. J., & Angold, A. (2007). Differences among children whose mothers have a history of arrest. *Women & Criminal Justice*, *17*(2/3), 45–63.

Phillips, S. D., Erkanli, A., Keeler, G. P., Costello, E. J., & Angold, A. (2006). Disentangling the risks: Parent criminal justice involvement and children's exposure to family risks. *Criminology and Public Policy*, *5*(4), 677–702.

Phillips, S. D., Leathers, S. J., & Erkanli, A. (2009). Children of probationers in the child welfare system. *Journal of Child & Family Studies*, *18*, 183–191.

Phillips, S. D., & Zhao, J. (2010). The relationship between witnessing arrests and elevated symptoms of posttraumatic stress: Findings from a national study of children involved in the child welfare system. *Children and Youth Services Review*, *32*, 1246–1254.

Poehlmann, J. (2005). Representation of attachment relationships in children of incarcerated mothers. *Child Development, 76*, 679–696.

Pratt, T. C. (2001). Assessing the relative effects of macro-level predictors of crime: A meta-analysis. *Dissertation Abstracts International, A: The Humanities and Social Sciences, 62*(5).

Puddefoot, G., & Foster, L. K. (2007). *Keeping children safe when their parents are arrested: Local approaches that work*. Sacramento: California Research Bureau, California State Library. Available from http://www.library.ca.gov/crb/07/07-006.pdf

Sack, W. H., Seidler, J., & Thomas, S. (1976). The children of imprisoned parents: A psychosocial exploration. *American Journal of Orthopsychiatry, 46*, 618–628.

Sampson, R. J. (1985). Neighborhoods and crime: The structural determinants of personal victimization. *Journal of Research in Crime and Delinquency, 22*, 7–40.

Sampson, R. J., & Groves, W. B. (1989). Community structure and crime: Testing social disorganization theory. *American Journal of Sociology, 94*, 744–802.

Sampson, R. J., & Laub, J. (1993). *Crime in the making*. Cambridge, MA: Harvard University Press.

Stanger, C., Higgins, S. T., & Bickel, W. K. (1999). Behavioral and emotional problems among children of cocaine- and opiate-dependent parents. *Journal of the American Academy of Child and Adolescent Psychiatry, 38*, 421–428.

Stanton, A. M. (1980). *When mothers go to jail*. Lexington, MA: Lexington Books.

U.S. Department of Health and Human Services. (2001). *Mental health: Culture, race, and ethnicity—A supplement to mental health*. A report of the Surgeon General. Rockville, MD: U.S. Department of Health and Human Services, Substance Abuse and Mental Health Services Administration, Center for Mental Health Services.

Visher, C., & Farrell, J. (2005). *Chicago communities and prisoner reentry*. Washington, DC: Urban Institute.

Wildeman, C. J. (2009). Parental imprisonment, the prison boom, and the concentration of childhood disadvantage. *Demography, 46*, 265–280.

Zalba, S. (1964). *Women prisoners and their families*. Sacramento, CA: Department of Social Welfare and Department of Corrections.

Chapter 6

The Impact of Reentry from Incarceration on the Health of African-American Men

Jean Bonhomme
Elisabeth Kingsbury

Learning Objectives

- Recognize the existing marked disparities in sentencing for African-American males, especially in the area of drug offenses.

- Appreciate hazards to the African-American ex-offender and the African-American community posed by blood-borne and sexually transmitted diseases, such as HIV and hepatitis, that may be contracted or transmitted during incarceration.

- Gain awareness of the negative effects of the incarceration of large numbers of African-American men on the health and stability of the African-American family and the African-American community.

- Be able to identify at least three resources that could potentially facilitate successful community reentry and health maintenance for African-American ex-offenders.

- Understand the role played by stigma against individuals with incarceration histories and how the effect of that stigma is compounded by existing racism against African Americans.

● ● ●

Social scientists have long acknowledged the detrimental effect of releasing inmates into the same environments that led to their initial incarceration. The continual incarceration and discharge of large numbers of disproportionately African-American male individuals has an especially deleterious effect on the health status of African-American communities already facing huge social and economic disadvantages. Ex-offenders typically reenter society beleaguered by untreated or inadequately treated substance use disorders, as well as physical and mental health problems. African-American releasees in particular more often suffer inadequate education, lack of marketable job skills, limited job opportunities, racism, unemployment and underemployment, classism, substandard housing (frequently in drug-infested locales), and pervasive, enduring stigma owing to their ex-convict status.

Tragically, nearly two-thirds of all prison releasees will re-offend within three years of release, frequently facing re-incarceration for new crimes or parole violations. This high rate of recidivism is clearly related to the ineffective transition of inmates back to community life, a process further compounded for African-American male ex-offenders by the institutionalized social and economic barriers faced by African Americans in general. These circumstances predictably predispose African-American releasees in particular to a vicious cycle that relegates them to a permanently marginalized status in society. The overall financial costs to society of this continuous cycle of incarceration and reentry are enormous, with national expenditures on corrections having increased from $9 billion in 1982 to $69 billion in 2006.

The authors aim to increase awareness of the specific barriers to successful community reintegration facing the African-American male ex-offender. In addition, the authors advocate intensive culturally sensitive and linguistically appropriate targeted intervention beginning well before release aimed at meeting the needs of this population, to include extensive prerelease planning, with intervention efforts intensifying through the 72 hours following release and continuing for months afterward. Specific services needed to improve community reintegration outcomes for African-American male ex-offenders include health care referrals, health care access, mental health counseling, client advocacy, substance abuse treatment and prevention, STD/HIV prevention education and treatment, housing support, family counseling, employment access, marketable job skills development, job training and preparation, as well as peer support groups. Vigorous intervention on these issues is essential to enabling the newly released African-American ex-offender to stabilize, maintain health, and successfully reintegrate into community life while consistently functioning in accordance with society's values.

Prisoner Reintegration and African-American Men: Scope of the Problem and Impact on Society

Every year, more than 700,000 individuals are released from state and federal prisons nationwide, usually to return to their communities of origin (West, Sabol, & Cooper, 2009). Approximately 9 million individuals are released from jails annually (Beck, 2006). Between 2000 and 2007, the average annual growth in the number of prison releasees was 2.5 percent, with the actual number in 2008 being 735,454 (West et al., 2009). African-American males are markedly disproportionately represented in America's jail and prison populations. The U.S. Bureau of Justice Statistics estimates that approximately 32 percent of African-American men born in 2001 and 17 percent of Latino men born that year will serve prison time at some point during their lives, while the corresponding number for white men is less than 6 percent (Uggen et al., 2006). Moreover, 9 percent of African-American males aged 25 to 29 were incarcerated in 1999, contrasted with 3 percent of Hispanic males and only 1 percent of white males in this age group (Beck, 2000). For African-American male high school dropouts born between 1965 and 1969, nearly 60 percent went to prison by 1999 (Western & Pettit, 2004). As releasees, African-American men in particular will reenter society beleaguered by untreated substance abuse, medical and psychiatric health problems, lack of marketable job skills, limited job prospects, unemployment and underemployment, classism, substandard housing (often in drug-infested locales), racism, and pervasive, enduring stigma as a result of ex-convict status.

For a number of years, social scientists have examined and acknowledged the detrimental impact of releasing inmates into the same environments that contributed substantially to their initial incarceration. From a number of policy perspectives, the longstanding issue of prisoner reintegration is taking on renewed importance. Greater numbers of prisoners are returning home following longer periods of incarceration, with minimal preparation for life on the outside and nominal assistance with the reintegration process. Owing to lack of adequate discharge planning, common difficulties include reconnecting with jobs, housing, and families. Unemployment and underemployment are strongly linked to lack of access to health insurance. Nearly two-thirds of people released from prison will be rearrested within three years of release, with approximately half returning to prison for either new crimes or parole violations (Langan & Levin, 2002). Rehabilitation and correctional personnel have recognized for decades that this high rate of recidivism is largely related to the ineffective transition of inmates back to community life. This "prison cycle"— the constant removal and return of large numbers of disproportionately African-American male individuals—is concentrated principally in urban African-American communities already facing enormous social and economic disadvantages. Predictably, these circumstances strongly predispose African-American male ex-offenders to a vicious cycle that relegates them to a permanently marginalized status in society, adversely impacting the overall health status and stability of African-American communities and the African-American family.

Physical and mental health concerns and substance abuse problems that remain unresolved at the time of release can diminish an individual's chances of successful reentry during this crucial point in time. Recent releasees with compromised health may be disabled with respect to work, and their families may be unable or unwilling to assist them (Mallik-Kane & Visher, 2008). Those without adequate treatment for mental health and substance abuse diagnoses are at especially high risk of re-offending. The chances of drug relapse and recidivism are exacerbated while facing the challenges of coping with illness and managing the tasks associated with transitioning back to community life (Mallik-Kane & Visher, 2008). Despite the fact that subsequent offenses by this population are frequently for minor, nonviolent crimes directly related to behaviors associated with mental illness and/or substance use, the rate of return to imprisonment is high. According to an Ohio-based study, nearly 75 percent of people with mental illness released from jail are rearrested within 36 months (Ventura, Cassel, Jacoby, & Huang, 1998). This problem is exacerbated by the response of law enforcement officials who have not received training in crisis intervention techniques, as well as judges and other decision makers who are not aware of or able to access suitable alternatives to incarceration.

Beyond physical and mental health implications, profound collateral consequences exist for nearly anyone who has had involvement with the criminal justice system. Legal and societal barriers may be present during reentry to obtaining affordable housing, employment, family reunification, parental rights, immigration status, and voting rights as well as eligibility for other public benefits such as federal student loans, and driver licenses among other essentials of life. Both job readiness and the ability to find and secure stable employment on release are critical both to successful reentry and access to health insurance. Unemployment, which is typically roughly twice the national average for African-Americans, is closely linked to recidivism. Wages on average are lower for African-Americans, and a 10 percent decrease in wages is associated with a 10 to 20 percent increase in criminal activity and likelihood of incarceration (Pager, 2008). The implications for family formation and stability in the African-American community are profound. Few married couples are able to endure the incarceration of a partner. Disproportionate incarceration of African-American males reduces the already limited number of marriageable African-American males available to African-American females, predicting family disruption and increased crime (Courtwright, 1996). The financial costs to society of this cycle of incarceration, release, and reentry are substantial from several perspectives. Expenditures on corrections alone increased from $9 billion in 1982 to $69 billion nationally in 2006 (Bureau of Justice Statistics, 2008). Significant portions of state budgets are now invested in criminal justice. Public safety is another major issue, as high recidivism rates translate into thousands of new crime victims yearly. Moreover, none of these figures take into account the costs of arrest and sentencing processes or the costs to victims. In addition, there are far-reaching social costs, including public health risks, disenfranchisement, homelessness, and weakened ties among families and communities. African-American families and communities in particular are negatively affected by failed reintegration, as well as African-American ex-offenders themselves.

Following release from prison, inmates are moved directly from a well-structured environment to a much lower level of supervision. They may be thrown suddenly into contact with high-risk places, persons, or situations, while few have developed the necessary skills during their incarceration to deal with these challenges. While facing release, prisoners often report feeling apprehensive about the imminent tribulation of reestablishing family ties, finding employment, and managing finances (Castellano & Soderstrom, 1997). For African Americans, these factors are undoubtedly compounded by the prospect of returning to the long-standing economic and social problems facing African-American communities. The term "Gate Fever" has been coined to refer to a psychological syndrome defined by increased anxiety and irritability at the time of a prisoner's release. Few empirical studies have investigated the phenomenon, although this syndrome is widely recognized among correctional workers. The limited research on this issue indicates that the documented heightened stress levels at the time of release reflect realistic concerns about successfully managing a return to the outside world and facing new problems that did not exist in the prison setting (Castellano & Soderstrom, 1997). Postrelease, maladaptive coping with the outside world is commonplace. Released offenders have a tendency to manage everyday problems in ineffective and at times destructive ways (Austin, Bruce, Carroll, McCall, & Richards, 2000; Stephan, 1999). Research aimed at understanding the postrelease coping process demonstrates that many ex-offenders are unable to successfully recognize and/or deal with problem situations, frequently leading to impulsive, physically hazardous, and often criminal behavioral choices (Zamble & Quinsey, 1997). However, there is a pervasive lack of resources aimed at helping the released prisoner cope successfully with life outside prison walls. Thus, effective management of reentry aimed at addressing health issues and achieving successful long-term reintegration would have substantial benefits for society.

African-American Men: Disparities in Legal Treatment under the U.S. Criminal Justice System

Considerable controversy exists as to how much of the demonstrable overrepresentation of African-American males in the criminal justice system actually represents a higher frequency of criminal behavior among African Americans as opposed to differential treatment in the criminal justice system based upon race. A specific health-related issue, drug addiction and abuse, exacerbates the existing racial disparities owing to sentencing policy changes adopted throughout the 1980s and early 1990s requiring mandatory minimum sentences for many drug-related offenses. A 1990 RAND study found that while African-American defendants in California received generally comparable sentences with other races for comparable offenses, this was not the case with respect to drug offenses (Klein et al., 1990). The referenced policy changes resulted in a significant increase in the number of drug offenders sentenced to prison as well as in longer prison terms. Between 1985 and 1995, the total number of African-American drug offenders sentenced to prison increased by 707 percent (Mumola & Beck, 1997), while the number of white drug offenders increased by only 306 percent during the same period. During that same 10-year period, drug offenders accounted for 42 percent of the rise in the African-American state prison population as compared with only 26 percent of the rise in the white state prison population. Current estimates reveal that the number of incarcerated drug offenders had increased a substantial 510 percent from 1983 to 1993 (U.S. Department of Justice, 1996). Also significant is the observation that 74 percent of the total inmate population (approximately 800,000 persons) during the same time period was in need of drug treatment, but only 15 percent (120,000) received the necessary treatment (U.S. Department of Justice, 1996).

U.S. District Judge Clyde S. Cahill of Missouri stated that the federal guidelines for possession of crack have "been directly responsible for incarcerating nearly an entire generation of young African-American men." Substantial disparities in sentencing for drug possession are based on the form of drug commonly used by specific ethnic groups, dramatically increasing the percentage of African Americans and other ethnic minorities in correctional facilities (Braithwaite & Arriola, 2008). African Americans and Latinos are more likely to use cocaine in smokeable "crack" form than as powder. Crack is merely cocaine powder with the chemical hydrochloride moiety removed by heating with common baking soda. However, possession of crack typically incurs a much harsher sentence under federal guidelines. A mandatory five-year minimum sentence, up to a possible maximum of 20 years, is levied for possession of five grams of crack (the weight of only two pennies). By contrast, five grams of powder cocaine is considered a misdemeanor with no mandatory minimum sentence and a maximum penalty of only one year in jail. One hundred times the weight of crack, or half a kilogram of powder cocaine, is necessary to carry the more severe crack penalty. In reality, 500 grams of powder cocaine has a far greater street value than five grams of crack, is much more likely to be sold or otherwise distributed, remains a highly addictive drug in any form, and could be converted easily into crack. Thus, this huge sentencing differential does not appear justifiable or reasonable.

According to the U.S. Sentencing Commission, the racial distribution of cocaine powder convictions in 2000 was as 17.8 percent white defendants, 30.5 percent African American, and 50.8 percent Latino. In the same year, the racial breakdown of crack cocaine convictions was 5.6 percent white defendants, 84.7 percent African American, and 9.0 percent Latino. These numbers represent a conviction rate 15 times greater for African Americans than for whites caught with the same basic drug. Advocates for social justice and equity regard these sentencing guidelines as a form of racial profiling.

Public Health and African-American Prisoner Reintegration

The postincarceration release of large numbers of individuals, disproportionately African-American men, is heavily concentrated in urban African-American communities already challenged severely by major social and economic disadvantages. Unique pitfalls exist in the immediate postrelease period. During the first 72 hours, ex-inmates are confronted with a myriad of choices that can lead to potentially health-damaging outcomes. Inmates readily fall prey to relapse into the use of illegal controlled substances during their first few days in transition. Newly released male ex-offenders will characteristically seek female companionship and intimacies from significant others, prostitutes, or young females soon after release. Being particularly anxious to engage in sexual intercourse, they are more likely to neglect safer sexual practices, often after having engaged in high-risk activities while incarcerated, with African Americans already suffering greatly disproportionate HIV infection rates. Many released inmates will be released beset by health problems, some directly related to their prison experience. Correctional systems are experiencing an increase in the number of older inmates, possibly due to a fundamental shift to a more retributive and punitive response to crime, an aging population, the previously referenced increase in prison capacity over the past two decades, and the previously discussed increase in prosecution of African Americans for drug offenses, with the attendant increase in the average expense of medical care due to the increased rates of age-associated chronic illness.

African Americans face markedly disproportionate rates of HIV and hepatitis C infection. High-risk activities for transmission of HIV as well as other sexually transmitted and blood-borne diseases are exceedingly prevalent among the incarcerated, magnifying the public health threat that African-American communities face from the newly released ex-offender (Chu, 2009; Turnbull, Power, & Stimson, 1996). High-risk sexual activities, injection drug use (IDU) with needle sharing (Stark, Bienzle, Vonk, & Guggenmoos-Holzmann, 1997; Valera, Epperson, Daniels, Ramaswamy, & Freudenberg, 2009), and tattooing (Braithwaite, Hammett, & Mayberry, 1996; Dolan, 1997) are unquestionably taking place in prisons and jails despite prohibitions against these activities. Recent national survey findings demonstrate that prison inmates have an AIDS rate nearly six times that of the general population (Braithwaite et al., 1996). A 2002 study using surveys and surveillance data to develop national estimates on the total burden of infectious diseases among the incarcerated concluded that between 20 percent and 26 percent of all persons living with HIV, between 29 percent and 43 percent of those living with hepatitis C, and 40 percent of those who had active tuberculosis in the entire United States had passed through the correctional system during calendar year 1997 alone (Hammett, Harmon, & Rhodes, 2002). Another study found that 70 percent of persons who had used heroin in the month prior to incarceration continued use of the drug even during incarceration (Strang et al., 2006).

Owing largely to inadequate intervention for existing health problems prior to release, reintegration is not only a challenging time for the ex-offender, but a dangerous one as well. A retrospective cohort study conducted on former inmates from Washington State prisons found that during the first two weeks after release, the risk of death among former inmates was 12.7 times that of other state residents. The most frequent contributors to this markedly increased mortality were drug overdoses, cardiovascular disease, homicides, and suicides (Binswanger, 2007).

HIV transmission in prison is exacerbated by institutional policies designating condoms as contraband. However, it is widely accepted that knowledge of safer sex practices does not automatically translate into risk-reduction practices, such as avoiding unprotected sex and not having sex with multiple partners (Weinhardt, Carey, Johnson, & Bickham, 1999). An estimated 4.4 percent of prison inmates and 3.1 percent of jail inmates reported at least one incident of sexual victimization either during the past 12 months or since admission to the facility (if admission was less than a year before the incident). These data suggest that roughly 88,500 adults of incarcerated individuals nationally have been victimized sexually (Beck & Harrison, 2010). However, IDU has always been the principal risk factor for AIDS among the incarcerated, even more than male homosexual activity. Estimates of prison HIV risk behavior hold that injection drug users may account for up to half the inmate population, and an estimated one-third or more of those who injected before incarceration will continue to do so while incarcerated (Dolan, 1997–1998). Prison tattooing is a well-known phenomenon, taking place in an environment offering no access to sterile tattoo equipment. Restriction on the availability of needles in prison, intended to reduce the prevalence of drug use, instead almost certainly promotes widespread sharing of the few available needles (Braithwaite et al., 1996). Sharing of needles includes not only passing needles between the incarcerated, but also used needles and syringes originating from outside. Pieces of pens and light bulbs are sometimes used by inmates to inject drugs (Mahon, 1996). Sharing of unclean or improperly cleaned paraphernalia, including injection solutions, containers, cotton, and other materials, also contributes to transmission of blood-borne disease. Hepatitis C becomes chronic in approximately 80 percent of infections and is primarily transmitted by IDU, but is believed also to be transmitted through the sharing of straws for intranasal inhalation of drugs. Long-term consequences of hepatitis C may include cirrhosis or liver cancer decades after the initial infection. Hepatitis B is easily transmitted through both IDU and sexual activity. Tattooing is often done in prison settings with nonsterile but expedient materials such as guitar strings (Braithwaite et al., 1996). Somewhat surprisingly, access to illegal drugs continues to be prevalent even within many U.S. correctional facilities.

Incarceration and Reentry of African-American Men: Impact on the African-American Family

The opportunity to participate in stable and supportive family life has clear implications for the chances of maintaining physical and mental health. However, the cycle of incarceration and reentry has a disproportionate impact on the African-American family (Johnston & Gabel, 1995). High rates of incarceration among African Americans may have transgenerational consequences, as children of incarcerated parents are at high risk of inappropriate and inconsistent discipline, problem behavior in youth, future delinquency, and/or criminal behavior in adulthood (Kjellstrand & Eddy, 2011). Parental incarceration was especially predictive of internalizing problems and antisocial behavior from ages 14 through 48 if the children were male (Murray & Farrington 2008). Separation because of parental imprisonment also predicted the co-occurrence of high rates of incarceration, homicide, and limited employment prospects among African-American males and have all contributed to an imbalance of marriageable African-American males to African-American females, with major implications for successful African-American family formation and stability (Dallao, 1997). Incarceration creates huge barriers against continued contact and involvement with the family, such as restricted visitation hours and long travel distances, and greatly undermines men's economic contribution to the family (Herman-Stahl, Kan, & McKay, 2008). Incarceration has been associated with a 30 percent decrease in the likelihood of marriage among African Americans. Men never incarcerated were found to be twice as likely to marry as ex-offenders (Western & McLanahan, 2000). At one year after the child's birth, ex-offenders were only half as likely to be involved with the mother of their child (Western & McLanahan, 2000). Among African-American male ex-offenders, only 8 percent were married to their partner a year after the birth of their child. Incarceration alone is estimated to cause 15 percent of the observed absenteeism among African-American fathers (Western, Lopoo, & McLanahan, 2004; Western & McLanahan, 2000). Already married men, once they are incarcerated, attain the national 50 percent divorce rate in a much shorter period of time (Western et al., 2004). A major factor negatively impacting family formation and stability is a history of incarceration characteristically leading to a future of reduced wages and impaired job stability (Western et al., 2004). An incarceration history has been associated with as much as a 66 percent decline in employment (Huebner, 2005). African-American ex-offenders, already facing handicaps finding stable employment due to existing racial biases coupled with frequent lack of education and marketable job skills, now face employment discrimination as ex-offenders as well (Visher & Travis, 2003).

Restricted Postincarceration Resources and the African-American Ex-Offender

Safe, affordable housing is fundamental to both health maintenance and stability in life. For individuals with a criminal record, however, the challenge of securing suitable accommodations is substantial. Public housing options, which in the African-American community are frequently the only affordable option, become limited for those with incarceration records. Racial disparities in the treatment of drug-related crimes for African Americans assume particular importance here, as public housing authorities (PHAs) are legally permitted to use their discretion to "deny public admission to or evict individuals who have engaged in criminal activity, especially drug-related criminal activity, on or off public housing premises, regardless of whether they were arrested or convicted for these activities." (Cooper, 2003). Despite the fact that PHAs may exercise discretion to rendering decisions, for example, by considering factors such as time since conviction and efforts made in furtherance of rehabilitation, PHAs generally disqualify people with criminal records (Travis, 2005). These same legal bars create significant barriers for formerly incarcerated individuals attempting to form or renew family ties and bond with children left behind during their prison terms. Research indicates that homelessness is also directly linked to the reincarceration of people who have served jail or prison sentences. For instance, homeless individuals on parole have been shown to be seven times more likely to abscond after the first month of release than those located in more stable housing (Brown, 2006).

Job readiness can be an obstacle for many people leaving incarceration. African-American males suffer unemployment rates far above the national average to start with, making access to health insurance and health care much more problematic. For those who have been incarcerated for a number of years, technological advances may render their skills uncompetitive in the current labor market. However, for too many African-American men, length of incarceration is not the source of the problem; instead, the difficulty lies in the fact that they have never held stable employment, which is frequently due to lack of opportunity in African-American communities. In these cases, becoming "job ready" may mean learning the basic tenets of holding a job, including appropriate attire, dealing with supervisors, and attendance and punctuality. A more significant obstacle to securing employment is the discrimination that past offenders face due to their criminal record. Stigmatization on the part of employers is rampant, just as it is among the general public. Research on the effect of a criminal record on employment opportunities show telling results regarding differences in effect magnitude between African Americans and whites. Thirty-four percent of whites without criminal records received callbacks, compared to only 17 percent of whites with criminal records, demonstrating that a criminal record reduced the likelihood of a callback by 50 percent. Among African-Americans without criminal records, only 14 percent received callbacks and only 5 percent of African-Americans with criminal records received callbacks (Pager, 2008). Moreover, employers who otherwise might be more forgiving may be concerned about the legal liability of knowingly hiring someone with a criminal record. Finally, state licensing boards often bar people with criminal records from obtaining licenses necessary for jobs such as nursing/caretaking, truck driving, and even hairdressing (Samuels & Miasmal, 2004).

Given the markedly disproportionate drug conviction rate of African Americans, it is especially significant that individuals convicted of any state or federal drug-related felony are barred for life from receiving assistance through the Temporary Assistance to Needy Families (TANF) and Supplemental Nutrition Assistance Program (SNAP, formerly known as *food stamps*), cutting off a small but often critical source of income for individuals in reentry. (Cooper, 2003; Fine, Ganong, & Demo, 2005). States have the choice to modify or opt out of the lifetime ban provisions. Nine states and the District of Columbia have opted out of the ban, 10 states have kept the ban in its entirety, and 31 states have modified it in some way. Although still helpful to some individuals, some states' modified policies have extremely limited applicability, such as states that lift the ban only for those people who have successfully completed drug court (Samuels & Miasmal, 2004).

Closing the Disparity Gap for the African-American Ex-Offender

A range of policy-based solutions exist to combat the devastating effects of cyclical incarceration and reentry for African-American men. These include:

- Investment in Crisis Intervention Training (CIT) for law enforcement
- Ensuring that judges have meaningful and reasonable alternatives to the excessive incarceration of African-American men, including specialty courts (e.g., drug and mental health courts) and enhanced community supervision options
- Making graduated sanctions available to parole and probation officers and encouraging their use, particularly in instances of minor parole or probation violations
- Training and use of community health workers, peer navigators, or discharge planners to provide strong continuity of care and assistance between prison and the African-American community for individuals as they are discharged
- Ensuring intensive community case management for individuals who may require it due to mental illness or substance use disorders and ensuring access to these services for African-American males
- Suspending, rather than terminating, Medicaid and Social Security benefits for individuals who are already receiving them upon incarceration in order to ensure immediate reinstatement on release
- Modification of hiring practices, such as eliminating criminal history questions on first-round job applications, and implementing employment discrimination standards that are especially relevant for African-American ex-offenders
- Ensuring that PHAs are culturally competent in issues pertaining to the African-American community and review applications on a case-by-case basis

In addressing the complex behavioral, drug use, and mental health challenges facing the recently released, potential therapeutic approaches which may be especially suited to the unique needs of African-American male ex-offenders include social cognitive theory, problem behavior theory, and motivational interviewing. Social cognitive theory is especially relevant for promoting behavioral change, for example, encouraging adaptive behaviors such as condom use. In applications aimed at reducing risky sexual behavior, social cognitive theory primarily emphasizes the concept of self-efficacy, while providing information that encourages preventive measures, such as the data on the benefits of condom use (Bandera, 2001). Problem behavior theory contends that the predisposition for social deviance is associated with specific psychosocial, interpersonal, and environmental risk factors, such as low self-esteem, low motivation for achievement in traditional domains (e.g., school, organized sports), unsupportive family relationships, and a deprived neighborhood. For this reason, behaviors such as delinquency, risky sex, and substance use tend to cluster among groups of high-risk individuals (Jessor, 2001). The theory calls for wide-ranging interventions that compensate for these risk factors by improving self-concept and enhancing achievement motivation while promoting family and community involvement. Motivational interviewing begins by developing a rapport with participants aimed at helping them to resolve ambivalence about their health care behaviors and to become aware of and act on their own motivations to change (Rollnick & Miller, 1995). A series of interventions is used to gradually increase awareness of the need to change, ultimately assisting individuals in attaining their behavioral goals and taking constructive action. Motivational interviewing has been shown to be effective in treating addiction, mental illness, smoking cessation, and compliance with antiretroviral medications.

Summary

Circumstances that undermine the stabilization and community reintegration of African-American ex-offenders include inadequate access to health care and social services, lack of information within the correctional system regarding client referral sources, inadequate discharge planning, lack of job-training opportunities during incarceration, negative attitudes toward ex-offenders, and communication difficulties (Gaiter & Doll, 1996). These adverse factors are superimposed on prevalent racist attitudes against African Americans. Participation of parole officers and development of a strong case management system with effective and efficient intra- and interagency referral capacity is vital to successful post release health care reintegration efforts. Mental health counseling, client advocacy, substance abuse treatment and prevention, employment access, marketable job skills development, job training and preparation, and peer support groups, all culturally sensitive to the challenges facing African Americans, are all vital issues for empowering the newly released African-American inmate to function in accordance with prevailing societal values.

The time of release presents opportunities for policy innovation aimed at developing strategies that create short-term links to provide assistance during the immediate transition. At present, released inmates are afforded few resources aimed at helping them to secure employment, access substance-abuse treatment, and reestablish family and community ties. African Americans are facing the additional challenges of returning to resource-poor communities. Implementing policies that provide inmates with prerelease preparations together with referral and follow-up on the outside would likely reduce the risks of drug relapse and recidivism while enhancing the odds of successful, sustained reintegration after release. Follow-up could be accomplished by referral and linkage to existing associations such as parole, transitional facilitators, peer educators, health care providers, nonprofit community organizations, faith institutions, and family or friends.

Newly released inmates are likely to be compromised in regard to health beliefs and practices. Newly released male inmates are typically anxious to engage in sexual intercourse owing to their renewed access to females, and thus likely to overlook the importance of safer sexual practices. Given that the majority of inmates will eventually be released, a unique opportunity exists to provide them information during incarceration and the prerelease phase of their transition back to community life on HIV, STDs and drug relapse prevention (Braithwaite et al., 1996). Such an intervention would prove potentially invaluable in protecting the health of the public and the community at large.

Programs are needed to work with inmates from months prior to release, upon release, during the first 72 hours following, and for several months thereafter. Any such program needs to intensely monitor, motivate, counsel, and assist releasees as they transition, referring and connecting them with needed human support services. Emphasis must be placed on the development of interventions for African-American male ex-offenders that are culturally competent, linguistically appropriate, gender-specific, realistic, and aware of the unique challenges that African-American ex-offenders will face on reentry to their communities. Responsiveness to the special needs of parolees and other released persons include providing educational and job-training opportunities, health and substance abuse treatment services, and safe, affordable housing options, with comprehensive discharge planning as an essential component. Maximizing the communication between the prison staff and parole officers would likely augment the efficacy of the overall system from a continuity of care perspective.

Finally, community-based education and follow-up is an essential component of reintegration. Substance use treatment and HIV risk-reduction interventions initiated in correctional facilities should include aftercare or booster services that will assist former inmates after they return to the community. Thus, community-based education and follow-up that builds on educational efforts and health treatment delivered during incarceration will assist former inmates in using disease prevention and health maintenance strategies as they inevitably encounter risk situations on the outside. The authors advocate vigorous interventions for African-American male ex-offenders that will likely promote stabilization and successful reintegration into community life including extensive prerelease planning, referral services, job training, housing, health care access job skills, health care referrals, as well as STD, HIV, and drug prevention and treatment (Braithwaite et al., 1996).

Key Terms

ex-offender

gate fever

mandatory minimum sentences

prison cycle

recidivism

reintegration

releasee

stigma

transition

Discussion Questions

1. We have discussed the benefit of reentry programs and policies to African-American ex-offenders in reentry. What would be the benefits to the African-American community as a whole to which the ex-offender is returning?

2. Describe some of the differences in the challenges faced by African-American men leaving jail or prison compared with the challenges faced by individuals who are not members of racial minority groups.

3. Describe how the lack of housing, employment, and a supportive family network following incarceration may impact the African-American male ex-offender's medical and psychiatric health status.

4. What is the role played by stigma against persons who have been incarcerated in hampering readjustment in the community, and how is this stigma compounded by racism for African-American men?

5. How and why do untreated substance use disorders and mental health problems affect recidivism rates among African-American ex-offenders?

References

Austin, J., Bruce, M. A., Carroll, L., McCall, P. L., & Richards, S. C. (2000). *The use of incarceration in the United States*. Paper prepared for the annual meeting of the American Society of Criminology, San Francisco.

Bandera, A. (2001). Social cognitive theory: An agentive perspective. *Annual Review of Psychology, 52*, 1–26.

Beck, A. J. (2000, April 13). *State and federal prisoners returning to the community: Findings from the Bureau of Justice Statistics*. Paper presented at the First Reentry

Courts Initiative Cluster Meeting, Washington, DC. Retrieved from http://www.ojp .usdoj.gov/bjs/pub/pdf/sfprc.pdf

Beck, A. J. (2006, June 27). *The importance of successful reentry to jail population growth*. Presented at the Urban Institute's Jail Reentry Roundtable.

Beck, A. J., & Harrison P. M. (2010). Sexual victimization in prisons and jails reported by inmates, 2008–09. National Inmate Survey, 2008–09.

Binswanger, I. A., Stern, M. F., Deyo, R. A., Heagerty, P. J., Cheadle, A., Elmore, J. G., & Koepsell, T. D. (2007). Release from prison—A high risk of death for former inmates. *New England Journal of Medicine, 356,* 157–165.

Braithwaite, R., Hammett, T., & Mayberry, R. (1996). *Prison and AIDS: A public health challenge*. San Francisco, CA: Jossey-Bass.

Braithwaite, R. L., & Arriola, K. J. (2008) Male prisoners and HIV prevention: A call for action ignored. *American Journal of Public Health, 98*(9 Suppl.), S145–149.

Brown, K. (2006). *Homelessness and prisoner re-entry*. Council of State Governments. Retrieved from http://reentrypolicy.org/jc_publications/homelessness_prisoner_ reentry;file

Bureau of Justice Statistics. (2008). *Justice expenditure and employment extracts, 2006*. NCJ 224394. Retrieved from http://bjs.ojp.usdoj.gov/index.cfm?ty= pbdetail&iid=1022

Bureau of Justice Statistics. (2010, August). NCJ 231169.

Castellano, T. C., & Soderstrom, I. R. (1997). Self-esteem, depression, and anxiety evidenced by a prison inmate sample: Interrelationships and consequences for prison programming. *Prison Journal, 77*(3), 259–280.

Chu, S. (2009). Clean switch: The case for prison needle and syringe programs. *HIV AIDS Policy Law Review, 14*(2), 5–19.

Cooper, C. S. (2003). Drug courts—Just the beginning: Getting other areas of public policy in sync. *Substance Use & Misuse, 42*(2–3), 243–256.

Courtwright, D. T. (1996). The drug war's hidden toll. *Issues in Science and Technology, 13*(2), 73.

Dallao, M. (1997). Coping with incarceration from the other side of the bars. *Corrections Today* (59), 96–98.

Dolan, K. (1997–1998). Evidence about HIV transmission in prisons. *Canada HIV AIDS Policy Law Newsletter, 3–4*(4–1), 32–38.

Fine, M. A., Ganong, L. G., & Demo, D. H. (2005). Divorce as a family stressor. In S. Price & P. McKenry (Eds.), *Families and change: Coping with stressful events and transitions* (3rd ed., pp. 227–252). Newbury Park, CA: Sage.

Gaiter, J., & Doll, L. (1996). Improving HIV/AIDS prevention in prisons is good public health policy. *American Journal of Public Health, 86,* 1201–1203.

Hammett, T. M., Harmon, M. P., & Rhodes, W. (2002). The burden of infectious disease among inmates of and releasees from US correctional facilities, 1997. *American Journal of Public Health, 92*(11), 1789–1794.

Herman-Stahl, M., Kan, M. L., & McKay, T. (2008). Incarceration and the family: A review of research and promising approaches for serving fathers and families, U.S. Department of Health and Human Services (HHS), September 2008.

Huebner, B. M. (2005). The effect of incarceration on marriage and work over the life course. *Justice Quarterly, 22*, 281–303.

Jessor, R. (2001). Problem-behavior theory. In J. Rathel (Ed.), *Adolescent risk behavior: Explanations, forms, and prevention*. Opladen, Germany: Leske + Budrich.

Johnston, D., & Gabel, K. (1995). Incarcerated parents. In D. Johnston & K. Gabel (Eds.), *Children of incarcerated parents*. New York, NY: Lexington Books.

Kjellstrand J. M., & Eddy, J. M. (2011). Parental incarceration during childhood, family context, and youth problem behavior across adolescence. *Journal of Offender Rehabilitation, 50*(1), 18–36.

Klein, S., Petersilia, J., & Turners, S. (1990). Race and imprisonment decisions in California. *Science* (247), 812–816.

Langan, P., & Levin, D. (2002). *Recidivism in prisoners released in 1994*. Washington, DC: Bureau of Justice Statistics.

Mahon N. (1996). New York inmates' HIV risk behaviors: The implications for prevention policy and programs. *American Journal of Public Health, 86*(9), 1211–1215.

Mallik-Kane, K., & Visher, C. A. (2008). *Health and prisoner reentry: How physical, mental, and substance abuse conditions shape the process of reintegration*. Washington, DC: Urban Institute, Justice Policy Center. Retrieved on April 28, 2010, http://www.urban.org/UploadedPDF/411617_health_prisoner_reentry.pdf

Mumola, C., & Beck, A. (1997). *Prisoners in 1996*. Washington, DC: U.S. Department of Justice, Bureau of Justice Statistics.

Murray J., & Farrington, D. P. (2008). Parental imprisonment: Long-lasting effects on boys' internalizing problems through the life course. *Development and Psychopathology, 20*(1), 273–90.

Pager, D. (2008, November 20). Statement of Devah Pager to the U.S. Equal Employment Opportunity Commission meeting regarding employment discrimination faced by individuals with arrest and conviction records. Retrieved from http://www.eeoc.gov/abouteeoc/meetings/11-20-08/pager.html

Rollnick S., & Miller, W. R. (1995). What is motivational interviewing? *Behavioural and Cognitive Psychotherapy* (23), 325–334.

Samuels, P., & Mukamal, D. (2004). *After prison: Roadblocks to reentry*. A report on state legal barriers facing people with criminal records. Legal Action Center.

Stark, K., Bienzle, U., Vonk, R., & Guggenmoos-Holzmann, I. (1997). History of syringe sharing in prison and risk of hepatitis B virus, hepatitis C virus, and human immunodeficiency virus infection among injecting drugs users in Berlin. *International Journal of Epidemiology, 26*(6), 1359–66.

Stephan, J. J. (1999, August). *State prison expenditures, 1996*. [NCJ 172211]. Washington, DC: U.S. Department of Justice, Bureau of Justice Statistics.

Strang J., Gossop M., Heuston J., Green J., Whiteley C., Maden, A. (2006). Persistence of drug use during imprisonment: relationship of drug type, recency of use and severity of dependence to use of heroin, cocaine and amphetamine in prison. *Addiction 101*(8), 1125–1132.

Travis, J. (2005). *But they all come back: Facing the challenges of prisoner reentry*. Washington, DC: Urban Institute Press.

Turnbull P. J., Power R., & Stimson, G. V. (1996) "Just using old works": Injecting risk behaviour in prison. *Drug and Alcohol Review*, *15*(3), 251–260.

Uggen C., Manza J., & Thompson M. (2006). Citizenship, democracy, and the civic reintegration of criminal offenders. *Annals of the American Academy of Political and Social Science* (605), 281–310.

U.S. Department of Justice. (1996). *Prisoners in 1996*. Bureau of Justice Statistics Bulletin. Washington, DC: U.S. Department of Justice.

Valera, P., Epperson, M., Daniels, J., Ramaswamy, M., & Freudenberg, N. (2009). Substance use and HIV-risk behaviors among young men involved in the criminal justice system. *American Journal of Drug and Alcohol Abuse*, *35*(1), 43–47.

Ventura L. A., Cassel C. A., Jacoby, J. E., & Huang, B. (1998). Case management and recidivism of mentally ill persons released from jail. *Psychiatric Services*, *49*, 10.

Visher, C. A., & Travis, J. (2003). Transitions from prison to community: Understanding individual pathways. *Annual Review of Sociology* (29), 89–113.

Weinhardt, L. S., Carey, M. P., Johnson B. T., & Bickham, N. L. (1999). Effects of HIV counseling and testing on sexual risk behavior: A meta-analytic review of published research, 1985–1997. *American Journal of Public Health*, *89*(9), 1397–1405.

West, H. C., Sabol, W., & Cooper, M. (2009). *Prisoners in 2008*. NCJ 228417. Washington, DC: U.S. Department of Justice, Bureau of Justice Statistics.

Western, B., Lopoo, L. & McLanahan, S. (2004). Incarceration and the bonds between parents in fragile families. In M. Patillo, D. Weiman, & B. Western (Eds.), *Imprisoning America: The social effects of mass incarceration* (pp. 21–45). New York, NY: Russell Sage Foundation.

Western, B., & McLanahan, S. (2000). Fathers behind bars: The impact of incarceration on family formation. *Contemporary Perspectives in Family Research* (2), 307–322.

Western, B., & Pettit, R. (2004). *Mass imprisonment and the life course: Race and class inequality in U.S. incarceration*. Retrieved from http://www.wjh.harvard.edu/soc/faculty/western/pdfs/ASRv69n2p.pdf

Zamble, E., & Quinsey, V. L. (1997). *The criminal recidivism process*. Cambridge, UK: Cambridge University Press.

Chapter 7

Life-Course Socioeconomic Position and Hypertension in African-American Men

The Pitt County Study

Sherman A. James
John Van Hoewyk
Robert F. Belli
David S. Strogatz
David R. Williams
Trevillore E. Raghunathan

Learning Objectives

- Understand the odds of **hypertension** among black men with reference to their **socioeconomic position (SEP)** in both childhood and adulthood.

- Appreciate the relevance of **life-course SEP** and **CVD** risk in relation to black men in America.

- Learn how a **community-based prospective study** can be utilized to explore the odds of hypertension among black men with reference to their socioeconomic position (SEP).

- Appreciate the relevance of access to material resources in both childhood and adulthood as protective factors against premature hypertension in black men.

• • •

This chapter reports on a community-based prospective study exploring the odds of hypertension for black men with reference to their socioeconomic position (SEP) in childhood and adulthood.

Objectives. We investigated the odds of hypertension for black men in relationship to their socioeconomic position (SEP) in both childhood and adulthood.

Methods. On the basis of their parents' occupation, we classified 379 men in the Pitt County (North Carolina) study into low and high childhood SEP. The men's own education, occupation, employment status, and home ownership status were used to classify them into low and high adulthood SEP. Four life-course SEP categories resulted: **low childhood/low adulthood, low childhood/high adulthood, high childhood/low adulthood**, and **high childhood/high adulthood**.

Results. Low childhood SEP was associated with 60 percent greater odds of hypertension, and low adulthood SEP was associated with twofold greater odds of hypertension. Compared with men of high SEP in both childhood and adulthood, the odds of hypertension were seven times greater for low/low SEP men, four times greater for low/high SEP men, and six times greater for high/low SEP men.

Conclusions. Greater access to material resources in both childhood and adulthood was protective against premature hypertension in this cohort of black men. Though some parameter estimates were imprecise, study findings are consistent with both pathway and cumulative burden models of hypertension.

Literature Review and Conceptual Framework

Studies documenting an association between low socioeconomic position (SEP) in childhood—or, alternatively, low SEP in both childhood and adulthood—and increased risk for morbidity and mortality from a variety of chronic diseases in adulthood are growing in number (Davey Smith, 2003; Galobardes, Lynch, & Smith, 2004; Kuh & Ben-Shlomo, 2004). A recent review (Pollitt, Rose, & Kaufman, 2005) focusing specifically on life-course socioeconomic factors and risk for cardiovascular disease (CVD) concluded that studies provide moderate support for an independent contribution of low SEP in early life and increased CVD risk factors, CVD morbidity, and CVD mortality in adulthood. Though the review found little support for an independent association between CVD risk and social mobility (i.e., movement from one SEP level in childhood to another in adulthood), fairly consistent support was observed for a positive association between lifelong socioeconomic disadvantage and adverse CVD outcomes in adulthood (Pollitt et al., 2005).

Three major conceptual models have been advanced (Ben-Shlomo & Kuh, 2002; Hertzman & Power, 2003) to organize the literature on life-course SEP and early versus late emergence of CVD and other chronic diseases in adulthood. The first is the **latency effects model** (Hertzman & Power, 2003), also called the *biological chains of risk* model (Ben-Shlomo & Kuh, 2002), which posits that early-life SEP can influence adult health independent of intervening changes in SEP. The second is the **pathway** (Hertzman & Power, 2003) or "social chains of risk" model (Ben-Shlomo & Kuh, 2002), which acknowledges the importance of early-life conditions for adult health, but stipulates that important intervening life events (like upward or downward social mobility) can alter health trajectories initiated in early childhood. Finally, the **cumulative burden model** (Hertzman & Power, 2003), also called the *accumulation of risk* model (Ben-Shlomo & Kuh, 2002), hypothesizes that health-damaging effects of socioeconomic deprivation in both childhood and adulthood aggregate over the life course to significantly undermine health by middle adulthood.

Because of the more widespread availability of epidemiological data on childhood SEP (most commonly measured by father's occupation) in western and northern Europe, the vast majority of studies dealing with life-course SEP and CVD have been conducted on the European continent (Galobardes et al., 2004; Pollitt et al., 2005). The number of U.S.-based studies is increasing (Galobardes et al., 2004; Pollitt, Rose & Kaufman, 2005), but to date these studies have focused largely on white Americans. Indeed, as others (Pollitt et al., 2005) have noted, the paucity of research on life-course SEP and CVD risk in U.S. racial and ethnic minorities represents a significant gap in the literature.

We found only one study dealing with life-course SEP and CVD risk in black Americans. This study (Broman, 1989), which used data from the National Survey of Black Americans, investigated associations between self-reported hypertension and **childhood SEP** (father's occupation), **adulthood SEP** (respondent's education and occupation), and **downward intergenerational social mobility** (i.e., father's occupation was higher than respondent's). Although adulthood SEP was inversely associated with self-reported hypertension, no associations were observed for childhood SEP or downward social mobility. Thus, neither the latency model nor the pathway effects model was supported in this study (Broman, 1989). It is not clear to what extent misclassification of respondents on childhood SEP (and, therefore, downward social mobility) or, alternatively, misclassification on hypertension status (because of reliance on self-report data) biased the findings toward the null in this study. Additional research on life-course SEP and hypertension risk in black Americans that builds on this initial effort (Broman, 1989) is clearly needed, given the well-documented excess prevalence, (Burt et al., 1995; Cooper et al., 1997; Hajjar & Kotchen, 2003) seriousness (Cooper, Liao &

Rotimi, 1996; Lopes, Hornbuckle, James, & Port, 1994; Wong, Shapiro, Boscardin, & Ettner, 2002), and earlier age of onset (Burt et al., 1995; Cooper et al., 1996) of hypertension in black Americans. The earlier onset of hypertension in black adults, relative to whites, suggests that the origins of the excess risk for this condition among blacks reside, at least in part, in the problematic social and material life conditions to which numerous black Americans are exposed in childhood (Aber, Bennett, Conley, & Li, 1997; Duncan & Rodgers, 1991; Proctor & Dalaker, 2003).

Using the three aforementioned conceptual models (Ben-Shlomo & Kuh, 2002; Hertzman & Power, 2003) of the relationship between life-course SEP and health in adulthood to frame the research questions, we investigated the contribution of relative socioeconomic deprivation—during childhood, adulthood, and over the life course—to risk for hypertension in a community probability sample of black men aged 25 to 50 years.

Methods

The following section reports the methods used in this study. It includes a description of the study participants, the measurement of blood pressure, the measurement of childhood SEP, the measurement of adulthood SEP, the measurement of life-course SEP, covariates, descriptive variables, and statistical analysis.

Study Participants

Data for this study come from the 2001 follow-up survey of participants in the Pitt County (North Carolina) Study, a community-based, prospective investigation of risk factors for hypertension and related disorders in blacks ages 25 to 50 years in 1988, the baseline year. Because a major objective of the Pitt County Study was to investigate differential risk for hypertension between working-class and middle-class blacks, individuals residing in middle-class neighborhoods were oversampled. The baseline sample, the sampling strategy, and the content of the baseline household interview are described elsewhere (James, Keenan, Strogatz, Browning, & Garrett, 1992; Strogatz et al., 1991).

Of the 2,225 race- and age-eligible individuals, 1,773 (661 men and 1,112 women), or 80 percent, were interviewed in 1988. In 2001, the cohort was reinterviewed to obtain information on the individuals' social and economic resources from early childhood to the date of the interview. The goal was to link this life-course information on socioeconomic resources to major CVD risk factors, such as hypertension, obesity (James et al., 2006), type-2 diabetes, and cigarette smoking, as recorded in 1988.

Interviews in 2001 were sought with all cohort members believed to be alive, noninstitutionalized, and residing within a 100-mile radius of Greenville, the county's principal city. Of the 1,540 individuals (543 men and 997 women) meeting these criteria, 1,221 (428 men and 793 women), or 79 percent, were reinterviewed. Of these, 43 were excluded because of significant discrepancies in birth year ($\geq$ 2 years) or height ($\geq$ 2 inches) when comparing 1988 and 2001 values. These exclusions resulted in 1,178 individuals (418 men and 760 women), or 77 percent of the 1,540 targeted interviews. This report focuses on the male respondents.

Measurement of Blood Pressure

Approximately 15 minutes into the 1988 baseline survey, trained interviewers used a standard mercury sphygmomanometer to measure three sitting blood pressures on the participant's right arm. Blood pressure was subsequently defined by the average of the second and third readings, with the fifth-phase Korotkoff's sound indicating diastolic blood pressure. An individual was classified as hypertensive if any one of three conditions was met: systolic blood pressure $\geq$ 140 mm Hg, diastolic blood pressure $\geq$ 90 mm Hg, or current use of antihypertensive medication.

Measurement of Childhood SEP

Data to measure childhood SEP were obtained with the assistance of a computerized **Event History Calendar** developed expressly for this study. This methodology enhances recall of information stored years or decades in the past by using more easily remembered events (e.g., where one lived and with whom at specific points in time) to stimulate the recall of events less easily remembered (Belli, 1998; Belli, Shay & Stafford, 2001; Freedman, Thornton, Camburn, Alwin, & Young-DeMarco, 1988). Study participants provided a brief description of the main job held by their family's primary breadwinner during their childhood years, defined as birth to 13 years of age. Each job description was coded to fit one of nine categories of the 1990 Census Occupational Classification: 1 = managerial and professional; 2 = technical, sales, and administrative support; 3 = protective services (including military); 4 = farm owners; 5 = precision production, craft, and repair; 6 = service occupations for private households; 7 = service occupations, except protective and households; 8 = operators, fabricators, assemblers, and laborers; and 9 = farm laborers. No code exists for life-long homemakers (i.e., persons who never worked outside the home for pay). In the case of two salaried working parents, the higher occupational rank, irrespective of gender, was used.

The above nine categories were subsequently collapsed into two broad job categories: skilled (Codes 1 to 5) versus semi-unskilled (Codes 6 to 8) or farm laborer (Code 9), and designated high and low childhood SEP, respectively. Childhood SEP could not be determined for 21 men because 6 were offspring of single (homemaker) mothers, and 15 had missing data on the family breadwinner variable.

Measurement of Adulthood SEP

Our prior work (James et al., 1992; Strogatz et al., 1997) indicated that education and occupation, taken alone or in combination, were weak predictors of hypertension in the Pitt County study population. Therefore, in this study we sought to minimize misclassification of respondents with respect to their "true" socioeconomic standing in the community by creating an index of adulthood SEP on the basis of four variables collected in 1988.

The first variable, education, had four levels: less than high school, high school, some college, and college graduate. The second variable, occupation, was based on nine Hollingshead job prestige (Ainsworth, Keenan, Strogatz, Garrett, & James, 1991) scores: 1 = farm laborer/menial service worker; 2 = unskilled worker; 3 = machine operator or semiskilled worker; 4 = skilled manual worker; 5 = clerical/sales worker; 6 = skilled technician/small business owner; 7 = manager/farm owner ($\geq$ 150 acres); 8 = administrator/registered nurse; and 9 = higher executive/major professional. These nine scores were subsequently collapsed into two broad occupational categories: "blue collar" if Hollingshead scores were from 1 to 4; and "white collar" if Hollingshead scores were from 5 to 9. The third variable, current employment status, had two levels: employed versus not employed, as did the fourth variable, homeowner: yes or no. Household income was not collected in 1988; hence, employment status and home ownership provided some indirect information on access to income and wealth.

Scores for the adulthood SEP index were produced with the following algorithm: education (less than high school = 0, high-school graduate but less than college = 0.5, college graduate = 1.0), occupation (blue collar = 0, white collar = 1), currently employed (no = 0, yes = 1), and home owner (no = 0, yes = 1). Thus, the highest possible score on the adulthood SEP index was 4.0. To identify individuals who could be plausibly designated as "socioeconomically advantaged," at least relative to other cohort members, persons scoring 3.0 or higher on the adult SEP index were categorized as "high"; those scoring less than 3.0 were categorized as "low."

Measurement of Life-Course SEP

Life-course SEP was determined by combining information on childhood and adulthood SEP. Four nonoverlapping life-course SEP categories were created:

low childhood/low adulthood, low childhood/high adulthood, high childhood/low adulthood, and high childhood/high adulthood.

Covariates

Results from earlier papers (Ainsworth et al., 1991; Croft et al., 1993; James et al., 1992; Strogatz et al., 1991; Strogatz, Croft & James, et al., 1997) indicated that the following variables could account for the association between life-course SEP variables and 1988 hypertension status: age (years), body mass index, waist-to-hip ratio, alcohol consumption (abstainer/drinker), cigarette smoker (yes/no), strenuous physical exercise (physical activity $\geq$ three times/week, $\geq$ 20 minutes per occasion, intense enough to breathe hard and perspire), currently married (yes/no), instrumental support (low/high), emotional support (low/high), perceived stress (low/high), and John Henryism (low-high), defined as a strong behavioral predisposition to engage in high-effort coping with social or economic adversity. These covariates were controlled in all analyses.

Descriptive Variables

Interviewers used the Event History Calendar to collect information on the study participants' material conditions of life during childhood; for example, whether their childhood home(s) had electricity (yes/no) and indoor plumbing (yes/no). In addition, to assess exposure to early childhood nutritional deprivation, interviewers recorded (in inches) respondents' leg length (Davey Smith et al., 2001; Wadsworth, Hardy, Paul, Marshall, & Cole, 2002), measured as the distance from the bony prominence at the top of the leg to the floor. These three descriptive variables were used primarily to assess whether the four life-course SEP categories captured differences among respondents concerning exposure to early life material deprivation.

Statistical Analysis

Analyses were weighted to take into account the oversampling of middle-class households in 1988 and nonresponse to both the 1988 and 2001 surveys. Multiple logistic regression was used to test latency effects by contrasting the odds of hypertension among men in the low versus high childhood SEP categories, after control for adulthood SEP and potential confounders. (Main effects for low versus high adulthood SEP, after control for childhood SEP, were also conducted.) When testing for cumulative burden and pathway effects, men in the high/high SEP group, or those "relatively advantaged" over the life course, were used as the referent category. The cumulative burden model was tested by comparing the odds of hypertension for men in the high/high SEP group and men in the low/low (or "chronically disadvantaged") SEP group. Two pathway models were tested. First, the odds of hypertension for men in the high/high SEP group were compared with those for men in the low/high SEP group; and second, the odds of hypertension for men in the high/high SEP group were compared with those for men in the high/low SEP group.

Hierarchical regression models were used to add potential confounders individually or as a block to isolate their unique contributions to the odds for hypertension. For example, when testing main effects for childhood or adulthood SEP, and similarly when testing additive effects for life-course SEP, the fully adjusted model controlled for potential confounders in the following order: age (Model 1); body mass index and waist-to-hip ratio (Model 2); smoking, alcohol consumption, and physical exercise (Model 3); marital status, instrumental and emotional support, perceived stress, and John Henryism (Model 4). For parsimony's sake, only the results for Models 1 and 4 will be presented.

All analyses were performed using SAS, Version 9.12 (SAS Institute Inc, Cary, NC) (Berglund, 2002). Weighted estimates of parameters, variances, and 95 percent confidence intervals were obtained using either linearization or Jackknife Repeated Replication techniques (Kish & Frankel, 1974). Analyses were restricted to the 379 men (70 percent of the initial target number) with no missing values on study variables.

Results

Table 7.1 summarizes differences in selected background characteristics of the men, stratified by life-course SEP. The overwhelming majority (307 of 379; 81 percent) grew up in low childhood SEP households, and only 22 percent (68 of 307) achieved substantial upward social mobility in adulthood. Consequently, most men (239 of 379; 63 percent) were assigned to the low/low SEP category. Correspondingly, the high/high SEP category had the smallest number of men (25 of 379; 7 percent).

Comparison of baseline demographic and behavioral characteristics by life-course SEP showed statistically significant differences only for age and marital status: High/low SEP men were youngest and least likely to be married whereas low/high SEP men were oldest and most likely to be married. Comparisons involving the three variables believed to reflect exposure to childhood material deprivation generally supported the validity of the life-course SEP categories. First, there was a tendency ($p < .09$) for men from slightly more advantaged childhood backgrounds (high/high and high/low SEP groups) to have grown up in homes with electricity. These men were also more likely ($p < .04$) to have grown up in homes with indoor plumbing. Interestingly, men

Table 7.1. Differences in Selected Characteristics of Black Men, by Life-Course Socioeconomic Position: The Pitt County (North Carolina) Study, 2001

| | Childhood/Adulthood Socioeconomic Position | | | | |
	Low/Low ($n = 239$)	Low/High ($n = 68$)	High/Low ($n = 47$)	High/High ($n = 25$)	p^a
Mean age (SE)	34.6 (0.51)	37.3 (0.86)	31.5 (0.92)	35.4 (1.28)	$< .01$
Mean waist–hip ratio (SE)	0.89 (0.00)	0.90 (0.01)	0.89 (0.01)	0.89 (0.02)	.13
Obese,[b] %	20.5	24.8	19.7	10.1	.35
Smoker, %	51.7	33.1	45.3	33.6	.56
Drinker, %	62.6	63.1	70.1	67.7	.98
Strenuous exerciser,[c] %	62.2	61.4	73.9	41.0	.13
Married, %	54.3	87.6	54.5	71.5	.01
Crowded households,[d] %	17.6	4.8	17.0	3.6	.17
Childhood[e] homes lacking, %					
Electricity	12.8	21.0	10.5	3.9	.09
Plumbing	74.1	77.6	48.8	49.9	.04
Mean leg length[f] (SE)	36.8 (0.18)	37.9 (0.41)	37.9 (0.48)	38.0 (0.66)	$< .01$

Note. Data were weighted for oversampling and nonresponse.

[a]F tests, two-tailed; all comparisons except age were age adjusted.

[b]Body Mass Index ≥ 30.0.

[c]Respondent exercises $\geq$ three times/week, ≥ 20 minutes per occasion, enough to breathe hard and perspire.

[d]Households with more than one person per room, on average.

[e]Childhood was defined as birth to 13 years old.

[f]Distance, in inches, between bony prominence at top of leg and floor.

The unadjusted, category-specific prevalence of hypertension is shown in Table 7.2. The prevalence was 14.1 percentage points higher (40.9 vs. 26.8) among men from low versus high childhood SEP backgrounds, and 11.4 percentage points higher (41.2 vs. 29.8) among men in the low versus high adulthood SEP groups. For life-course SEP, the differences were more marked: 42.3 % of men in the low/low SEP group were hypertensive compared with 10.9 % of men in the high/high SEP group. Interestingly, hypertension prevalence for men in the low/high SEP (35.8 %) and high/low SEP (35.1 %) categories were virtually identical.

in the low/low SEP group had a significantly ($p < .01$) shorter mean leg length (about 1 inch shorter) than men in the other three groups. Furthermore, when mean leg length was compared for men in the low versus high childhood SEP groups, ignoring adulthood SEP, the 372 men in the former group had a significantly ($p < .05$) shorter mean leg length (37.05 inches) than the 72 men in the latter group (37.90 inches) (data not shown).

Table 7.2. Unadjusted Prevalence of Hypertension among Black Men, by Childhood, Adulthood, and Life-Course Socioeconomic Position: The Pitt County (North Carolina) Study, 2001

Socioeconomic Position	n	Percentage Hypertensive[a]	p[b]
Childhood[c]			
Low	307	40.9	< .14
High	72	26.8	
Adulthood[d]			
Low	286	41.2	< .02
High	93	29.8	
Life-course[e]			
Low/low	239	42.3	< .04
Low/high	68	35.8	
High/low	47	35.1	
High/high	25	10.9	

[a]Hypertension = systolic blood pressure $\geq$ 140 mm Hg, or diastolic blood pressure $\geq$ 90 mm Hg, or currently taking antihypertensive medication.
[b]Likelihood ratio tests, 2-tailed; data are weighted for oversampling and nonresponse.
[c]Low = parent's occupation: unskilled worker/farm laborer; high = skilled worker.
[d]Low = respondent's SEP index score < 3; high = SEP index score $\geq$ 3.
[e]Low/low = low childhood/low adulthood SEP.
low/high = low childhood/high adulthood SEP.
high/low = high childhood/low adulthood SEP.
high/high = high childhood/high adulthood SEP.

Table 7.3 presents the odds ratios and 95 percent confidence intervals for hypertension by childhood, adulthood, and life-course SEP. The odds ratios in the first column are adjusted for age only; those in the second column are adjusted for age plus the indicated covariates. In general, the two sets of estimates are very close in value. A modest, non–statistically significant "latency effect" was observed for childhood SEP: Men from low childhood SEP backgrounds had a 60 percent greater odds of hypertension (multivariable adjusted OR = 1.60; 95 percent CI = 0.75, 3.38) than their higher childhood SEP counterparts. In contrast, a fairly robust association for adulthood SEP was observed: men in the low adulthood SEP category had a twofold greater odds (multivariable adjusted OR = 2.25; 95 percent CI = 1.15, 4.40) of hypertension than their higher SEP counterparts. (The inclusion of mean leg length as a covariate did not alter the findings for childhood and adulthood SEP; data not shown.) Finally, though the parameter estimate was imprecise, strong support for the cumulative burden model was observed: Men in the low/low SEP group had a sevenfold greater odds of hypertension (multivariable adjusted OR = 7.27; 95 percent CI = 1.91, 27.51) than men in the high/high SEP group.

Table 7.3. Relative Odds of Hypertension among Black Men, by Childhood, Adulthood, and Life-Course Socioeconomic Position: The Pitt County (North Carolina) Study, 2001

Socioeconomic Position	n	Odds Ratios (95% Confidence Interval)	
		Age-Adjusted	Multivariable-Adjusted[a]
Childhood[b]			
Low	307	1.67 (0.82, 3.38)	1.60[c] (0.75, 3.38)
High	72	Referent	Referent
Adulthood[d]			
Low	286	2.02 (1.09, 3.72)	2.25[e] (1.15, 4.40)
High	93	Referent	Referent
Life-course[f]			
Low/low	239	6.52 (1.48, 28.63)	7.27 (1.91, 27.51)
Low/high	68	4.14 (0.86, 19.82)	3.85 (0.91, 16.13)
High/low	47	5.85 (1.14, 29.94)	5.87 (1.25, 27.49)
High/high	25	Referent	Referent

[a]Adjusted for age, body mass index, waist–hip ratio, marital status, alcohol, smoking, strenuous exercise, perceived stress, John Henryism, instrumental support, emotional support; data weighted for oversampling and nonresponse.
[b]Low = parent's occupation: unskilled worker/farm laborer; high = skilled worker.
[c]Also adjusted for adulthood SEP.
[d]Low = respondent's SEP index score < 3; high = SEP index score ≥ 3.
[e]Also adjusted for childhood SEP.
[f]Low/low = low childhood/low adulthood SEP.
low/high = low childhood/high adulthood SEP.
high/low = high childhood/low adulthood SEP.
high/high = high childhood/high adulthood SEP.

Study findings also pointed to potential pathway effects as indicated, for example, by a nearly fourfold greater odds (multivariable adjusted OR = 3.85; 95 percent CI = 0.91, 16.13) of hypertension among low/high SEP men compared with high/high SEP men. Though sizeable, this odds ratio was actually 47 percent lower than the odds ratio of 7.27 observed for low/low SEP men, suggesting the potential importance of substantial upward social mobility in mitigating risk for hypertension among black men who grew up poor. Potential pathway effects are similarly suggested by the multivariable adjusted odds ratio of 5.87 (95 percent CI = 1.25, 27.49) observed for men in the high/low SEP group. Despite having presumably comparable childhood material life conditions, as adults, the high/low SEP men had a sixfold greater odds of hypertension than their high/high SEP counterparts. Parameter estimates for both pathway models were imprecise, however, because of small sample sizes.

Discussion

Our study findings indicate that socioeconomic conditions in childhood and adulthood, separately and in combination, influenced the hypertension status of black men aged 25 to 50 years at the time of their enrollment, in 1988, in the Pitt County study. The somewhat modest (and non-statistically significant) 60 percent excess odds for hypertension associated with low childhood SEP was nevertheless in the direction predicted by the latency effects model (Ben-Shlomo & Kuh, 2002; Hertzman & Power, 2003).

This study provided stronger support for the cumulative burden model, as evidenced by the sevenfold greater odds of hypertension among men who were relatively disadvantaged in both childhood and adulthood compared with men who were relatively advantaged at both time points. Formal tests of the cumulative burden model, with a specific focus on CVD risk factors, such as hypertension, are still few (Pollitt et al., 2005). Our positive findings for black men in Pitt County agree with evidence supporting a cumulative burden model of hypertension in British women (Lawlor, Ebrahim, & Davey Smith, 2002) and Scottish men (Smith, Hart, Blane, Gillis, & Hawthorne, 1997).

We also found some evidence supporting the pathway model, though relevant associations could not be estimated with precision because of small numbers. Membership in the low/high SEP group, which, in this study, represents substantial upward social mobility, was associated with a 47 percent reduction in the odds of hypertension compared with men who remained relatively disadvantaged in both childhood and adulthood. Whether this is a solid clue regarding the cardiovascular health benefits of significant upward social mobility for black men, or a chance finding, is a question for future studies to answer.

Similar reservations apply to the highly suggestive sixfold greater odds of hypertension among men in the high/low SEP group, relative to their high/high SEP counterparts. Strictly speaking, of course, men in the high/low SEP group are not necessarily downwardly mobile, as many of these men may have acquired more socioeconomic resources (e.g., more education and better-paying jobs) in adulthood than the adults who raised them. The only thing that can be said with confidence is that although the high/low SEP men and the high/high SEP men may have had comparable material resources in childhood, the former had fewer such resources in adulthood. The only other known study of intergenerational social mobility and hypertension in black Americans (Broman, 1989) found no association between downward social mobility and self-reported hypertension. Our study findings cannot be directly compared with that study, (Broman, 1989) however, because of major differences in how the two studies defined adulthood SEP.

Though most other studies also report weak childhood SEP main effects on CVD risk factors in adulthood (Pollitt et al., 2005), our study may have underestimated the association between childhood SEP and hypertension status because of either measurement error or limited variation on the exposure variable. Even if the Event History Calendar (Belli, 1998; Belli et al., 2001; Freedman et al., 1988) succeeded in improving respondents' recollection of distant life experiences, including the family breadwinner's primary occupation, differences in the material well-being of men from low and high childhood SEP backgrounds in the Pitt County study population may have been too small to predict larger differences in long-term risk for hypertension. Future studies that include a larger number of blacks with explicit variation in social class backgrounds will be able to avoid this limitation.

Our adulthood SEP index incorporated information on respondents' home ownership and current employment status as well as their education and occupation. Although respondent occupation (e.g., manual vs. nonmanual job) is the most common measure of adulthood SEP used in life-course health research (Broman, 1989; Galobardes et al., 2004; Pollitt et al., 2005), some investigators (Lynch, Kaplan, Salonen, & Salonen, 1997) used an index that included income, housing, material possessions, and job security. Incorporating this kind of "economic security" information in indices of adulthood SEP for research with black populations could be especially important because a growing literature (Blank, 2001; Collins, 1997; Council of Economic Advisers for the President's Initiative on Race, 1998; Davern & Fisher, 1995; Oliver & Shapiro, 1995; Shapiro, 2004; Williams & Collins, 1995) indicates that blacks, even those with college degrees or white-collar jobs, have very little wealth (and therefore little real economic security) as measured by net worth or net financial assets (Blank, 2001; Council of Economic Advisers for the President's Initiative on Race, 1998; Davern & Fisher, 1995; Oliver & Shapiro, 1995; Shapiro, 2004). Hence, measures of adulthood SEP that include easily collected wealth data, such as home ownership (the most common form of wealth owned by blacks) (Davern & Fisher, 1995; Oliver & Shapiro, 1995; Shapiro, 2004) could minimize misclassification on adulthood SEP, thereby enhancing the study's validity for blacks. The robust, twofold excess odds for hypertension observed for men in the low as opposed to high adulthood SEP category in the current study contrasts with the weaker education (and occupation) main effects on hypertension in our earlier work (James et al., 1992; Strogatz et al., 1991). This difference is most likely caused by our use of a more informative measure of adulthood SEP for blacks in this study.

The rather large odds ratios observed for the three life-course SEP comparisons were attributable to the unusually low prevalence (10 percent) of hypertension among men in the high/high SEP group. The prevalence for men in the other three groups was comparable to the national average (about 34 percent) for black men (Burt, et al., 1995; Hajjar & Kotchen, 2003). Though replication is clearly called for, this unusually low prevalence of hypertension for men in the high/high SEP group points to the potential importance of stable access to adequate socioeconomic resources *across the life course* for preventing hypertension in black men.

Limitations of our study include a small sample size, which decreased the precision of some parameter estimates; an overrepresentation of respondents in low SEP categories, a legacy of the historically high poverty rates among blacks in the Southeastern United States (MDC, 2004; Proctor & Dalaker, 2003); and our reliance on retrospective childhood SEP data, which, along with limited variation in the childhood SEP measure, could have produced an underestimate of childhood SEP main effects. Although the 30 percent nonresponse to the 2001 interview is also a limitation, our analyses were weighted to account for nonresponse; thus, the findings apply to all black men ages 25 to 50 years residing in Pitt County in 1988.

Strengths of our study include the following: It is the first fully integrated (Pollitt et al., 2005) examination of latency, pathway, and cumulative burden SEP models of hypertension in a U.S. black population; the observed associations involving life-course SEP and hypertension status were largely unaffected by known correlates (Ainsworth et al., 1991; Croft et al., 1993; James et al., 1992; Strogatz et al., 1991; Strogatz et al., 1997) of hypertension in this study population; a computerized Event History Calendar (Belli, 1998; Belli et al., 2001; Freedman et al., 1988) was used to improve respondents' recall of distant life experiences; and, finally, the research utility of an adulthood SEP index that addressed fundamental economic security issues for blacks was demonstrated.

More research on life-course SEP and CVD risk in blacks and other U.S. populations of color is clearly needed (Pollitt et al., 2005). However, our success in laying a solid empirical foundation in support of multisectoral interventions to eliminate racial and ethnic inequalities in CVD will likely require the development of research models that are attentive to the unique features of a given group's history and standing in America.

Policy Implications

There are a number of policy implications that can be drawn from this study. First, incorporating economic security information in indices of adulthood SEP for research with black populations may be important due to the relative lack of wealth among African Americans as compared to their white counterparts. Second, the unusually low prevalence of hypertension in the high/high SEP group is indicative of the potential importance of stable access to adequate socioeconomic resources *across the life course* for preventing hypertension in black men. Finally, the study demonstrates the need for more research, and also interventions relating to life-course SEP and CVD risk in blacks and other U.S. populations of color.

Summary

This chapter has described a community-based prospective study exploring the odds of hypertension for black men with reference to their socioeconomic position (SEP) in childhood and adulthood. The authors used a community probability sample of black men ages 25 to 50 years to investigate the role of relative social deprivation in the development of hypertension. A key objective of the study was the measurement of differential risk of hypertension among working class and middle class blacks.

The results of the study demonstrate an association between hypertension and low SEP:

- Low childhood SEP was associated with a 60 percent higher probability of having hypertension.
- Low adulthood SEP was associated with a twofold higher probability of having hypertension.
- Low childhood/low adulthood SEP was associated with a sevenfold higher probability of having hypertension as compared with men of high SEP in both childhood and adulthood.
- Low childhood/high adulthood SEP was associated with a fourfold higher probability of having hypertension as compared with men of high SEP in both childhood and adulthood.
- High adulthood/low childhood SEP was associated with a sixfold higher probability of having hypertension as compared with men of high SEP in both childhood and adulthood.

Despite noted limitations, the study made a clear contribution to the literature on the relationship between SEP and cardiovascular disease given the prior lack of work on this issue relating to the black population. It also highlighted the relationship between access to socioeconomic resources *across the life course* and hypertension in black men.

Key Terms

adulthood SEP

cardiovascular disease (CVD)

childhood SEP

community-based prospective study

cumulative burden model

downward intergenerational social mobility

Event History Calendar

high childhood/high adulthood

high childhood/low adulthood

hypertension

latency effects model

life-course SEP

low childhood/high adulthood

low childhood/low adulthood

pathway model

socioeconomic position (SEP)

Discussion Questions

1. Discuss the three major conceptual models that have been advanced to organize the literature on life-course SEP and early versus late emergence of CVD. Consider possible strengths versus weaknesses of the various approaches.

2. Were you surprised to learn the extent of hypertension disparities among working class and middle class black men? Why/Why not?

3. The authors suggest that access to adequate socioeconomic resources *across the life course* may be necessary for preventing hypertension in black men. Do you agree with this view? Why/Why not?

References

Aber, L., Bennett, N., Conley, D., & Li, J. (1997). The effects of poverty on child health and development. *Annual Review of Public Health, 18*, 463–483.

Ainsworth, B. E., Keenan, N. L., Strogatz, D. S., Garrett, J. M., & James, S.A. (1991). Physical activity and hypertension in black adults: The Pitt County study. *American Journal of Public Health, 81*, 1477–1479.

Belli, R. (1998). The structure of autobiographical memory and the event history calendar: Potential improvements in the quality of retrospective reports in surveys. *Memory, 6*, 383–406.

Belli, R. F., Shay, W. L., & Stafford, F. P. (2001). Event history calendars and question list surveys: A direct comparison of interviewing methods. *Public Opinion Quarterly, 65*, 45–74.

Ben-Shlomo, Y., & Kuh, D. (2002). A life course approach to chronic disease epidemiology: Conceptual models, empirical challenges and interdisciplinary perspectives. *International Journal of Epidemiology, 31*, 285–293.

Berglund, P. A. (2002). *Analysis of complex sample survey data using the SURVEYMEANS and SURVEYREG procedures and macro coding.* Ann Arbor: Institute for Social Research, University of Michigan.

Blank, R. M. (2001). An overview of trends in social and economic well-being, by race. In N. J. Smelser, W. J. Wilson, & F. Mitchell (Eds.), *Racial trends and their consequences* (Vol. 1, pp. 21–39). Washington, DC: National Academy Press.

Broman, C. L. (1989). Social mobility and hypertension among blacks. *Journal of Behavioural Medicine, 12*(2), 123–134.

Burt, V. L., Cutler, J. A., Higgins, M., Horan, M. J., Labarthe, D., Whelton, P., . . . Roccella, E. J. (1995). Trends in the prevalence, awareness, treatment, and control of hypertension in the adult US population. Data from the health examination surveys, 1960 to 1991. *Hypertension*, *26*(1), 60–69.

Collins, S. M. (1997). Black mobility in white corporations: Up the corporate ladder but out on a limb. *Social Problems*, *44*, 55–67.

Cooper, R., Rotimi, C., Ataman, S., McGee, D., Osotimehin, B., Kadiri, S., . . . Wilks, R. (1997). The prevalence of hypertension in seven populations of West African origin. *American Journal of Public Health*, *87*, 160–168.

Cooper, R. S., Liao, Y., & Rotimi, C. (1996). Is hypertension more severe among US blacks, or is severe hypertension more common? *Annals of Epidemiology*, *6*, 173–180.

Council of Economic Advisers. (1998). *Changing America: Indicators of social and economic well-being by race and Hispanic origin*. Washington, DC: U.S. Government Printing Office.

Croft, J. B., Strogatz, D. S., Keenan, N. L., James, S. A., Malarcher, A. M., & Garrett, J. M. (1993). The independent effects of obesity and body fat distribution on blood pressure in black adults: The Pitt County study. *International Journal of Obesity and Related Metabolic Disorders*, *17*, 391–397.

Davern, M. E., & Fisher, P. J. (1995). *Household net worth and asset ownership*. Washington, DC: U.S. Census Bureau.

Davey Smith, G. (Ed.). (2003). *Health inequalities: Lifecourse approaches*. Bristol, UK: Policy Press.

Davey Smith, G., Greenwood, R., Gunnell, D., Sweetnam, P., Yarnell, J., & Elwood, P. (2001). Leg length, insulin resistance, and coronary heart disease risk: The Caerphilly study. *Journal of Epidemiology and Community Health*, *55*, 867–872.

Duncan, G., & Rodgers, W. (1991). Has children's poverty become more persistent? *American Sociological Review*, *56*, 538–550.

Freedman, D., Thornton, A., Camburn, D., Alwin, D., & Young-De-Marco, L. (1988). The life history calendar: A technique for collecting retrospective data. *Sociological Methodology*, *18*, 37–68.

Galobardes, B., Lynch, J. W., & Smith, G. D. (2004). Childhood socioeconomic circumstances and cause-specific mortality in adulthood: Systematic review and interpretation. *Epidemiologic Reviews*, *26*, 7–21.

Hajjar, I., & Kotchen, T. A. (2003). Trends in prevalence, awareness, treatment, and control of hypertension in the United States, 1988–2000. *Journal of the American Medical Association*, *290*, 199–206.

Hertzman, C., & Power, C. (2003). Health and human development: Understandings from life-course research. *Developmental Neuropsychology*, *24*, 719–744.

James, S. A., Keenan, N. L., Strogatz, D. S., Browning, S. R., & Garrett, J. M. (1992). Socioeconomic status, John Henryism, and blood pressure in black adults: The Pitt County study. *American Journal of Epidemiology*, *135*, 59–67.

James, S. A., Van Hoewyk, J. V., Belli, R. F., Strogatz, D. S., Williams, D. R., & Raghunathan, T. E. (2006). Life-course socioeconomic position and hypertension in African American men: The Pitt County study. *American Journal of Public Health*, *96*(5), 812–817.

Kish, L., & Frankel, M. R. (1974). Inference from complex samples. *Journal of the Royal Statistical Society, B 36*, 1–37.

Kuh, D., & Ben-Shlomo, Y. (2004). *A life course approach to chronic disease epidemiology* (2nd ed). Oxford, UK: Oxford University Press.

Lawlor, D. A., Ebrahim, S., & Davey Smith, G. (2002). Socioeconomic position in childhood and adulthood and insulin resistance: cross sectional survey using data from British women's heart and health study. *British Medical Journal, 325,* 805–807.

Lopes, A. A., Hornbuckle, K., James, S. A., & Port, F. K. (1994). The joint effects of race and age on the risk of end-stage renal disease attributed to hypertension. *American Journal of Kidney Diseases, 24,* 554–560.

Lynch, J., Kaplan, G. A., Salonen, R., & Salonen, J. T. (1997). Socioeconomic status and progression of carotid atherosclerosis. Prospective evidence from the Kuopio ischemic heart disease risk factor study. *Arteriosclerosis, Thrombosis, and Vascular Biology, 17,* 513–519.

MDC. (2004). *The state of the south: Fifty years after Brown v. Board of Education.* Chapel Hill, NC: MDC.

Oliver, M. L., & Shapiro, T. M. (1995). *Black wealth/white wealth: A new perspective on racial inequality.* New York, NY: Routledge.

Pollitt, R. A., Rose, K. M., & Kaufman, J. S. (2005). Evaluating the evidence for models of life course socioeconomic factors and cardiovascular outcomes: A systematic review. *BMC Public Health, 5,* 7.

Proctor, B. D., & Dalaker, J. (2003). *Poverty in the United States: 2002* (Current Population Reports, P60–222). Washington, DC: U.S. Census Bureau.

Shapiro, T. M. (2004). *The hidden cost of being African American: How wealth perpetuates inequality.* New York, NY: Oxford University Press.

Smith, G.D., Hart, C., Blane, D., Gillis, C., & Hawthorne, V. (1997). Lifetime socioeconomic position and mortality: Prospective observational study. *British Medical Journal, 314,* 547–552.

Strogatz, D. S., Croft, J. B., James, S. A., Keenan, N. L., Browning, S. R., Garrett, J. M., & Curtis, A. B. (1997). Social support, stress, and blood pressure in black adults. *Epidemiology, 8,* 482–487.

Strogatz D. S., James, S. A., Haines, P. S., Elmer, P. J., Gerber, A. M., Browning, S. R., . . . Keenan, N. L. (1991). Alcohol consumption and blood pressure in black adults: The Pitt County study. *American Journal of Epidemiology, 133,* 442–450.

Wadsworth, M. E. J., Hardy, R. J., Paul, A. A., Marshall, S. F., & Cole, T. J. (2002). Leg and trunk length at 43 years in relation to childhood health, diet and family circumstances: Evidence from the 1946 national birth cohort. *International Journal of Epidemiology, 31,* 383–390.

Williams, D. R., & Collins, C. (1995). U.S. socioeconomic and racial differences in health: Patterns and explanations. *Annual Review of Sociology, 21,* 349–386.

Wong, M. D., Shapiro, M. F., Boscardin, W. J., & Ettner, S. L. (2002). Contribution of major diseases to disparities in mortality. *New England Journal of Medicine, 347,* 1585–1592.

Part Two

Social Determinants of Health Behavior

Chapter 8

Social Determinants of Medical Mistrust among African-American Men

Wizdom Powell Hammond
Arjumand A. Siddiqi

Learning Objectives

- Appreciate the significance and sociohistorical underpinnings of medical mistrust among African-American men.
- Understand theoretical frameworks used to conceptualize medical mistrust among African-American men.
- Assess direct and indirect associations between social determinants and African-American men's mistrust of medical organizations.
- Recognize the potential role of policy to address social determinants of medical mistrust.

• • •

This chapter proposed and tested a conceptual model of medical mistrust in a sample of African-American men recruited primarily from barbershops in the North, South, Midwest, and West regions of the United States. Potential social determinants were grouped into factors outlined by the World Health Organization (WHO) Commission on Social Determinants of Health; key determinants include social constructions of masculinity, socioeconomic position, racial discrimination, and health care access/delivery. Consistent with the WHO model and past research, the authors consider perceived racism in health care as a psychosocial mediator of racial discrimination. Our results suggest that, in every socioeconomic stratum, experiences of everyday racial discrimination serve as a fundamental cause of medical mistrust, and that this association is mediated by perceived racism in health care.

Significance and Sociohistorical Underpinnings of Medical Mistrust among African-American Men

Several studies have documented higher levels of **medical mistrust**, the lack of trust someone has in the health care system, including providers, facilities, and insurers, among African Americans (Armstrong et al., 2008; LaVeist, Nickerson, & Bowie, 2000). Most often, researchers have associated African Americans' mistrust of health care organizations to past and present incidents of medical malice (Gamble, 1997). For some time, the Tuskegee Study of Untreated Syphilis in the Negro Male (TSUS), which took place between 1932 and 1972, was presumed to be the primary source of African Americans' disproportionately higher medical mistrust (Gamble, 1997). Yet this presumption has been recently challenged by researchers who observed no significant relationship between knowledge of the TSUS and medical mistrust in a random sample of Baltimore residents (Brandon, Isaac, & LaVeist, 2005). This finding suggests that the TSUS may not be the sole source of medical mistrust among African Americans and thus investigations that consider the role played by other determinants are needed.

Undoubtedly, occurrences of medical malice itself have occurred in the context of other broad forms of structural discrimination exhibited by society in the United States over the course of its history—from the practice of slavery, to Jim Crow Era legislation, to present day systematic racial disparities in socioeconomic resources such as income, education, and housing and neighborhood conditions, to name only a few—which themselves manifest also in everyday experiences of discrimination. Moreover, it is arguable that, because African-American men were the primary subjects for the TSUS, report greater exposure to racial discrimination than African-American women (Banks, Singleton, & Kohn-Wood, 2008; Sellers & Shelton, 2003), *and* bear a disproportionate burden of socioeconomic disadvantage, medical mistrust may be a particularly salient issue amongst this group. In this study, the social and psychosocial determinants of African-American men's mistrust in health care organizations are explored.

Motivations for the current chapter also stem from data indicating that medical mistrust plays a prominent role in how individuals utilize and assess health care experiences. For example, lower levels of health care system trust are associated with less satisfaction with care, treatment adherence, and health services use (Altice, Mostashari, & Friedland, 2001; Hammond, Matthews, & Corbie-Smith, 2010; LaVeist et al., 2000; LaVeist, Isaac, & Williams, 2009). Researchers have found that men report more medical mistrust than women (Altice et al., 2001; Armstrong, Ravenell, McMurphy, & Putt, 2007) and others affirm that men are overrepresented among adults who fail to use preventive health services (Cherry, Woodwell, & Rechtsteiner, 2007).

African-American men are less likely than non-Hispanic white men to attend annual preventive health visits, are less likely to know their cholesterol levels, have poorer BP control, and experience greater morbidity and premature mortality from conditions generally amenable to early interventions (such as cardiovascular disease, stroke, hypertension, and heart failure) (Arias, 2007; Hertz, Unger, Cornell, & Saunders, 2005; Thom et al., 2006). When compared to African-American women, African-American men are also less likely to seek help from physicians regardless of problem severity (Neighbors & Howard, 1987). These findings suggest that this group may face unique barriers to health care utilization and help-seeking. Rooted partly in the historical legacy of medical malice, this study proposes medical mistrust as one such barrier.

Although medical mistrust may not solely explain men's tendency to forgo help-seeking, the findings described above suggest that it is a barrier worthy of further investigation. We specifically explore the antecedents of African-American men's trust in the medical system as a whole, which we believe lie primarily in socioeconomic and psychological factors, as they relate to both the health care system and broader life experiences. This assertion arises logically from connecting understandings arising from the literature on social determination of health (see Berkman, 2009) and the large body of research on the psychological underpinnings of trust-mistrust (Rotter, 1971). In this chapter we examine medical mistrust among African-American men. We propose a model of medical mistrust based on present conceptual and empirical understandings, describe a study to test this model, and conclude by offering a discussion of our study results in the context of the existing literature.

Theoretical Frameworks and Conceptual Model

Mistrust is defined as a general lack of trust in the motives of individuals and organizations (Omodei & McLennan, 2000). In this chapter, we depend largely on theories of organizational trust, which posit that trust is multidimensional (Bromiley & Cummings, 1995), relational (Tyler & Kramer, 1996), state-specific (Lewis & Weigert, 1985), and history-based (Boon & Holmes, 1991). Together, these theories make a departure from those that frame trust as a trait or purely character-driven attitude (Rotter, 1971). Instead, theorists in this vein stress the role played by cumulative social transactions, drawing our attention to the way that they can cause trust to "thicken" or "thin" (Kramer, 1999).

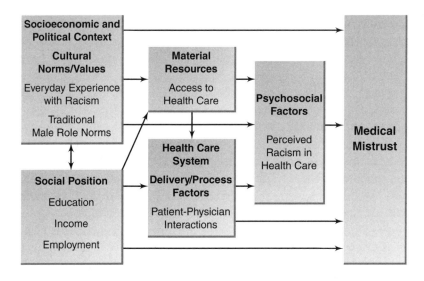

Figure 8.1. Conceptual Model of African-American Men's Medical Mistrust

Note: Adapted from the World Health Organization Commission on Social Determinants of Health (Irwin & Sandler, 2007)

We also draw on a framework for understanding social determinants of health produced by the World Health Organization (WHO) Commission on Social Determinants of Health (Commission of Social Determinants of Health, 2008; Solar & Irwin, 2007). Our study proposes a conceptual model (Figure 8.1) that elaborates on the WHO framework by explicating the interdependency of socioeconomic and psychological factors that lead to medical mistrust as a key barrier to use of health care systems.

Our conceptual model views medical mistrust among African-American men as a phenomenon fundamentally produced by three main factors: (1) societal constructions of masculinity (traditional male role norms), (2) everyday experiences of racial discrimination, and (3) one's own socioeconomic position in society. Together, these factors may determine the extent of perceived racism in the health care system, and ultimately the extent of medical mistrust.

We focus on societal constructions of masculinity because other researchers (Mansfield, Addis, & Courtenay, 2005) have framed mistrust as a consequence of **traditional male role norms**, or cultural belief systems about what men should do and feel (Levant, Hirsch, Celentano, & Cozz, 1992). African-American men's medical mistrust has also been linked to traditional male norms in a more recent study (Hammond, 2010). Traditional male role norms are socially constructed (Connell, 1995) and direct men to display strength, restrict emotion, and to be relentlessly self-reliant, thereby weakening norms of reciprocity that may facilitate trust building. Further, health care system transactions can require men to relinquish power and control and to let down emotional defenses. Such requirements are in direct opposition with culturally valued norms of masculinity. Although African-American men define masculinity in ways that differ from dominant men (Hammond & Mattis, 2005), we anticipate that traditional male role norms (such as those related to disclosing vulnerability) will be associated with greater medical mistrust.

Racial discrimination, or "differential treatment on the basis of race that disadvantages a racial group" (National Research Council, 2004), is included as a feature of the socioeconomic and political context because racial discrimination has been noted to be a persistent feature of African-American life (Williams, Neighbors, & Jackson, 2003) and researchers have found associations between racial discrimination and medical mistrust (Hammond, 2010; LaVeist et al., 2000). Taking the suggestions made by Smedley, Stith, and Nelson (2003), we suggest that racial discrimination in the broader social environment cumulates as interactional histories or scripts that get carried over to health care system interactions. Our model focuses specifically on subtle experiences of **everyday racism,** or repeated, systematic occurrences of racism based on prevailing societal attitudes (Essed, 1991), because of their potential to chronically diminish health care system trust.

We also consider the contributions made by health insurance and usual source of care. These factors facilitate health care access and thus afford opportunities for African-American men to establish relationships with physicians that could enhance or diminish medical mistrust. These health care resources also impact and shape evaluations of patient-physician interaction quality. Patient-centeredness is one marker of health care interaction quality (Institute of Medicine, 2001) and is characterized by mutuality (Roter & Hall, 1992), as well as empathic and responsive communication. Investigators have found that patient-centered interactions are associated with higher patient trust (Fiscella et al., 2004; Halbert, Armstrong, Gandy, & Shaker, 2006) and are less commonly reported by African-American patients (Johnson, Roter, Powe, & Cooper, 2004). We view patient-centered health care delivery in our model as a structural opportunity to "thicken" or "thin" patient trust.

Our key psychosocial variable of interest is **perceived racism in health care**, defined as participants' views on the presence and extent of racism in health care, including determination of medical treatment on the basis of race. Perceived racism in health care has been cited as an important determinant of African Americans' trust in medical organizations and willingness to utilize services (Greene, 1995; LaVeist et al., 2000). Hammond (2010) found that perceived racism in health care was a significant predictor of African-American men's medical mistrust even after controlling for other factors. In addition, Hammond (2010) found that perceived racism in health care mediated the relationship between racial discrimination and medical mistrust. Our model also accounts for this possibility.

We believe that medical mistrust will vary as a function of one's social position. This premise follows from studies indicating that individuals with lower socioeconomic status (Armstrong et al., 2007; Doescher, Saver, Franks, & Fiscella, 2000; Halbert et al., 2006) report more medical mistrust. The literature also suggests that traditional male role norms (Levant et al., 2007; Ojeda, Rosales, & Good, 2008) and racial discrimination (Gee, 2008) are socioeconomically patterned. It is well-known that individuals with lower income and education also have access to fewer health care specific material resources. Thus, our approach is to determine whether patterns of associations between our model determinants and medical mistrust vary across income and education strata.

Methods

Data for the current study were drawn from a cross-sectional investigation of African-American men's health and social lives conducted in three independent waves from 2003 to 2009. The majority of participants (77.9 percent) were recruited from seven barbershops in Michigan, Georgia, California, and North Carolina, and a smaller percentage (22.1 percent) from two academic institutions and events. The academic institutions were a community college located in Southeastern Michigan, and a historically black university (HBU) located in central North Carolina. Fifty percent of the community college population was male and 22 percent were members of ethnic minority groups. African Americans constituted 77 percent of the HBU population where 33 percent of the student body was male. The academic event was a conference for African-American male law enforcement professionals held in Miami, Florida, in 2003.

Recruitment Procedure and Research Settings

Participants were recruited through flier advertisements, direct contact, and by word-of-mouth. Barbershops were chosen as primary recruitment sites because they are noted as key locales for interpersonal exchange among African-American men from various socioeconomic backgrounds and have been successfully targeted in health promotion interventions with this population (Hart & Bowen, 2004; Hess et al., 2007). Eight barbershops characterized by key African-American male community informants as popular, "high-volume" businesses were approached about potential participation. "High-volume" shops were preferred because men could use their wait time to complete the surveys. Initial contact with barbershop owners was made in person or by telephone and followed-up with a study brochure, copy of the survey, and consent forms. Of the eight barbershop owners approached, only one declined to participate in the study citing past negative experiences with research investigators. Barbershop owners and barbers were invited to provide feedback about the survey content, length, and form, which was subsequently incorporated. Following this process, the receptionist or barber invited patrons to participate in a study about African-American men's health; participants 18 years or older and who self-identified as African American were eligible to complete the survey.

Ninety percent of the men approached in the barbershops verbally consented to participate. The most frequently cited reason for nonparticipation was time constraints. Although men were given the option of dropping off the survey at a later date, most completed the survey on site and received a gift certificate for a free haircut valued at $25 in exchange for their participation. Similar procedures were used for participants recruited at academic institutions and events who were approached by African-American research assistants during lunch hours or meal breaks in places of high congregation (student unions, cafeterias, conference exhibit halls, etc.). At academic institutions and events, 86 percent of the men approached agreed to complete the survey and received a $25 gift card in exchange for their participation. All study procedures were approved by the University of Michigan, California, and North Carolina Institutional Review Boards.

Measures

Socio-demographic, economic, and material resource factors assessed were age, level of education ($\leq$ high school, some college, and college/graduate or professional degree), marital status (currently married or unmarried), participant annual income ($<$ $20,000, $20,001–$39,999, $\geq$ $40,000), and employment status (employed full or part-time versus unemployed). Health care access factors assessed were health insurance status (has health insurance versus no health insurance), and usual source of care (has a usual source of care versus no usual source of care).

Traditional Male Role Norms

We used the restrictive emotionality subscale of the Male Role Norms Inventory (MRNI), a seven-item measure that assesses traditional masculinity norms around emotional disclosure (for example, "a man should never reveal worries to others" and "One should not be able to tell how a man is feeling by looking at his face"). A mean score was computed from responses ranging from 1 ("strongly disagree") to 7 ("strongly agree"), with higher scores indicating a greater endorsement of traditional male norms around emotion disclosure (Cronbach's $\alpha = .79$).

Quality of Recent Patient–Physician Interactions

We assessed the quality of recent patient–physician interactions with the four-item *Patient-Centeredness Scale* from the Medical Expenditure Panel Survey (MEPS) (Agency for Healthcare Research and Quality, 2000). This measure assesses the degree to which individuals feel that physicians have conveyed empathy, responsiveness to needs, and respect during health care visits. Participants responded to each of the four items: "How often in the past 12 months did physicians: (1) listen carefully, (2) explain things clearly, (3) show respect for what you had to say, and (4) spend enough time with you?" using a scale anchored with "never" (1) and "always" (4). Internal consistency was good ($\alpha = .92$) and a mean score was computed so that higher scores would indicate having experienced a recent higher quality or "patient-centered" interaction.

Racial Discrimination

We assessed racial discrimination experiences with the 18-item Daily Life Experience (DLE) subscale of the Racism and Life Experiences Scales (RaLes) (Harrell, 2000). This measure assesses the frequency with which particular race-related "micro-aggressions" (such as being ignored, overlooked, or not given service) occurred over the past year. Participants responded to each item using a scale anchored with "never" (0) and "once a week or more" (6). Internal consistency was good ($\alpha = .95$) and a mean score was computed so that higher scores on this measure would indicate more frequent occurrences of discrimination experiences.

Perceived Racism in Health Care

Perceived racism in health care was assessed with 16 items of an adapted version of the *Perceptions of Racism Scale* developed by Greene (1995). The measure assesses perceptions of race-based disparities in treatment by health care professionals. The original scale contained 20 items and was developed for African-American women. Hence, references to "women" in the item wording had to be changed to "men." The four excluded items assessed racism in educational opportunities, the receipt of public assistance, and general social mobility. Participants responded to each item (for example, "Doctors treat white men with more respect than African-American men" and "Racial discrimination in a doctor's office is common") using a scale anchored with "strongly disagree" (1) and "strongly agree" (4). Seven items were reverse coded and a mean score was computed so that higher scores on this scale would reflect more perceived racism in health care. The internal consistency for this scale was acceptable ($\alpha = .83$).

Medical Mistrust

Medical mistrust was assessed with the 14-item *Medical Mistrust Index* (MMI) (LaVeist et al., 2000; LaVeist et al., 2009), which assesses an individual's degree of mistrust in health care organizations as a whole. Participants responded to each item (for example, "When dealing with the health care system, one better be cautious," "Health care organizations have sometimes done harmful experiments on their patients without their knowledge," and "Health care organizations often want to know more about your business than they need to know"), using a scale anchored with "strongly disagree" (1) and "strongly agree" (4). Six items were reverse coded and a mean score was computed so that higher scores on this scale would indicate greater levels of medical mistrust. The internal consistency for this scale was acceptable ($\alpha = .71$).

Data Analytic Strategy

We conducted simple (unadjusted) bivariate analyses (chi-square and ANOVA) to describe sample characteristics and assess their association with medical mistrust. To examine associations between medical mistrust and variables outlined in our conceptual model, we used hierarchical regression analyses stratified by income and education, allowing us to compare results across sub-populations reflecting social position. Determinants were entered into the model starting with those we expected to have the least direct impact on medical mistrust and ending with those presumed to have the most direct effect. Accordingly, the determinants reflecting cultural norms and values (traditional male role norms) are entered in Step 1. In Step 2, the determinant reflecting the socioeconomic and political context (racial discrimination) is entered. Health care system access determinants (such as health insurance status and usual source of care) are entered in Step 3. The determinant reflecting the process of health care delivery (patient-centered care) is considered in Step 4. Our psychosocial factor of interest (perceived racism in health care) was entered in Step 5. In each of our models, we adjusted for age, marital status, and recruitment site. We investigated the overall model fit (Adjusted R^2's) and the change in model fit (R^2 change). We also conducted mediation analyses using classic procedures (Baron & Kenny, 1986). Finally, a Sobel Test (Sobel, 1982) was performed to confirm the presence of indirect effects. The **Sobel Test** confirms the presence of mediation by comparing the strength of the indirect effect of the independent variable on the outcome to the null hypotheses that this same effect equals zero (Preacher & Hayes, 2004).

Multiple imputation procedures (Allison, 2000) were used to account for missing data. **Multiple imputation** (MI) is a strategy of filling in missing data (generally when ≤ 5 percent are missing) with values calculated from observed participant responses (see Schafer, 1999). Singularly imputed datasets can overstate the precision of estimates. Thus, values are generated for more than one dataset (typically five). Values from the datasets are pooled and analyzed. MI requires data to be **missing at random** (MAR). Data are said to be MAR when the probability of variables being missing can be predicted from other variables in the dataset. In the current study, ≤ 5 percent of the variables except for income (missing for 8.0 percent), health insurance (missing for 10.4 percent), usual source of care (missing for 6.5 percent), and patient-centered care (missing for 11.0 percent); this confirmed the data were likely to be missing at random.

Results

Characteristics of the study participants are presented in Table 8.1. Participant ages ranged from 18 to 78 ($M = 32$, $SD = 11.10$), and the largest single percentage of men were concentrated in the 18- to 29-year-old age group (48.1 percent). Most participants were unmarried, residents of the South, employed at least part time, insured, and reported having insurance and a usual source of care. Participant incomes and levels of education were equally distributed across the sample.

Bivariate and Correlational Analyses

Bivariate analyses suggested significant differences in most socio-demographic variables by recruitment site. Therefore, recruitment site was included as a control variable in our subsequent multivariate analyses. In correlation analyses (table not shown) we found medical mistrust was positively related to racial discrimination ($r = .20$, $p < .001$) and perceived racism in health care ($r = .51$, $p < .001$) and negatively related to the quality of recent patient–physician interactions ($r = -.14$, $p < .01$). Age was negatively related to racial discrimination ($r = -.17$, $p < .001$) and positively related to the quality of recent patient–physician interactions ($r = .16$, $p < .001$). Traditional male role norms were positively related to racial discrimination ($r = .12$, $p < .01$). Racial discrimination was negatively related to the quality of patient–physician interactions ($r = -.25$, $p < .001$) and positively related to perceived racism in health care ($r = .25$, $p < .001$). Perceived racism in health care was negatively related to the quality of recent patient–physician interactions ($r = .12$, $p < .01$). The patterns of correlations were fairly similar across recruitment site and in the expected direction. Therefore we only display results for the full sample.

Table 8.1. Study Sample Characteristics by Recruitment Site

Characteristic	Total (N = 674)* % (n) or Mean (±SD)		Barbershops (n = 524) % or Mean (±SD)	Academic Institutions/ Events (n =150) % Or Mean (±SD)	p Value
Age continuous (years)	32.00	(±11.10)	33.28 (±10.71)	27.58 (±11.37)	<.001
Age categories					<.001
18–29	(321)	48.1	41.6	70.3	
30–39	(180)	26.9	31.8	10.1	
≥40	(167)	25.0	26.6	19.6	
Education					<.001
≤High school	(214)	32.4	36.3	19.2	
Some college	(247)	37.4	31.6	58.2	
College/graduate/professional degree	(199)	30.2	32.2	22.6	
Marital status					<.001
Married	(175)	26.0	30.4	13.6	
Unmarried	(483)	71.7	69.6	86.4	
Income					<.001
<$20,000	(238)	28.4	32.2	60.6	
$20,000-$39,999	(193)	31.1	35.3	16.1	
≥$40,000	(189)	30.5	32.6	23.4	

(continued)

Table 8.1. (Continued)

Characteristic	Total (N = 386) % (n) or Mean (±SD)		Barbershops (n = 252) % or Mean (±SD)	Academic Institutions/ Events (n = 134) % Or Mean (±SD)	p Value
Employment status					
Employed full or part-time	82.0	(539)	85.6	69.6	
Unemployed	18.0	(118)	14.4	30.4	**<.001**
Health insurance status					
Has health insurance	68.7	(415)	69.3	66.4	
No health insurance	31.3	(189)	30.7	33.6	.526
Usual source of care					
Has a usual source of care	57.6	(363)	59.2	48.2	
No usual source of care	42.4	(267)	40.8	51.8	.120
Geographic region					
North	2.4	(16)	0.0	10.8	
South	6.2	(502)	75.3	16.2	**<.001**
Midwest	74.4	(42)	3.3	72.3	
West	16.8	(113)	21.4	0.7	
Racial discrimination[a]	1.74	(±.05)	1.70 (±1.17)	2.79 (±.69)	.095
Traditional male role norms[a]	4.02	(±.06)	4.06 (±1.14)	3.87 (±1.16)	**.004**
Quality of patient-physician interactions[a]	2.95	(±.04)	2.93 (±1.01)	2.98 (±.90)	.665
Perceived racism in healthcare	2.54	(±.02)	2.54 (±0.43)	2.52 (±.32)	.499
Medical mistrust	2.54	(±.44)	2.51 (±.39)	2.61 (±.31)	**.005**

Note. Some cells may not add up to total N due to missing data.

*Variables with missing data and percentage of missing values age (1.5), education (2.1), marital status (2.4), income (8.0), employment status (2.5), health insurance status (10.4), usual source of care (6.5), racial discrimination (4.2), traditional male role norms (4.7), quality of patient-physician interactions (11.0), perceived racism in healthcare (6.8), medical mistrust (1.3). Comparisons for between-group differences, based on χ2 tests for categorical variables and *F*-tests for continuous variables.

[a]Higher scores indicate more medical mistrust, racial discrimination experiences, traditional male role norms, patient-centered interactions, and perceived racism in health care.

Results from the one-way ANOVAs and planned comparisons (tables not shown) indicated education and income differences in mean scores on some of our study variables. When examining mean differences by education, we found men with a college, graduate, or professional degrees reported lower mean traditional male role norms scores than men in each of the other education groups, F (2, 629) = 6.9, $p < .01$, $\eta^2 = .14$. Men with an HS or less education reported lower mean quality of patient-physician interactions F (2, 588) = 3.4, $p < .05$, $\eta^2 = .11$ and perceived racism in health care F (2, 614) = 7.7, $p < .001$, $\eta^2 = .16$ scores than men with a college, graduate, or professional degree. Our evaluation of income differences revealed that men with incomes of $< \$20,000$ reported higher mean racial discrimination F (2, 597) = 8.7, $p < .001$, $\eta^2 = .17$ and lower traditional male role norms scores F (2, 562) = 6.5, $p < .01$, $\eta^2 = .15$ than men in all of the other income groups. Men with incomes between $\$20,000$ and $\$39,000$ reported higher mean patient-physician interaction quality scores F (2, 591) = 3.9, $p < .05$, $\eta^2 = .11$.

Hierarchical Regression Analyses

Results of the stratified hierarchical regression analysis are presented in Table 8.2 (stratification by education) and Table 8.3 (stratification by income).

The hierarchical multiple regression stratified by education indicated that 36 percent (HS or less), 16 percent (some college), and 46 percent (college, graduate, or professional degree) of the variance was accounted for by all the model determinants. Traditional male role norms (Step 1) did not account for a significant amount of the variance in either education strata. Racial discrimination (Step 2) was positively associated with medical mistrust and accounted for a significant increase in the variance explained across all three education strata (HS or less: $\Delta R^2 = .04$, p = $< .05$; some college $\Delta R^2 = .06$, p $< .01$; college, graduate, or professional degree: $\Delta R^2 = .09$, p = $< .001$).

Health insurance status and usual source of care (Step 3) were not significantly associated with medical mistrust and did not contribute significantly to the overall variance explained in either of the education strata. The quality of recent patient–physician interactions were significantly and negatively associated with medical mistrust for men in the highest education strata. For this group, the inclusion of this variable resulted in a significant increase in the overall variance explained ($\Delta R^2 = .05$, p $< .01$). Perceived racism in health care (Step 5) was positively and significantly associated with medical mistrust across all three education strata. However, the strength of this association varied by stratum, with those in the high school or less stratum ($\beta = 0.62$, p $< .001$) and college or more stratum ($\beta = 0.62$, p $< .001$) demonstrating a stronger effect than the some college

Table 8.2. Summary of Hierarchical Regression Analyses Predicting Medical Mistrust Stratified by Education ($n = 674$)

Variables	Step 1 β (SE)[†]	Step 2 β (SE)[†]	Step 3 β (SE)[†]	Step 4 β (SE)[†]	Step 5 β (SE)[†]
HS or less					
Traditional male role norms	.04(.03)	.02(.03)	.01(.03)	.03(.03)	.03(.02)
Racial discrimination	—	.19(.02)*	.18(.02)*	.17(.02)	.09(.02)
Health insurance status (ref., no insurance)	—	—	−.00(.06)	.01(.06)	−.00(.05)
Usual source of care (ref., no usual source)	—	—	−.14(.06)	−.13(.06)	−.16(.04)*
Quality of patient–physician interactions	—	—	—	−.09(.03)	−.02(.02)
Perceived racism in healthcare	—	—	—	—	.62(.06)***
Adjusted R²=	−.00	.03	.03	.03	.41***
ΔR²=	—	.04*	.02	.01	.36***
Some college					
Traditional male role norms	.05(.03)	.02(.03)	.02(.03)	.01(.03)	−.03(.03)
Racial discrimination	—	.26(.03)**	.23(.03)**	.22(.03)*	.11(.03)
Health insurance status (ref., no insurance)	—	—	−.12(.07)	−.11(.07)	−.10(.06)
Usual source of care (ref., no usual source)	—	—	−.06(.07)	−.05(.07)	−.08(.07)
Quality of patient–physician interactions	—	—	—	−.06(.04)	−.03(.03)
Perceived racism in healthcare	—	—	—	—	.33(.07)***
Adjusted R²=	.00	.06*	.07*	.06*	.16***
ΔR²=	—	.06**	.02	.00	.10***
College, graduate, or professional degree					
Traditional male role norms	.15(.03)	.12(.03)	.11(.03)	.13(.03)	.09(.02)
Racial discrimination	—	.31(.03)***	.31(.03)***	.25(.03)**	.04(.03)
Health insurance status (ref., no insurance)	—	—	.01(.12)	.06(.12)	.03(.09)
Usual source of care (ref., no usual source)	—	—	−.02(.09)	.03(.09)	−.03(.07)
Quality of patient–physician interactions	—	—	—	−.24(.04)**	−.16(.03)
Perceived Racism in Healthcare	—	—	—	—	.62(.06)***
Adjusted R²=	.01	.09**	.08*	.12**	.46***
ΔR²=	—	.09***	.00	.05**	.32***

Note: *p < .05. **p < .01. **p < .001.

[†]Represents standardized regression coefficient estimates after adjusting for age, marital status, and recruitment site.

Table 8.3. Summary of Hierarchical Regression Analyses Predicting Medical Mistrust Stratified by Income ($n = 674$)

Variables	Step 1 β (SE)[†]	Step 2 β (SE)[†]	Step 3 β (SE)[†]	Step 4 β (SE)[†]	Step 5 β (SE)[†]
Less than $20,000					
Traditional male role norms	.16 (.02)*	.13 (.03)	.12 (.03)	.12 (.03)	.10 (.03)
Racial discrimination	—	.17 (.02)*	.15 (.02)	.15 (.02)	.10 (.02)
Health insurance status (ref., no insurance)	—	—	−.14 (.05)	−.14 (.05)	−.14 (.05)
Usual source of care (ref., no usual source)	—	—	−.05 (.05)	−.05 (.06)	−.07 (.05)
Quality of patient–physician interactions	—	—	—	−.00 (.03)	.01 (.03)
Adjusted R²=	.04*	.06**	.07**	.07*	.10**
ΔR²=		.03*	.02	.00	.04*
$20,000–39,000					
Traditional male role norms	.12 (.03)	.10 (.03)	.09 (.03)	.12 (.03)	.04 (.02)
Racial discrimination	—	.45 (.03)***	.44 (.03)***	.41 (.03)***	.22 (.02)**
Health insurance status (ref., no insurance)	—	—	−.05 (.07)	−.03 (.07)	−.02 (.06)
Usual source of care (ref., no usual source)	—	—	−.06 (.07)	−.01 (.07)	−.06 (.06)
Patient-centered care	—	—	—	−.14 (.04)	−.09 (.03)
Perceived racism in healthcare	—	—	—	—	.58 (.05)***
Adjusted R²=	−.00	.19***	.19***	.19***	.50***
ΔR²=		.20***	.01	.01	.29***
$40,000+					
Traditional male role norms	−.05 (.04)	−.05 (.04)	−.05 (.04)	−.04 (.03)	.03 (.03)
Racial discrimination	—	.28 (.04)**	.25 (.04)**	.22 (.04)	−.07 (.03)
Health insurance status (ref., no insurance)	—	—	.10 (.15)	.12 (.15)	.07 (.12)
Usual source of care (ref., no usual source)	—	—	−.18 (.10)	−.16 (.10)	−.15 (.08)
Quality of patient–physician interactions	—	—	—	−.22 (.04)*	−.04 (.03)
Perceived racism in healthcare	—	—	—	—	.69 (.07)***
Adjusted R²=	−.01	.06*	.07*	.12**	.48***
ΔR²=		.08**	.02	.05*	.34***

Note: *p < .05, **p < .01, ***p < .001.
[†]Represents standardized regression coefficient estimates after adjusting for age, marital status, and recruitment site.

stratum ($\beta = 0.33$, p < .001). The inclusion of this variable resulted in a significant increase in the variance explained across all three education strata (HS or less: $\Delta R^2 = .36$, p = < .001; some college $\Delta R^2 = .10$, p < .001; college, graduate, or professional degree: $\Delta R^2 = .32$, p = < .001).

Analyses stratified by income (Table 8.3) yielded somewhat similar results. Thus, we only summarize the findings here. Traditional male role norms (Step 1) were positively associated with medical mistrust only for men reporting incomes of less than $20,000. Racial discrimination (Step 2) was consistently associated with medical mistrust and contributed to a significant increase in the variance across all income strata. Neither health insurance nor usual source of care (Step 3) was significantly associated with medical mistrust. The quality of patient–physician interactions (Step 4) was negatively associated with medical mistrust among men in the highest income strata, increasing the overall variance explained for that group. Perceived racism in health care was also positively associated with medical mistrust across all income strata (Step 5). However, unlike for education, the strength of the association between perceived racism in health care and medical mistrust increased progressively across income strata, with those earning less than $20,000 exhibiting the weakest association ($\beta = 0.20$, p < .05), followed by those earning between $20,000 and $39,000 ($\beta = 0.50$, p < .001), and those earning $40,000 or more demonstrating the strongest association ($\beta = 0.69$, p < .001). The inclusion of perceived racism in health care resulted in the most significant increase in the overall variance in medical mistrust across all income strata.

Mediation Analyses

In the series of regression analyses conducted to evaluate mediation, we controlled for age, marital status, recruitment site, health insurance, usual source of care, and the quality of patient–physician interactions. First, medical mistrust was regressed on discrimination experiences. Second, perceived racism in health care was regressed on discrimination experiences. A final regression analysis was conducted in which medical mistrust was regressed on perceived racism in health care and discrimination. In this final regression analysis, the introduction of perceived racism in health care resulted in a relative decrease in the beta coefficient associated with discrimination experiences. The results from these regression analyses satisfied the conditions of mediation outlined by Baron and Kenney (1986) and indicate that perceived racism in health care serves as a mediator between racial discrimination and medical mistrust. However, this mediated relationship was only present for men in the highest and lowest income strata (Figure 8.2) and men in the some college and college degree or more strata (Figure 8.3).

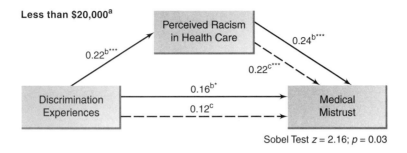

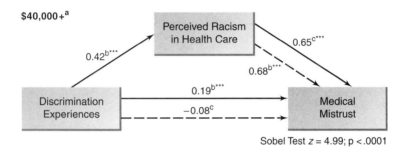

Figure 8.2. Perceived Racism in Health Care as a Mediator of the Racial Discrimination–Medical Mistrust Relationship (by Income)

[a]Note: *p < .05; **[c]p < .01; ***p< .001.

Mediation analyses controlled for participant age, marital status, recruitment site, health insurance status, usual source of care, and quality of patient-physician interactions.

[b]Unmediated standardized beta coefficients

[c]Mediated standardized beta coefficients

Discussion

In this cross-sectional study of African-American men, we proposed and tested a conceptual model of medical mistrust. Our conceptual model suggested that, along with experiences of everyday discrimination, African-American men's socioeconomic resources would be part of the broader social context in which psychological processes leading to medical mistrust could best be understood. Specifically, we imagined that the pathways leading from racial discrimination to medical mistrust might hold different valence in different socioeconomic strata. The results we obtained confirmed that socioeconomic status does affect the relationships we have explored, but in ways that vary by socioeconomic indicator. However, the pattern of variation across socioeconomic groups and socioeconomic indicators is rather perplexing.

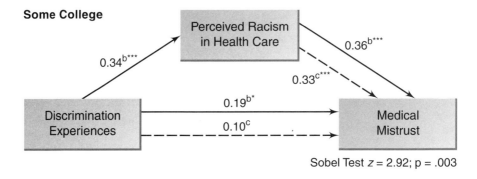

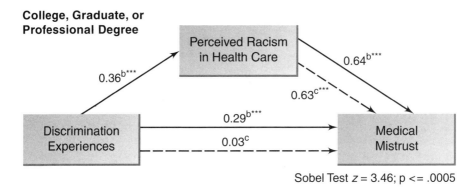

Figure 8.3. Perceived Racism in Health Care as a Mediator of the Racial Discrimination–Medical Mistrust Relationship (By Education)

[a]Note: *p < .05; **[c]p < .01; ***p< .001. Mediation analyses controlled for participant age, marital status, recruitment site, health insurance status, usual source of care, and quality of patient–physician interactions.

[b]Unmediated standardized beta coefficients

[c]Mediated standardized beta coefficients

We did not find a consistent or sustained effect for traditional male role norms. In fact, traditional male role norms were only significantly associated with more medical mistrust among men in the lowest income strata, who also had the lowest mean scores on this measure. This effect disappeared when racial discrimination was entered in the model, suggesting that this factor may mediate the association between traditional male role norms and medical mistrust. We were limited by the chapter focus from formally exploring this possibility. Nonetheless, we speculate that this initial effect was produced because men with less income may feel more bound by cultural prescriptions for masculinity. The relatively lower social position occupied by this group may increase their desire to conform to traditional male role norms because doing so may allow them to diminish their sense of vulnerability. In other words, withholding trust among this group may be viewed as a symbolic attempt to recoup power, autonomy, and control. Our results indicate that, in every income stratum, everyday experiences of racial discrimination are significantly associated with medical mistrust, and that this relationship is mediated by perceived discrimination in the health care system. These findings are consistent with previous research (Hammond, 2010; LaVeist et al., 2000). However, our study further implies that there is a socioeconomic gradient in the strength of this relationship, such that higher income levels demonstrated a stronger association between perceived racism in health care and medical mistrust.

Previous literature on the interdependencies between these factors is scant, but there seem to be two particularly compelling possible explanations: (1) Our results suggest that, as income levels rise, the sense of expectations, or entitlement, regarding fair treatment increase. (2) Due to differences in the setting in which people from different socioeconomic strata receive health care (for example, community health clinics versus major medical centers), the *relative differential* between African-American men and their health care providers increases as income level increases.

However, analyses stratified for education were not consistent with those stratified for income. That is, a gradient effect was not observed; instead a U-shape relationship emerged, such that those with high school diplomas or less and those with college degrees or more demonstrated a stronger association between perceived racism in health care and medical mistrust than those with some college, in whom the effect size was halved. Again, there is a dearth of prior literature to guide interpretation; however, it is clear that our results paint a complex picture. Indeed there may be different reasons for the association between perceived racism in health care and medical mistrust within each educational stratum. In the highest stratum, the association may be due to the "relative differential" argument presented earlier. In the lowest stratum, the association may be due to overall poor quality of health care, including clinical facilities, interactions with health care providers, and the like. The middle educational stratum may be somewhat buffered either because (due to younger age) they have fewer or less involved interactions with the health care system, or because they are more likely to interact with smaller student health facilities, in which the relative differential in status between African-American men and their health care providers is smaller.

We also hypothesized that perceived racism in health care would mediate the relationship between racial discrimination and medical mistrust. Affirming propositions made by others about the carryover effects of racial discrimination (Smedley et al., 2003), our findings imply that everyday racial discrimination experiences elicit perceptions of discrimination in health care that, in turn, lead African-American men to have more medical mistrust. Extending previous research (Hammond, 2010), we also found a stronger mediation effect for men at the highest income and education strata. Preliminary analyses revealed that men with more education had higher perceived racism in health care scores. Although it is difficult to confirm with our data, we believe that this pathway was more significantly mediated among African-American men with more years of education because of increased expectations for fair treatment within the health care system.

Study Limitations and Strengths

Our cross-sectional study design limits us from making causal inferences. Longitudinal studies that assess changes in social determinants and medical mistrust over time would remedy this issue. Our recruitment strategy did not allow us draw a random sample of the population. Hence, our results may not be generalizable to other African-American men. Reporting biases may have led some African-American men to overestimate reports of racial discrimination. However, given the tendency for minimization of racial discrimination by minority group members (Ruggiero & Taylor, 1997), we believe this bias to be less probable. Similar biases may have led participants to negatively assess the quality of their interactions with physicians. Yet, data suggest that African Americans are more likely to receive lower quality health care (Smedley et al., 2003). Thus, we believe these assessments to accurately reflect the processes governing care delivery among our participants.

Despite these limitations, this chapter advances our current understanding by moving the discourse beyond purely trait-based conceptualizations of medical mistrust towards the consideration of how medical mistrust among African-American men might be patterned by broader social conditions. To our knowledge, this study represents only the second investigation of factors associated with medical mistrust among African-American men. With one exception (Hammond, 2010), studies have not simultaneously considered the role played by traditional male role norms and racial discrimination experiences in African-American men's mistrust of health care organizations. This study offers a preliminary look at these relationships. The conceptual model presented in the current chapter offers insights about the factors associated with African-American men's medical mistrust, which might explain their higher levels of disengagement from health care organizations. These insights might be applied to the development of interventions for this population in health care and community settings.

Policy Implications

Our study suggests several areas of potential policy solutions. However, we emphasize the need for additional policy-related inquiry due to the relative novelty of the relationships we explored. At the most fundamental level, our findings indicate that improving the socioeconomic circumstances of African-American males is a key avenue for reducing experiences of racial discrimination and medical mistrust, because it may induce increased expectations of fair treatment, and because this strategy can reduce the socioeconomic differential between African-American men and their care providers. From this it follows that such policies should be mindful not only of improving the absolute socioeconomic circumstances of African-American men, but also of their *relative* position in society. Thus, policies that lift socioeconomic resources by small increments (for example, a policy that moves an individual from below the poverty line to just above the poverty line) are likely to be insufficient. Rather, policies should consider the socioeconomic distribution of society as a whole, and aim to narrow, for example, the societal distribution of income. This is also intimately tied to providing greater employment opportunities to African-American males. Finally, policies should be considered to improve the outreach of the health care system to African-American males, and to improve their experience with health care professionals. In part, systematic ways to increase the supply of African-American physicians are likely to be very effective. However, physicians of all races must be sensitized and given guidance regarding the potential for medical mistrust as a critical part of caring for African-American males.

Summary

In this chapter, we learned that in every socioeconomic stratum, experiences of everyday racial discrimination serve as a fundamental cause of medical mistrust, and that this association is mediated by perceived racism in health care. However, the strength of the mediation varies by position in the socioeconomic hierarchy, and by indicator of socioeconomic status. Our study establishes the need for further research to understand the mechanisms through which socioeconomic resources condition perceptions of racism in health care and medical mistrust. Moreover, the noted discrepancies in results between income and education also deserve further examination. There is a well-known racial difference in income returns to education (U.S. Census Bureau, 2004), which provides a basis for making sense of divergent results by these two indicators of socioeconomic resources. However, this is only a starting point and more direct investigation regarding implications of income and education for medical mistrust (and its antecedents) is necessary in order to fully comprehend the social and psychological determination of medical mistrust.

Key Terms

everyday racism	perceived racism in health care
medical mistrust	racial discrimination
mistrust	traditional male role norms

Discussion Questions

1. Everyday racial discrimination experiences appeared to serve as a potential catalyst for medical mistrust. How can this relationship be further explained?

2. In this chapter, we observed a gradient effect for income and a U-shaped pattern for education. Why did these differential patterns emerge?

3. What other strategies can public health professionals and policy makers employ to address social determinants of medical mistrust?

References

Agency for Healthcare Research and Quality. (2000). *Your health and health opinions, a self administered supplement to the MEPS*. Rockville, MD: Agency for Healthcare Research and Quality.

Allison, P. D. (2000). Multiple imputation for missing data: A cautionary tale. *Sociology Methods Research*, *28*(3), 301–309.

Altice, F. L., Mostashari, F., & Friedland, G. H. (2001). Trust and the acceptance of and adherence to antiretroviral therapy. *Journal of Acquired Immune Deficiency Syndromes*, *28*(1), 47.

Arias, E. (2007). United States life tables, 2004. *National Vital Statistics Report*, *56*(9), 1–39.

Armstrong, K., McMurphy, S., Dean, L., Micco, E., Putt, M., Halbert, C., . . . Shea, J. (2008). Differences in the patterns of health care system distrust between blacks and whites. *Journal of General Internal Medicine*, *23*(6), 827–833.

Armstrong, K., Ravenell, K. L., McMurphy, S., & Putt, M. (2007). Racial/ethnic differences in physician distrust in the United States. *American Journal of Public Health*, *97*(7), 1283–1289.

Banks, K. H., Singleton, J. L., & Kohn-Wood, L. P. (2008). The influence of hope on the relationship between racial discrimination and depressive symptoms. *Journal of Multicultural Counseling and Development*, *36*(4), 231–244.

Baron, R., & Kenny, D. (1986). The moderator-mediator variable distinction in social psychological research: Conceptual, strategic, and statistical considerations. *Journal of Personality and Social Psychology*, *51*(6), 1173–1182.

Berkman, L. F. (2009). Social epidemiology: Social determinants of health in the United States: Are we losing ground? *Annual Review of Public Health*, *30*(1), 27–41.

Boon, S., & Holmes, J. (1991). The dynamics of interpersonal trust: Resolving uncertainty in the face of risk. In R. A. Hinde & J. Groebel (Eds.), *Cooperation and prosocial behaviour* (pp. 190–211). New York, NY: Cambridge University Press.

Brandon, D., Isaac, L., & LaVeist, T. (2005). The legacy of Tuskegee and trust in medical care: Is Tuskegee responsible for race differences in mistrust of medical care? *Journal of the National Medical Association*, *97*(7), 951.

Bromiley, P., & Cummings, L. (1995). Transactions costs in organizations with trust. In R. Bies, R. Lewicki, & B. Sheppard (Eds.), *Research on negotiation in organizations* (Vol. 5, pp. 219–250). Greenwich, CT: JAI.

Cherry, D. K., Woodwell, D. A., & Rechtsteiner, E. A. (2007). National Ambulatory Medical Care Survey: 2005 summary. *Advance Data*, *2007*(387), 1–39.

Commission of Social Determinants of Health. (2008). *Closing the gap in a generation: Health equity through action on the social determinants of health*. Final report of the Commission on Social Determinants of Health. Geneva, Switzerland: World Health Organization.

Connell, R. (1995). *Masculinities*. Berkeley: University of California Press.

Doescher, M. P., Saver, B. G., Franks, P., & Fiscella, K. (2000). Racial and ethnic disparities in perceptions of physician style and trust. *Archives of Family Medicine*, *9*(10), 1156–1163.

Essed, P. (1991). *Understanding everyday racism: An interdisciplinary theory*. Newbury Park, CA: Sage.

Fiscella, K., Meldrum, S., Franks, P., Shields, C., Duberstein, P., McDaniel, S., . . . Epstein, R. M. (2004). Patient trust: Is it related to patient-centered behavior of primary care physicians? *Medical Care*, *42*(11), 1049–1055.

Gamble, V. (1997). Under the shadow of Tuskegee: African Americans and health care. *American Journal of Public Health*, *87*(11), 1773–1778.

Gee, G. C. (2008). A multilevel analysis of the relationship between institutional and individual racial discrimination and health status. *American Journal of Public Health*, 98(Suppl. 1), S48–S56.

Greene, N. (1995). Development of the perceptions of racism scale. *Journal of Nursing Scholarship*, *27*, 141–146.

Halbert, C. H., Armstrong, K., Gandy, O. H., Jr., & Shaker, L. (2006). Racial differences in trust in health care providers. *Archives of Internal Medicine*, *166*(8), 896–901.

Hammond, W. P. (2010). Psychosocial correlates of medical mistrust among African American men. *American Journal of Community Psychology*, *45*(1–2), 87–106.

Hammond, W. P., Matthews, D., & Corbie-Smith, G. (2010). Psychosocial factors associated with routine health examination scheduling and receipt among African American men. *Journal of the National Medical Association*, *102*(4), 276–289.

Hammond, W. P., & Mattis, J. S. (2005). Being a man about it: Manhood meaning among African American men. *Psychology of Men & Masculinity*, *6*(2), 114–126.

Harrell, S. (2000). A multidimensional conceptualization of racism-related stress: Implications for the well-being of people of color. *American Journal of Orthopsychiatry, 70*(1), 42–57.

Hart, A., & Bowen, D. J. (2004). The feasibility of partnering with African-American barbershops to provide prostate cancer education. *Ethnicity and Disease, 14*(2), 269–273.

Hertz, R. P., Unger, A. N., Cornell, J. A., & Saunders, E. (2005). Racial disparities in hypertension prevalence, awareness, and management. *Archives of Internal Medicine, 165*(18), 2098–2104.

Hess, P. L., Reingold, J. S., Jones, J., Fellman, M. A., Knowles, P., Ravenell, J. E., . . . Victor, R. G. (2007). Barbershops as hypertension detection, referral, and follow-up centers for black men. *Hypertension, 49*(5), 1040–1046.

Institute of Medicine (2001). *Crossing the quality chasm: A new health system for the 21st century.* Washington, DC: National Academies Press.

Johnson, R., Roter, D., Powe, N., & Cooper, L. (2004). Patient race/ethnicity and quality of patient-physician communication during medical visits. *American Journal of Public Health, 94*(12), 2084–2090.

Kramer, R. (1999). Trust and distrust in organizations: Emerging perspectives, enduring questions. *Annual Review of Psychology, 50*(1), 569–598.

LaVeist, T. A., Isaac, L. A., & Williams, K. P. (2009). Mistrust of health care organizations is associated with underutilization of health services. *Health Services Research, 44*(6), 2093–2105.

LaVeist, T. A., Nickerson, K., & Bowie, J. (2000). Attitudes about racism, medical mistrust, and satisfaction with care among African American and white cardiac patients. *Medical Care Research and Review, 57*(2), 146–161.

Levant, R. F., Hirsch, L. S., Celentano, E., & Cozz, T. M. (1992). The male role: An investigation of contemporary norms. *Journal of Mental Health Counseling, 14*(3), 325–337.

Levant, R. F., Smalley, K., Aupont, M., House, A., Richmond, K., & Noronha, D. (2007). Initial validation of the male role norms inventory-revised (MRNI-R). *Journal of Men's Studies, 15*(1), 83–100.

Lewis, J., & Weigert, A. (1985). Trust as a social reality. *Social forces, 63*(4), 967–985.

Mansfield, A., Addis, M., & Courtenay, W. (2005). Measurement of men's help seeking: Development and evaluation of the barriers to help seeking scale. *Psychology of Men & Masculinity, 6*, 95–108.

National Research Council. (Ed.). (2004). *Measuring racial discrimination. Panel on methods for assessing discrimination.* Washington, DC: National Academies Press.

Neighbors, H., & Howard, C. (1987). Sex differences in professional help seeking among adult black Americans. *American Journal of Community Psychology, 15*(4), 403–417.

Ojeda, L., Rosales, R. O., & Good, G. E. (2008). Socioeconomic status and cultural predictors of male role attitudes among Mexican American men: Son mas machos? *Psychology of Men & Masculinity, 9*(3), 133–138.

Omodei, M., & McLennan, J. (2000). Conceptualizing and measuring global interpersonal mistrust-trust. *Journal of Social Psychology, 140*(3), 279–294.

Preacher, K. J., & Hayes, A. F. (2004). SPSS and SAS procedures for estimating indirect effects in simple mediation models. *Behavior Research Methods, Instruments, and Computers*, 36(4), 717–731.

Roter, D., & Hall, J. (1992). *Doctors talking with patients, patients talking with doctors: Improving communication in medical visits*. Westport, CT: Auburn House.

Rotter, J. (1971). Generalized expectancies for interpersonal trust. *American Psychologist*, 26(5), 443–452.

Ruggiero, K., & Taylor, D. (1997). Why minority group members perceive or do not perceive the discrimination that confronts them: The role of self-esteem and perceived control. *Journal of Personality and Social Psychology*, 72, 373–389.

Schafer, J. L. (1999). Multiple imputation: A primer. *Statistical Methods in Medical Research*, 8, 3–15.

Sellers, R. M., & Shelton, J. N. (2003). The role of racial identity in perceived racial discrimination. *Journal of Personality and Social Psychology*, 84(5), 1079–1092.

Smedley, B., Stith, A., & Nelson, A. (Eds.). (2003). *Unequal treatment: Confronting racial and ethnic disparities in health care*. Washington, DC: National Academy of Science

Sobel, M. (1982). Asymptotic confidence intervals for indirect effects in structural equation models. In S. Lienhart (Ed.), *Sociological Methodology* (Vol. 13, pp. 290–312). San Francisco, CA: Jossey-Bass.

Solar, O., & Irwin, A. (2007). A conceptual framework for action on the social determinants of health. *Discussion paper for the Commission on Social Determinants of Health*. Geneva, Switzerland: World Health Organization.

Thom, T., Haase, N., Rosamond, W., Howard, V. J., Rumsfeld, J., Manolio, T., . . . American Heart Association Statistics Committee and Stroke Statistics Subcommittee. (2006). Heart disease and stroke statistics—2006 update: A report from the American Heart Association Statistics Committee and Stroke Statistics Subcommittee. *Circulation*, 113(6), e85–151.

Tyler, T., & Kramer, R. (1996). Whither trust. In R. Kramer & T. Tyler (Eds.), *Trust in organizations: Frontiers of theory and research* (pp. 1–15). Thousand Oaks, CA: Sage.

U.S. Census Bureau. (2004). *Monthly income by education level and race*. Retrieved from http://www.census.gov/population/socdemo/education/sipp2001/tab2B.xls

Williams, D. R., Neighbors, H. W., & Jackson, J. S. (2003). Racial/ethnic discrimination and health: Findings from community studies. *American Journal of Public Health*, 93(2), 200–208.

Author Note

Wizdom Powell Hammond, Department of Health Behavior and Health Education, The University of North Carolina at Chapel Hill Gillings School of Global Public Health.

Arjumand Siddiqi, Dalla Lana School of Public Health, University of Toronto.

Correspondence should be sent to Wizdom Powell Hammond, Department of Health Behavior and Health Education, University of North Carolina, 334B Rosenau Hall, CB #7440, Chapel Hill, NC 27599. Email: wizdom.powell@unc.edu. (Tel): 919–962–9802. (Fax): 919–966–2921.

This research was supported by a Student Award Program award to the first author from the Blue Cross and Blue Shield of Michigan Foundation (Grant # 657.SAP), The Robert Wood Johnson Foundation Health & Society Scholars Program, and the University of North Carolina Cancer Research Fund. Additional research and salary support during the preparation of this manuscript was provided to the first author from the National Center for Minority Health and Health Disparities (Award # 1L60MD002605–01), and National Cancer Institute (Grant # 3U01CA114629–04S2).

Chapter 9

Beyond Gay, Bisexual, or DL

Structural Determinants of HIV Sexual Risk among Black Men in the United States

David J. Malebranche
Lisa Bowleg

Learning Objectives

- Understand the current HIV epidemiology among U.S. black men.
- Realize the limitations of sexuality orientation labels in HIV research.
- Identify common social contextual factors influencing HIV risk.
- Highlight future directions for HIV prevention and research targeting black men.

> Being a Black man is a hard struggle. Not just being gay, being straight—being a general Black man is an everyday struggle. I don't care how you put it, White America either wants me in a cell or in a grave.
>
> (Adrian, 21)

• • •

Since the beginning of the HIV and **AIDS (Acquired Immune Deficiency Syndrome)** epidemic in the United States in the early 1980s, public health and policy approaches to prevention efforts have been intricately interwoven with the Gay Civil Rights movement. This history makes perfect sense given the disproportionate burden borne by white gay men as the first wave of HIV/AIDS deaths hit major U.S. metropolitan areas such as New York and San Francisco. The early reaction from the white gay community successfully launched social marketing initiatives that coupled HIV education efforts with encouraging pride in sexual orientation, coming out, and identifying as "gay." The gay community was also instrumental in organizing sit-ins and marches to bring attention to political apathy and discriminatory public policies such as expensive markups on HIV/AIDS medications. These initiatives posited combating HIV/AIDS not only as a moral obligation but more importantly, as an act of social justice. By the mid-1990s, however, the HIV/AIDS epidemic had shifted from one that predominantly affected white gay men to one that exacted a disproportionate toll on black communities, particularly black gay and bisexual men. U.S. public health officials and media outlets alike, however, have been reluctant to fully acknowledge the changing winds of this stark demographic reality by expanding the focus of HIV prevention efforts to anything beyond those emphasizing sexual orientation categories. This intellectual and social inertia threatens to define us in the history books as the generation that stood idly by, focusing exclusively and myopically on sexual identity politics, while a preventable disease took a stranglehold on the collective neck of the black community in this country.

In a departure from the convention of focusing on black men's HIV risk solely through the prism of sexual orientation, our goal in this chapter is to broaden understanding about HIV/AIDS in black communities by exploring the larger structural context of black men's lives (regardless of sexual orientation) and its implications for HIV risk and prevention. We focus on presenting qualitative studies with black men of diverse sexualities, in an effort to allow their voices to be heard beyond the grim statistics, while also demonstrating the similar structural contexts that influence their lived experiences. To help readers understand how the **HIV (Human Immunodeficiency Virus)** epidemic has disproportionately impacted all black men in the United States, this chapter begins by reviewing the current HIV epidemiology and literature demonstrating the inconclusive role that **sexual orientation** labels and identities have in predicting risky sexual behavior in this population. We then present both quantitative and qualitative research highlighting the important yet overlooked role of larger social and structural determinants on the sexual behavior of black men. Finally, the chapter concludes by identifying future directions in social and HIV prevention research and interventions targeting black men.

Sexual Orientation over Structure: A Critical Mistake

We use the term *black men* to refer to men of African descent regardless of nationality. Thus, this term encompasses African-American men, Africans, Caribbean, and black Latino men. When it comes to general public and media conversations about black men and HIV/AIDS in the United States, terms such as *down low, gay,* **men who have sex with men** **(MSM),** and *closeted* are used so ubiquitously and carelessly that the disparate impact of the disease among black men regardless of sexual orientation is greatly obscured (Denizet-Lewis, 2003; King, 2004; Wright, 2001). By focusing exclusively on sexual orientation label categories at the expense of acknowledging larger **structural factors** that may better explain HIV risk in black communities, however, many HIV prevention theorists and researchers have also fallen into the same cognitive trap of compartmentalizing the HIV/AIDS epidemic as a "gay" disease (Galatzer-Levy & Cohler, 2002; Grov, Bimbi, Nanin, & Parsons, 2006).

So pervasive is the perspective that black MSM are the sexual vectors of HIV transmission in black communities that theory and research on black heterosexual men pales in comparison to the vast literature base of theory and research on black MSM. Although the disproportionate rates of HIV/AIDS among black MSM in the United States more than justify the abundant theory and research dedicated to this subpopulation, we decry the often sensationalistic and obsessive preoccupation with black male same-sex behavior that characterizes so much of the media and public health discourse on HIV/AIDS in black communities. The consequences of this misplaced focus are dire. At the theoretical and empirical level, it means that attempts to understand the broader structural contexts of black men's lives and implications for HIV risk are undermined by the "blame game" of HIV transmission culpability. This game segregates the black community into the "HIV guilty" (e.g. MSM, sex workers, IV drug users) and the "HIV innocent" (e.g., heterosexual women), and does nothing to unify the black community at-large against this disease. Additionally, at the applied level, black MSM and bisexual men are often portrayed as mere vectors of HIV transmission, but black heterosexual men are lured into a false sense of security about their own risk behaviors. Consequently, the epidemic rolls on through black communities unabated and incompletely addressed by public health officials.

The stark reality is that black men in the United States, regardless of the gender of their sexual partners, bear the disproportionate burden of HIV/AIDS compared with men of other races and ethnicities. Black men represent just 13 percent of the U.S. male population, but have rates of HIV/AIDS (cases per 100,000) that are more than seven times the rates of white men, and twice that of Latino men (Centers for Disease Control and Prevention [CDC], 2009). The primary exposure categories for black men include: MSM (48 percent), "high-risk" heterosexual contact (24 percent); and injection drug use (21 percent) (CDC, 2009). Rates of HIV in prisons are five times that of the general population, and black men constitute up to three-quarters of many prison populations (CDC, 2006). The fact that rates of HIV/AIDS among both black MSM and heterosexual men exceed that of men from other racial and ethnic groups suggests that factors other than sexual orientation may better explain risk in this population.

Structural factors include "physical, social, cultural, organizational, community, economic, legal and policy forces that can influence individual health behaviors" (Sumartojo, 2000; Sumartojo, Doll, Holtgrave, Gayle, & Merson, 2000). Indeed, it is these structural factors that can define and shape risk environments (e.g., social situations, structures, and places) that influence sexual HIV protective or risk behavior, instead of a traditional conception that individual cognitive decision making is the sole driver of risk behaviors (Rhodes, Singer, Bourgois, Friedman, & Strathdee, 2005). Risk environments may include, but are not limited to, physical spaces, peer norms, cultural beliefs, federal/regional laws and policies, as well as discrimination or inequality based on race, gender, or sexual orientation. Although the international HIV prevention community, particularly in sub-Saharan Africa, has embraced the idea of structural factors influencing sexual risk or protective behavior among sexually active black men (Vonarx & De Koninck, 2003; International HIV/AIDS Alliance, 2003; Vonarx & De Koninck, 2003), much of the U.S. public health approach appears to still be firmly rooted in a myopic focus on sexual identification as the primary aspect of HIV risk among black men. In fact, even when developing behavioral HIV prevention initiatives for heterosexual black Americans, the emphasis is squarely on heterosexual women and individual behavioral-level interventions, at the expense of acknowledging the role of black men other than MSM in this epidemic (Darbes, Crepaz, Lyles, Kennedy, & Rutherford, 2008). The manner in which the HIV/AIDS epidemic has evolved over the past three decades begs for a paradigm shift that prioritizes examining the role all sexually active black men play in transmission dynamics.

Gay, Heterosexual, and Bisexual: Labels and Limitations

HIV prevention research with black men often utilizes risk categories based on the self-described sexual identities (e.g., gay, heterosexual, bisexual). The terms *sexual identity* and *sexual orientation* are often used interchangeably, but orientation traditionally refers to the attraction of someone to a certain gender (e.g., homosexual, heterosexual, bisexual), while identity refers to how one identifies his or her own sexuality, which may or may not relate to his or her orientation (Laumann, Gagnon, Michael, & Michaels, 1994). In the 1990s, recognizing the limited utility of a sexual identification approach, CDC officials developed the "men who have sex with men (MSM)" label to account for men who engaged in same-sex behavior but did not identify as gay or bisexual (Young & Meyer, 2004). Although the move signaled a pragmatic and linguistically accurate approach, relying solely on the MSM designation fails to adequately explain the higher rates of HIV among sexually active black men.

Reviews exploring the potential factors driving the racial disparity among black MSM have noted that: (1) rates of **unprotected anal intercourse (UAI)** among black MSM are comparable to those of white and Latino MSM; (2) adopting the sexual identification label of *gay* does not increase condom use; and (3) high co-prevalence of **sexually transmitted infections (STI)** and late HIV testing practices partially contribute to higher HIV rates (Millett, Flores, Peterson, & Bakeman, 2007; Millett, Peterson, Wolitski, & Stall, 2006). However, these facts still do not explain what structural forces may be influencing some if not all of these behaviors. Moreover, neither disclosure of same-sex behavior nor discordance between sexual identification labels and sexual behavior among black MSM predict higher rates of UAI with male sexual partners (CDC, 2003; Essien, Meshack, Peters, Ogungbade & Osemene, 2005; Millett, Malebranche, Mason, & Spikes, 2005; Wohl et al., 2002). These findings highlight that while many studies have attempted to explain the relatively higher rates among black MSM compared with MSM of other ethnicities, variables highlighting individual risk behaviors, same-sex disclosure, and sexual identity labels provide an incomplete picture of understanding the factors driving this racial disparity.

In contrast to the recent increase in HIV prevention research addressing black MSM, studies targeting black heterosexual men in the United States are significantly fewer, and often focus solely on theoretical and "deficit-model" conceptual frameworks proposing how incarceration, low SES, substance abuse, STI prevalence and "hyper-masculinity" influence unsafe sexual behavior (Bogart & Thorburn, 2005; Crosby, Graham, Yarber, & Sanders, 2004; Essien et al., 2005; Payn, Tanfer, Billy, & Grady, 1997; Wang, Collins, Kohler, DiClemente, & Wingood, 2000: Wolfe, 2003). Moreover, unlike multicity studies examining quantitative predictors of risk among black MSM in major metropolitan areas, such as the Young Men's Study (YMS), similar studies addressing sexual risk among heterosexual black men are lacking (Valleroy et al., 2000). In short, HIV research with black MSM has abundant quantitative assessments of predictors of risk, but lacks explorations of theory and structural context, while studies on black heterosexual men rely heavily on theory, but pay little attention to either quantitative assessments of risk predictors or richer explorations of structural contexts.

Structural Considerations of HIV Sexual Risk among Black Men

Epidemiological studies demonstrate the relationship between low socioeconomic status (SES) and higher HIV/AIDS rates (Hu, Frey, & Costa, 1994; Simon, Hu, Diaz, & Kerndt, 1995; Zierler et al., 2000). A study with black heterosexual men and MSM found that low SES predicted higher sexual risk behavior (Myers, Javanbakht, Martinez, & Obediah, 2003), while SES problems associated with poverty, including limited access to high-quality health care, housing, and HIV prevention education, may directly or indirectly increase sexual HIV risk behavior (CDC, 2009). Some have suggested that black men of lower SES who fail to meet the economic and social requirements for "traditional" masculinity develop a "fragmented masculinity" that may encourage behaviors such as sex with multiple partners and attempts to father children to affirm their manhood (Whitehead, 1997).

We do know that samples of HIV-positive adults in the Southeast, the current U.S. epicenter of the epidemic, are predominantly male, black, and may be exposed through concurrent sexual partnerships with multiple partners and inconsistent condom use practices, likely influenced by larger structural forces of racism, poverty, and income inequality (Adimora et al., 2006; Lansky, Fleming, Byers, Koran, & Wortley, 2000; Stephenson, 2000). The relationship between these structural forces and sexual risk behavior among black men may be mediated by higher levels of psychological distress amid adverse social conditions, similar to findings with Latino MSM (Diaz, Ayala, & Bein, 2004; Diaz, Ayala, Bein, Henne, & Marin, 2001), but have yet to be fully explored in the literature. Moreover, qualitative data among rural African Americans in North Carolina suggests that themes of racial oppression, boredom, and lack of community recreation may be promoting sexual risk behaviors in ways that differ from those in urban metropolitan areas (Adimora et al., 2001). Little is known about how sexual risk differs between black men in urban and rural areas, however, because most of the HIV prevention research focused on black men focuses almost exclusively on black MSM in major metropolitan areas such as New York, Washington, DC, and Miami (CDC, 2005; Valleroy et al., 2000)

Gaps in knowledge also exist about the structural context of racial discrimination and HIV risk for black men. An abundant empirical literature documents the relationship between black people's experiences of racial discrimination and adverse health outcomes such as high rates of hypertension (Klonoff & Landrine, 2000), psychiatric symptoms (Klonoff, Landrine, & Ullman, 1999), mortality (Collins & Williams, 1999; Fang, Madhavan, Bosworth, & Alderman, 1998), and overall diminished physical and mental health (Jackson et al., 1996; Williams, Neighbors, & Jackson, 2008), but research on the link between racial discrimination and HIV risk in black communities is virtually nonexistent. An exception is a study with black patients at an STI clinic in North Carolina that found perceived racism to be associated with higher odds of HIV testing after controlling for other factors such as coping mechanisms (Ford et al., 2009). Research with Latino MSM, the first to investigate racial discrimination and risk, documents that those who had experienced more racial discrimination were more likely than those who had not experienced discrimination to engage in risky sexual and drug use behaviors (Diaz et al., 2001; Diaz et al., 2004). The disproportionately high rates of HIV/AIDS among black men regardless of sexual orientation attest to the need to understand how structural factors such as racial discrimination may be associated with HIV risk.

Black Men Speak about the Structural Contexts of Their Lives

Qualitative methods such as interviews and focus groups are ideal for exploring the structural context of black men's lives and the implications for HIV risk and protective behaviors. To this end, we present findings from qualitative studies that we have conducted with black men representing diverse sexual behavioral and identification categories. These studies include: (1) focus groups with 81 predominantly gay-identified black MSM in upstate New York and New York City (Malebranche, Peterson, Fullilove, & Stackhouse, 2004); (2) in-depth interviews with 30 black heterosexual men in Philadelphia, Pennsylvania (Bowleg, Teti, Malebranche, & Tschann, 2010); (3) in-depth interviews with 13 black heterosexual men in Washington, DC (Bowleg, 2004); (4) semi-structured interviews with 29 black MSM in Atlanta, Georgia (Malebranche, Fields, Bryant, & Harper, 2009); and (5) semi-structured interviews with 39 bisexually active black men in Atlanta, Georgia (Malebranche, Arriola, Jenkins, Dauria, & Patel, 2010). Although these studies differ in terms of objectives and participants' sexual orientation categories, they highlight the similar and overlapping structural contexts of black men's lives. Common threads in the qualitative themes include: (1) masculinity and gender role pressure; (2) experiences with various forms of trauma; and (3) larger cultural beliefs and practices influencing choice of sexual partners and condom use. We use pseudonyms to protect the confidentiality of the participants.

Provide, Hustle, and Survive: Masculinity and Gender Role Pressure

Historically, **black masculinity** has been defined by physical and heterosexual prowess, reflecting the historical context of slavery and focus on the expectations of black men to "work and breed" (Whitehead, 1997). These gender role norms differed from the more Eurocentric masculine attributes of competition, individualism, aggression, and paternalism, which may be denied to black men by racist and classist structural institutions (Harris, 1992; Hunter & Davis, 1994; Jackson, 1997; Staples, 1978; Whitehead, 1997). Although it has been suggested that these differing definitions of masculinity for black men may be instrumental in HIV risk behavior (Wolfe, 2003), virtually no studies have tested this potential relationship. Although not specifically focused on HIV/AIDS, the **"Cool Pose"** conceptual framework attempts to explain the masculinity ideologies of low-income urban black men (Majors & Billson, 1992). This framework asserts that black men, in response to larger institutional and environmental racially driven pressures, adopt coping behavior such as aloof posturing, violence, hustling, and an overemphasis on physical and sexual prowess to compensate for the denial of masculine attainment through traditional means (e.g., education, jobs). In this context, some black men may attempt to prove their manhood through multiple sexual conquests and fathering children.

Qualitative studies have demonstrated similar definitions of masculinity and gender role pressures among black men of various sexual orientations. In a study of predominantly gay-identified black MSM in Atlanta, participants recounted that they had had few black male role models in their formative years, and often discussed gender role-related pressure to always be the provider, "hustling" (e.g., doing whatever needed to be done) to survive, and the inherent issues of societal or institutional racism and racial differences in societal expectations of manhood (Malebranche et al., 2009). To Kwame, a 34-year-old participant, survival and fatherhood were the key masculine indicators that he learned when he was a boy: "Survive. To survive, get what you want, getting what you want, how to survive, making it. That's what I learned. All the male role models around me either sold drugs or just made babies." Echoing this theme, Chris, a 43-year-old participant, reflected that: "White men are taught to be the provider, just to get a good job, get educated. Black men have been taught, 'Hey, hustle, make it any way you can.' I mean, that's the perception we've been taught."

Participants in this study, such as Jeffery, a 32-year-old man, also described the social context of slavery, race, and racism in America, and how these factors had influenced his perceptions of opportunities for black men: "I guess it goes back to history. I guess by [white people] having the power to do what they wanna do versus black people or minorities having the power such as they do [in terms of money or politics]. It just seems easier for [white people]."

Many also perceived that as black men, they lacked the financial privilege and access that many white men enjoyed. Denied the opportunities to achieve financially in the workplace, some respondents described hustling, the practice of selling either legal or illegal merchandise or drugs, to survive. Hustling also provided men with financial success and respect, and as such allowed them to assert an alternative form of masculinity (Whitehead, 1997). Additionally, many described their perceptions that society had lower expectations for black men. Descriptions of relative disempowerment and restricted masculine expectations for black males in the United States were a recurrent theme in many of the interviews.

Consistent with our chapter's title that black men's lives in the context of HIV risk often transcend their sexual orientation, several of the black MSM in this study noted that their race rather than their sexuality often shaped how others responded to them. Such was the case with John, a 40-year-old gay-identified man who expressed a conscious choice to prioritize his racial identity over a sexual identity, a common sentiment among the vast majority of participants: "When I walk into a room and no one knows me they know that I'm black, but they don't know that I'm gay. Or, I don't tell them, 'I'm gay.' So I think it's more important for me to be a good black man than it is to be a good gay. You can hide being gay, but I can't hide being black."

Findings from this study also mirror results from a study on health care experiences among 81 black MSM in upstate New York and New York City (Malebranche et al., 2004). Many men in this study described how their experiences with rigid gender role norms had influenced how they perceived themselves as men, utilized medical services, and communicated with medical providers, particularly about their sexuality. On the influence of gender norms in his life and the internal strife it caused for him, Lonnie, a 49-year-old divorced father of two, described his difficulty in reconciling definitions of masculinity with his current same-sex behavior and orientation:

> You know, that's the way I was brought up: grow up, go to high school, go to college, marry a woman, then you have children. And you had a house, the dog, and I grew up like that, and I did that. I did the marriage thing, and the children, and the wife. You know, but that's because that's what was instilled in me. And I remember on my wedding day my big brother said to me, "You know you don't have to do this." He saw something in me [that] I didn't wanna see in myself. So, I said, "You're crazy, I gotta do this. Everybody's watching." And it was always about everybody, you know, pleasing everybody instead of dealing with inner self.

Findings from a recent qualitative study exploring issues of same-sex disclosure and sexual risk behavior among 39 bisexually active black men in Georgia (Malebranche et al., 2010) echo many of the findings among MSM samples. Fred, a 37-year-old participant, for example, described how he hustled to make money: "[I've got] a lot a ways I make money. I got a brain to work. I always know peoples who are working in the streets. I know people who do a lot of stuff. I know a lot of people so and I just sometimes eventually hook up with peeps and do work. I would make money like that being in the streets." Central to many of the narratives about hustling and providing financially for one's loved ones was the notion that being able to provide financially is a key masculinity norm for black men. John, a 28-year-old participant, reflected on how commonplace this norm was: "Just being like able to provide for your family if you're a father . . . everybody looks at that. A man is supposed to provide so that's always how I've raised: to provide for your woman." Dwayne, a 43-year-old with a steady girlfriend, echoed John's perception of these expectations: "I think what's expected is to go back to the value system: take care of your family, take care of what's yours. I think that's expected within the black race."

Faced with the lack of opportunities, particularly opportunities for employment, many bisexual black men in this study also described how they had to hustle just to survive. Michael, 23, passionately described all of the obstacles that he faced to survive: "It's hard, man, but you got to survive, so you got to push it to the limit. It's just like being a black man you got to . . . I mean it's hard, now it's really hard to get a job places now. I ain't trying to work for nobody no more anyway; get my own shit, fuck that. [Hustling is] easy money that's quicker than working for McDonald's and some shit like that, you know, bullshit like that. Just being a black man, its hard man."

The challenges of being a black man and particularly the struggle to provide financially for one's loved ones were also key themes among the black hetero-sexual men in the Philadelphia study (Bowleg et al., 2010). In response to the study's interview question about society's expectations for black men, many interviewees responded with answers such as "Be protectors and providers of family," and "Take care of my family." Men such as Rob, a 40-year-old married man who could not easily provide for his family, expressed substantial stress: "I mean, it seem like, you know, sometime I feel like, you know, I'm lettin' my family down. You know. Like I'm not, you know, holdin' up the part o' my end o' the bargain. Supposed to be there for my wife, you know. She ain't supposed to be out there strugglin' durin' all the time and all the other stuff. You know?"

Taken together, the findings from these different studies suggest that, regardless of sexual orientation, many black men feel the pressure to comply with the gender role norm that men should be financial providers. Our findings also show that the structural context of black men's lives, namely that black men do not share the same access to financial success that their white counter-parts do, means that often low-income black men, regardless of sexual orientation, feel like they must resort to hustling to survive. Nor is the struggle to achieve financial success without a psychological toll. As Rob described, not being able to provide for oneself and family can be considerably stressful, and demonstrates how pervasive and intense masculinity and gender role pressures are in the lives of many black men.

Trauma: "I remember him beating the hell out of us." The role that situational, structural, and personal trauma plays in the lives of black men is understudied, but a small literature attests to its prevalence and impact on black men's mental and physical health. (Rich, 2010; Rich & Grey, 2005). This trauma includes, but is not limited to, conditions such as neighborhood, familial, and interpersonal violence, **childhood sexual abuse (CSA)**, experiences with racial discrimination, and police harassment/profiling. Although this is an emerging field of study as related to individual health behaviors of black men, its relevance to the mental health, health behaviors, and current racial HIV disparity among black men in the United States has not been fully elucidated.

Struggling and Being a Target: Protecting Black Men against Racism

For many black men, the daily experience of interacting in environments in which many people perceive them to be criminals, fear them, and/or have low expectations for them constitutes a baseline level of trauma. To deal with this trauma, Peter, a 20-year-old black MSM student in Rochester, New York, noted that "We [black men] have to wake up in the morning and put on armor every day." Indeed, the struggle inherent in being a black man in the United States was a common theme among black MSM focus group participants in New York (Malebranche et al., 2004) and black heterosexual men in Philadelphia (Bowleg et al., in press). Typical of this view was that of Adrian, a 21-year-old gay man in Buffalo: "Being a black man is a hard struggle. Not just being gay, being straight, being a general black man is an everyday struggle. I don't care how you put it, white America either wants me in a cell or in a grave."

Struggle was also the word that Anthony, a 40-year-old MSM in Albany, New York, used to describe his life: "Well, what it means being a black man in America is struggling. Struggling, you know, no unity, you know, like being a black man in America it is hard for a black man in America to maintain [unity]." Black bisexual men in Atlanta (Malebranche et al., 2008) also echoed Peter's notion of the inherent challenges and difficulties of just living as a black man every day. For example, Carl, a 25-year-old participant, observed, "[Being a black man in the U.S. is] hard. . . . It's like we have so many opportunities for us but it's like it's so hard to get them in some areas."

Men's narratives about their struggles reflect the challenges of how race, class, and gender intersect in the lives of black men in the United States. Their accounts also highlight how structural factors such as lack of education, poverty, racism, unemployment, and a dearth of social opportunities affect many black men regardless of sexual orientation. For example, several of the black bisexual interviewees in the Atlanta study (Malebranche et al., 2010) recounted frequent lifetime incidents of racial prejudice and discrimination. Among them was John, 51, who recalled a lifetime of being called racial epithets and described how he learned to cope with these repetitive experiences: "I've been called nigger. I mean I've been called a coon by old ass white folks but it doesn't bother me because I know me. I know that's not who I am. So you know words . . . I learn[ed] how to deal with words. I hear them and they go in one ear and go out the other one you know."

Respondents' accounts of racial prejudice and discrimination transcended socioeconomic status, sexual orientation, and occupation. Eddie, a 23-year-old medical student in Atlanta (Malebranche et al., 2009), recounted an experience while he was being interviewed for medical school: "One of the interviewers asked me a question and he was thinking . . . I guess he was trying to use the affirmative action thing against me. He was like, 'So how do you feel that your quality and your standing in school, and your GPA in school will get you here; not just the color of your skin?'"

From the same study, Gary, a 39-year-old Caribbean man living with HIV, said that he had never experienced overt racism growing up until he joined the United States Navy. He recalled an incident when he went to a white barbershop to get a haircut: "And [the white barber] said, 'Look, we don't touch your kind in here, you need to leave this store. There's a place down the street, where they do your kind of hair but your kind is not welcome in here.' And I was stunned, in this Navy uniform, like here I am in this Navy uniform ready to go to war to die for this fat fucker, and they can't even cut my hair. I thought, 'Oh my God, it's true what they say.' And that blew me away."

These accounts reflect common life experiences described by many black men in our research, regardless of sexual orientation or identity (Williams et al., 2008). These racial microaggressions may have profound cumulative implications for the mental health, HIV-risk behaviors, and health care utilization practices of black men (Malebranche et al., 2004; Sue et al., 2007; Sue, Capodilupo, & Holder, 2008). Although racial discrimination and HIV risk is an understudied topic with black men, a study with Latino gay men found that those who had experienced more racial discrimination, more financial hardship, and homophobia were also more likely to report engaging in risky behaviors compared with those with few or no experiences of social discrimination (Diaz et al., 2004). Similar assessments of these relationships among black men of all sexualities are needed.

Racial discrimination was also a key theme among the black heterosexual men in the Philadelphia study (Bowleg et al., in press). For example, Tony, a 22-year-old unemployed man, described his life as a black man as "challenging. It's tough. Tougher than it would be if, you know, I was another race, I think." And as was the case with many of the black MSM (Malebranche et al., 2009) and bisexual men (Malebranche et al., 2010) in the Atlanta studies, racial discrimination experiences were mundane and persistent life stressors, but more commonly in the form of police surveillance and harassment (Bowleg et al., in press). Participants recounted numerous instances in which the police had targeted them for questioning or searches without cause. Such was the case with Steve, a 23-year-old man who recalled walking to a restaurant to get something to eat and encountering police who demanded of him, "'What you doing and what you out here for?' [Then they] frisk me down to see if I've got any guns . . . drugs . . . they just let you go if you don't have any."

"You're always a target," was how Wayne, a 26-year-old, described his frequent interactions with the police: "And it happens over and over . . . Just getting the once over [by police], just being harassed by cops [who are] always looking [at me] like I'm suspicious . . . like a suspect or something, a criminal or something."

Childhood Sexual Abuse (CSA) among Black MSM

Among black MSM in particular, experiences with CSA have emerged as a unique aspect of trauma that had profound influences on individuals' lives.

Fields, Malebranche, and Feist-Price (2008) found a 33 percent prevalence of CSA among three diverse samples of black MSM in different geographical areas (Atlanta, Lexington, Kentucky, and Rochester, New York). Men across the three samples described their experiences with sexual abuse as repetitive, like Xavier, who stated: "I was 7 or 8. He [male cousin] molested me all the way up until I was like 17 or something." Others described being sexually abused by a male family member or trusted male role model, such as Norm, who was molested by his father:

> Well my actual first time, I was molested, so it was with a guy [his biological father] . . . I was maybe five or six. I was coming out of kindergarten and going into the first grade and part of my second grade year. It stopped like [during] my third grade year totally . . . We actually got into a fight . . . It got to . . . most of it was oral, but when it came to penetration, I tried to fight him off and my uncle actually stopped it and he overheard it and he walked in and was like, "What are you doing to your son?"

Similarly, Raymond, a 22-year-old-gay-identified man in Rochester, described being sexually molested by the deacon in his church, and never telling anyone about the incident:

> It was . . . it was one day after Sunday school, he . . . he used to always take all the kids out anyway, so . . . But, um, this one day after Sunday school, he took me out, we got somethin' to eat and he was . . . comin' on to me and things and it just happened. He was threatening and told me not to tell. At the time, which I thought, you know, I did not know, so, I thought I was gonna get in trouble and things and stuff like that. So, I kept it in my whole life.

Notably, these CSA experiences often led to self-reported feelings of depression, despair, anxiety, low self-esteem, and difficulty with personal and sexual intimacy, as was the case with Victor, a 31-year-old musician in Lexington, who stated: "I did him [had insertive penetrative sex], came in him and everything. He's like 'Man, you too good to be young.' And after that, it was like nothing but suicidal thoughts. I wanted to kill myself." Sam, a 19-year-old participant in Rochester, echoed these sentiments of how CSA affected his mental health, to the point of diagnosing his own behavior as an adult: "I think I'm bipolar. Sometimes I feel happy, then the next second, I'm totally pissed off."

These experiences shared by black MSM in varied geographic settings and of diverse claimed sexual identities (gay, heterosexual, bisexual) were characterized by secrecy and associations with close male relatives, were repetitive in nature, and ultimately had a negative influence on their mental health as adults. And while the men did not say directly that these experiences with CSA led to choices to have unprotected sex with future male partners as adults, there is sufficient literature evidence among general samples of predominantly white MSM to suggest that this is an area of research deserving of future exploration among sexually diverse samples of black men (Bartholow et al., 1994; Doll et al., 1992).

The broader context of condom use and sexual partners. Reviews of black MSM risk behaviors demonstrate that comparisons of "gay" versus "non-gay-identified" samples erroneously remain at the forefront of inquiry, despite no conclusive proof that claiming a gay identity is associated with increased condom use practices (Millett et al., 2006; Millett et al., 2007). Implicit in this approach is that it is the sexual identification in and of itself that drives risk. Interviews with black MSM in Atlanta (Malebranche et al., 2009), however, suggest that broader contextual and interpersonal factors such as trust and avoiding riskier behaviors (i.e., engaging in insertive anal sex instead of receptive anal sex) shape black MSM's decision making about condom use. In his description for not using condoms with his partner, for instance, Greg, a 29-year-old participant, recalled: "I think when we didn't use a condom, the first time, was our year anniversary. I think I felt really comfortable with him. I felt like I could trust him." Others, like Ivan, a 23-year-old student, strategically employed certain sexual behaviors so as to ensure decreased risk: "Well, I feel as though like, with me fuckin' somebody, I can see my condom and I know what's going on, you know what I'm saying, as opposed to somebody doin' me, so it's like that does play a role into it. I feel as though I'm a little bit more safe that way."

These examples suggest that decisions to forego condoms or engage in perceived safer behaviors constitute internal negotiations of potentially risk situations that are not solely linked to specific sexual identification labels. Moreover, they may more adequately reflect the intersection of larger structural contexts such as class, cultural beliefs, relationship modeling, and education that factor into individual level beliefs regarding trust, control, and condom use. For other participants in the same study, the choice to use condoms or not was simply related to "heat of the moment" sex or fear of contracting HIV. Again, decisions to use condoms during intercourse appeared to be personal decisions influenced by external experiences such as condom availability or risk perception, rather than being a direct byproduct of claiming a certain sexual identity or label.

Several of the men in the Atlanta MSM study (Malebranche et al., 2009) posited possible contextual factors linking racial discrimination experiences and HIV risk for black MSM. Their narratives cited the legacy of racism and negative experiences with being black in the United States as driving high rates of depression and low self-esteem. Negative mental health outcomes such as these could constrain their ability to make safer decisions in instances where they had to make choices about whether to use condoms with sexual partners, a finding affirmed in empirical research with Latino gay men (Diaz et al.,

2004). For example, Doug, a 36-year-old participant, noted that some black men may use sex as an ameliorative for the stressors in their lives: "And I know people use sex as an outlet. I don't know if that's because white people don't have as many problems as black folks or I don't know; this is my theory. And even though a scar can disappear but the hurt and the pain and the anguish are still here."

Will, 23, suggested that self-esteem might be at the root of some black MSM's risk taking: "If you loved yourself enough to live, you'll have more respect for yourself. You wouldn't be out there, throwing yourself around there and not protecting yourself, that's crazy."

Bisexually active black men in Atlanta (Malebranche et al., 2010) also reported contextual factors that decreased their likelihood of condom use such as being "caught up in the moment," being intoxicated, or after trust had been established and both partners had been HIV-tested. These risk environments were influenced by a paucity of affirming social outlets, broader cultural beliefs, and sometimes reflected personal assumptions of risk based on societal gender-related stereotypes and implications of fatherhood. Brian, a 38-year-old bisexual man, explained that the sex of his partners determined whether or not he used a condom: "I would always use a condom with a woman, but as far as a guy, because a guy can't get pregnant [I would be less likely to use a condom]. But I mean if we are both okay, and we got [HIV] tested and both are clean, and after a certain amount of time, I would say a year, and trust has been built and we trust each other and we just know that we'll be faithful to each other and not go out and do nothing crazy, I wouldn't use condoms."

Different approaches to condom use were common among the bisexual men in this study. Some men, for example, stated that they would be less likely to use condoms with women than men because of the perception that women are safer than men, while others noted that they would be more inclined to use condoms with casual partners rather than primary partners because sex without a condom is an expression of love or trust. The most commonly cited incentive for consistent condom use among the participants, however, was fear of contracting a disease (both male and female sexual partners) or pregnancy (female sexual partners). A qualitative study in New York City found similar influences on condom choice among black bisexual men, including sex being more enjoyable without condoms, lack of availability, perceived trust and "heat of the moment." (Dodge, Jefferies IV, & Sandfort, 2008).

Because there is such a dearth of HIV prevention research with black heterosexual men, empirical knowledge about the social factors that shape black heterosexual men's condom use decision making is scarce. A handful of studies suggest, however, that black heterosexual men cite many of the same reasons that black MSM in the aforementioned studies do for not using condoms, such as that condoms decrease sensitivity and are not necessary after partners have established trust in an intimate relationship (Bowleg, 2004; Crosby et al., 2004; Essien et al., 2005; Wang et al., 2000). Regardless, perhaps Reggie, a 32-year-old construction worker and MSM in Atlanta (Malebranche et al., 2009), most accurately stated how structural factors affecting black people transcend sexual orientation: "I think that some of the problems that we're experiencing in the black gay community it's because of what we have went through in the black community."

A Common Ground Approach to HIV Prevention for Black Men

The concept of highlighting the structural determinants of black men's HIV risk, regardless of sexual orientation, identity, or label, represents a relatively new and perhaps even radical approach to HIV prevention. Findings from our qualitative studies with sexually diverse black men illustrate that viewed through a structural lens, black men share more in common than the exclusive focus on sexual orientation reveals. Moreover, our collective studies' findings about the similarities between black MSM and heterosexual men are bolstered by empirical evidence that compartmentalizing black men's HIV risk merely in terms of sexual identification risk groups or labels fails to accurately reflect behavioral risk (Dodge et al., 2008; Millett et al., 2005; Millett et al., 2006; Pathela, Blank, Sell, & Schillinger, 2006).

Presumably because of the inextricable link between Gay Civil Rights efforts in the United States and HIV prevention advocacy, there remains an emphasis on sexual orientation approaches to current HIV prevention intervention efforts focused on black men. Although this approach has been successful in reducing HIV rates in white gay male communities, it has not been similarly effective among black men. Thus, the challenge that now faces the public health community is how to ascertain the exact pathways that link these similar contexts to the risk behaviors driving the epidemic in black communities. Only then can we develop more culturally appropriate HIV prevention initiatives that reflect the structural realities of black men's lives in the United States, regardless of the sex or gender of their sexual partners.

Our research demonstrates at least five key take-home lessons to guide future HIV prevention theory, research, policy, and interventions for black men. First, there is a critical need for more research focused on the structural contexts of masculinity, racism, trauma, CSA, and broader factors influencing condom use decisions for black men and their HIV risk. Second, additional qualitative and quantitative research is desperately needed exploring how black men's shared lived experiences and contexts are associated with their mental health, and in turn sexual risk and protective behavior. Third, HIV-prevention interventions grounded in the common structural experiences and contexts of black men's lives in the United States may be a much more fruitful place to begin addressing HIV risk rather than homing in exclusively on sexual identities and labels. Fourth, approaches seeking to understand health and disease in the context of larger structural factors may hold more promise for interventions for black men than those that simply pathologize individual-level behaviors as if they emerge from a vacuum.

Finally, perhaps the most important lesson gleaned from listening to the voices of black men in our HIV prevention research is the need to abandon the pervasive deficits-model approach and embrace an assets-model approach to black men's health (Utsey, 1997; Utsey, Bolden, Lanier, & Williams, 2007). We concede that although our qualitative approaches to understanding black men's experiences provide us with the benefit of hearing and learning from the voices of black men themselves, invariably our work persists in highlighting the many negative aspects of black men's lives. An assets approach would involve an exploration of the structural contexts in black men's lives that affirm and support ways that they create and maintain healthy lives. Such an approach would also involve the development of culturally grounded interventions that foster environments in which black men feel empowered to make decisions that lead to prosperity, upward mobility, and healthy minds and bodies, in spite of facing adverse structural contexts. Interventions that emphasize factors, including but not limited to, employment, job training, educational advancement, religion and spirituality, cultural diversity, family, fatherhood responsibilities, mentorship and role models, resiliency, and high expectations, should take center stage in our future public health discussions, research, and practice interventions for black men.

Summary

Our research with black men of all sexualities attests that HIV-prevention researchers, public health officials, and health care providers have much to learn from an examination of the relationships between the structural contexts of black men's lives and their sexual health. Understanding the relationship between structural contexts and sexual behavior is a public health imperative, as is the subsequent development of structurally based interventions that create environments in which black men can truly be healthy in mind, body, and spirit, regardless of the gender of their sexual partners.

Key Terms

acquired immune deficiency syndrome (AIDS)

black masculinity

childhood sexual abuse (CSA)

cool pose

human immunodeficiency virus (HIV)

men who have sex with men (MSM)

sexual orientation

sexually transmitted infections (STI)

structural factors

unprotected anal intercourse (UAI)

Discussion Questions

1. What is the current HIV epidemiology among various risk categories among black men in the United States?

2. How are sexual orientation or identity labels related to sexual risk behavior among black men?

3. Name three structural factors that are documented influences in the lives of black men and may be linked to individual behavioral choices driving HIV transmission.

References

Adimora, A. A., Schoenbach, V. J., Martinson, F. E., Coyne-Beasley, T., Doherty, I., Stancil, T. R., & Fullilove, R.E. (2006). Heterosexually transmitted HIV infection among African Americans in North Carolina. *Journal of Acquired Immune Deficiency Syndromes*, *41*(5), 616–623.

Adimora, A. A., Schoenbach, V. J., Martinson, F. E., Donaldson, K. H., Fullilove, R. E., & Aral, S. O. (2001). Social context of sexual relationships among rural African Americans. *Sexually Transmitted Diseases*, *28*(2), 69–76.

Bartholow, B. N., Doll, L. S., Douglas, J. M., Bolan, G., Harrison, J. S., Moss, P. M., & McKirnan, D. (1994). Emotional, behavioral, and HIV risks associated with sexual abuse among adult homosexual and bisexual men. *Child Abuse & Neglect*, *18*(9), 747–761.

Bogart, L. M., & Thorburn, S. (2005). Are HIV/AIDS conspiracy beliefs a barrier to HIV prevention among African Americans? *Journal of the Acquired Immune Deficiency Syndrome*, *38*(2), 213–218.

Bowleg, L. (2004). Love, sex, and masculinity in sociocultural context: HIV concerns and condom use among African American men in heterosexual relationships. *Men & Masculinities*, *7*, 166–186.

Bowleg, L., Teti, M., Malebranche, D. J., & Tschann, J. M. (in press). It's an uphill battle everyday: Exploring structural factors and implications for sexual HIV risk among black heterosexual men. *Psychology of Men and Masculinity*.

Centers for Disease Control and Prevention. (2003). HIV/STD risks in young men who have sex with men who do not disclose their sexual orientation—Six US cities, 1994–2000. *Monthly Morbidity & Mortality Report*, *52*, 81–86.

Centers for Disease Control and Prevention. (2005). HIV prevalence, unrecognized infection, and HIV testing among men who have sex with men—Five U.S. cities, June 2004—April 2005. *Monthly Morbidity & Mortality Report*, *54*(24), 597–601.

Centers for Disease Control and Prevention. (2006, April 21). HIV transmission among male inmates in a state prison system—Georgia, 1992–2005. *Monthly Morbidity & Mortality Report*, *55*(15), 421–426.

Centers for Disease Control and Prevention. (2009, February 18). *HIV/AIDS surveillance report 2007*. Vol. 19. Retrieved from http://www.cdc.gov/hiv/topics/surveillance/ resources/reports/2007report/pdf/2007SurveillanceReport.pdf

Centers for Disease Control and Prevention. (2010, July 19). Division of HIV/AIDS Prevention. Presented at the International AIDS Conference, Vienna, Austria. Retrieved from http://www.cdc.gov/nchhstp/newsroom/povertyandhivpressrelease. html

Collins, C. A., & Williams, D. R. (1999). Segregation and mortality: The deadly effects of racism? *Sociological Forum*, *14*(3), 495–523.

Crosby, R. A., Graham, C. A., Yarber, W. L., & Sanders, S. A. (2004). If the condom fits, wear it: A qualitative study of young African American men. *Sexually Transmitted Infections*, *80*, 306–309.

Darbes, L., Crepaz, N., Lyles, C., Kennedy, G., Rutherford, G. (2008). The efficacy of behavioral interventions in reducing HIV risk behaviors and incident sexually transmitted diseases in heterosexual African Americans. *AIDS*, *22*, 1177–1194.

Denizet-Lewis, B. (2003). Living (and dying) on the down low: Double lives, AIDS and the black homosexual underground. *New York Times Magazine*, *Section 8*: 28–33, 48, 52–53.

Diaz, R. M., Ayala, G., & Bein, E. (2004). Sexual risk as an outcome of social oppression: Data from a probability sample of Latino gay men in three U.S. cities. *Cultural Diversity & Ethnic Minority Psychology*, *10*(3), 255–267.

Diaz, R. M., Ayala, G., Bein, E., Henne, J., & Marin, B. V. (2001). The impact of homophobia, poverty, and racism on the mental health of gay and bisexual Latino men: Findings from 3 US cities. *American Journal of Public Health*, *91*(6), 927–932.

Dodge, B., Jeffries IV, W. L., & Sandfort, T. G. (2008). Beyond the down low: Sexual risk, protection, and disclosure among at-risk black men who have sex with both men and women (MSMW). *Archives of Sexual Behavior*, *37*(5), 683–696.

Doll, L. S, Joy, D., Bartholow, B. N, Harrison, J. S, Bolan, G., Douglas, J. M., . . . Delgado, W. (1992). Sexual reported childhood and adolescent sexual abuse among adult homosexual and bisexual men. *Child Abuse and Neglect*, *16*(6), 855–864.

Essien, E. J., Meshack, A. F., Peters, R. J., Ogungbade, G. O., & Osemene, N. I. (2005). Strategies to prevent HIV transmission among heterosexual African American men. *BMC Public Health*, *5*(3), 1–10.

Fang, J., Madhavan, S., Bosworth, W., & Alderman, M. H. (1998). Residential segregation and mortality in New York City. *Social Science & Medicine*, *47*(4), 469–476.

Fields, S. D., Malebranche, D., & Feist-Price, S. (2008). Childhood sexual abuse in black men who have sex with men: Results from three qualitative studies. *Cultural Diversity and Ethnic Minority Pscyhology*, *14*, 385–390.

Ford, C. L., Daniel, M., Earp, J. A., Kaufman, J. S., Golin, C. E., & Miller, W. C. (2009). Perceived everyday racism, residential segregation, and HIV testing among patients at a sexually transmitted disease clinic. *American Journal of Public Health*, *99*(Suppl. 1), S137–S143.

Galatzer-Levy, R., & Cohler, B. (2002). Making a gay identity: Coming out, social context, and psychodynamics, in rethinking psychoanalysis and the homosexualities. In J. Winer & W. Anderson (Eds.), *Annual of Psychoanalysis* (Vol. *XXX*, pp. 255–286). Hillsdale, NJ: Analytic Press.

Grov, C., Bimbi, D. S., Parsons, J. T., & Nanin, J. E. (2006). Layer upon layer: The coming out process as it relates to generations, race and gender. *Journal of Sex Research, 43*, 115–121.

Harris, S. M. (1992). Black male masculinity and same-sex friendships. *Western Journal of Black Studies, 16*(2), 74–81.

Hu, D. J., Frey, R., & Costa, S. J. (1994). Geographical AIDS rates and sociodemographic variables in Newark, New Jersey metropolitan area. *AIDS Public Policy Journal, 9*, 20–25.

Hunter, A. G., & Davis, J. E. (1994). Hidden voices of black men: The meaning, structure, and complexity of manhood. *Journal of Black Studies, 25*(1), 20–40.

International HIV/AIDS Alliance. (2003). *Working with men, responding to AIDS: Gender, sexuality and HIV—A case study collection*. U.S. Agency for International Development (USAID). Award number HRN-G-00-98-00010-00.

Jackson, R. L. (1997). Black manhood as xenophobe: An ontological exploration of the Hegelian dialectic. *Journal of Black Studies, 27*(6), 731–750.

Jackson, J. S., Brown, T. N., Williams, D. R., Torres, M., Sellers, S. L., & Brown, K. (1996). Racism and the physical and mental health status of African Americans: A thirteen year national panel study. *Ethnicity and Disease, 6*(1–2), 132–147.

King, J. L. (2004). *On the down low: A journey into the lives of "straight" black men who sleep with men*. New York, NY: Broadway Books.

Klonoff, E. A., & Landrine, H. (2000). Is skin color a marker for racial discrimination? Explaining the skin color-hypertension relationship. *Journal of Behavioral Medicine, 23*(4), 329–338.

Klonoff, E. A., Landrine, H., & Ullman, J. B. (1999). Racial discrimination and psychiatric symptoms among blacks. *Cultural Diversity and Ethnic Minority Psychology, 5*(4), 329–339.

Lansky, A., Fleming, P. L., Byers, R. H., Karon, J. M., & Wortley, P. M. (2001). A method for classification of HIV exposure category for women without HIV risk information. *Morbidity and Mortality Weekly Report* (Centers for Disease Control), 50(RR061), 29–40.

Laumann, E. O., Gagnon, J. H., Michael, R. T., & Michaels, S. (1994). *The social organization of sexuality: Sexual practices in the United States*. Chicago, IL: University of Chicago Press.

Majors, R., & Billson, J. M. (1992). *Cool pose: The dilemmas of black manhood in America*. New York, NY: Lexington Books.

Malebranche, D. J., Arriola, K. J., Jenkins, T. R., Dauria, E., & Patel, S. N. (2010). Exploring the "bisexual bridge": A qualitative study of risk behavior and disclosure of same-sex behavior among black bisexual men. *American Journal of Public Health, 100*(1), 159–164.

Malebranche, D. J., Fields, E. L., Bryant, L. O., & Harper, S. R. (2009). Masculine socialization and sexual risk behaviors among black men who have sex with men: A qualitative exploration. *Men and Masculinities, 12*(1), 90–112.

Malebranche, D. J., Peterson, J. L., Fullilove, R. E., & Stackhouse, R. W. (2004). Race and sexual identity: Perceptions about medical culture and healthcare among black men who have sex with men. *Journal of the National Medical Association*, *96*(1), 97–107.

Millett, G. A., Flores, S. A., Peterson, J. L., & Bakeman, R. (2007). Explaining disparities in HIV infection among black and white men who have sex with men: A meta-analysis of HIV risk behaviors. *AIDS*, *21*, 2083–2091.

Millett, G. A., Malebranche, D. J., Mason, B., & Spikes, P. (2005). Focusing "down low": Bisexual black men, HIV risks and heterosexual transmission. *Journal of the National Medical Association*, *97*(7), 52S–59S.

Millett, G. A., Peterson, J. L., Wolitski, R. J., & Stall, R. (2006). Greater risk for HIV infection of black men who have sex with men: A critical literature review. *American Journal of Public Health*, *96*(6), 1007–1019.

Myers, H. F., Javanbakht, M., Martinez, M., & Obediah, S. (2003). Psychosocial predictors of risky sexual behaviors in African American men: Implications for prevention. *AIDS Education & Prevention*, *15*(Suppl. 1), 66–79.

Pathela, P., Blank, S., Sell, R. L., & Schillinger, J. A. (2006). The importance of both sexual behavior and identity. *American Journal of Public Health*, *96*(5), 765.

Payn, B., Tanfer, K., Billy, J. O. G., & Grady, W. R. (1997). Men's behavior change following infection with a sexually transmitted disease. *Family Planning Perspectives*, *29*(4), 152–157.

Rich, J. A. (2010). *Wrong place, wrong time: Trauma and violence in the lives of young black men*. Baltimore, MD: Johns Hopkins University Press.

Rich, J. A., & Grey, C. M. (2005). Pathways to recurrent trauma among young black men: Traumatic stress, substance use, and the "code of the street." *American Journal of Public Health*, *95*(5), 816–824.

Rhodes, T., Singer, M., Bourgois, P., Friedman, S. R., & Strathdee, S. A. (2005). The social structural production of HIV risk among injecting drug users. *Social Science & Medicine*, *61*, 1026–1044.

Simon, P. A., Hu, D. J., Diaz, T., & Kerndt, P. R. (1995). Income and AIDS rates in Los Angeles County. *AIDS*, *9*(3), 281–284.

Staples, R. (1978). Masculinity and race: The dual dilemma of black men. *Journal of Social Issues*, *34*(1), 169–183.

Stephenson, J. (2000). Rural HIV/AIDS in the United States: Studies suggest presence, no rampant spread. *Journal of the American Medical Association*, *284*(2): 167–168.

Sue, D. W., Capodilupo, C. M., & Holder, A. M. (2008). Racial microaggressions in the life experience of black Americans. *Professional Psychology: Research and Practice*, *39*(3), 329–336.

Sue, D. W., Capodilupo, C. M., Torino, G. C., Bucceri, J. M., Holder, A. M., Nadal, K. L., & Esquilin, M. (2007). Racial microaggressions in everyday life: Implications for clinical practice. *American Psychologist*, *62*(4), 271–286.

Sumartojo, E. (2000). Structural factors in HIV prevention: Concepts, examples, and implications for research. *AIDS*, *14S*(1), S3–S10.

Sumartojo, E., Doll, L., Holtgrave, D., Gayle, H., & Merson, M. (2000). Enriching the mix: Incorporating structural factors into HIV prevention. *AIDS*, *14S*(1), S1–S2.

Utsey, S. O. (1997). Racism and the psychological well-being of African-American men. *Journal of African American Studies*, *3*(1), 69–87.

Utsey, S. O., Bolden, M. A., Lanier, Y., & Williams, III, O. (2007). Examining the role of culture-specific coping as a predictor of resilient outcomes in African Americans from high-risk urban communities. *Journal of Black Psychology*, *3*(1), 75–93.

Valleroy, L. A., MacKellar, D. A., Karon, J. M., Rosen, D. H., McFarland, W., Shehan, D. A., . . . Janssen, R. S. (2001). For the young men's survey study group HIV prevalence and associated risks in young men who have sex with men. *JAMA*, *284*(2): 198–204.

Vonarx, N., & De Koninck, M. (2003). *Taking action with reference to masculinity in West Africa: A training model*. Abstract presented at the XV International Conference on HIV/AIDS, Bangkok, Thailand.

Wang, M. Q., Collins, C. B., Kohler, C. L., DiClemente, R. J., & Wingood, G. (2000). Drug use and HIV risk-related sex behaviors: A street outreach study of black adults. *Southern Medical Journal*, *93*(2), 186–190.

Whitehead, T. L. (1997). Urban low-income African American men, HIV/AIDS, and gender identity. *Medical Anthropology Quarterly*, *11*(4), 411–447.

Williams, D. R., Neighbors, H. W., & Jackson, J. S. (2008). Racial/ethnic discrimination and health: Findings from community studies. *American Journal of Public Health*, *98* (Suppl. 1), S29–S37.

Wohl, A. R., Johnson, D. F., Lu, S., Jordan, W., Beall, G., Currier, J., & Simon, P. A. (2002). HIV risk behaviors among African American men in Los Angeles County who self-identify as heterosexual. *Journal of Acquired Immune Deficiency Syndrome*, *31*, 354–360.

Wolfe, W. (2003). Overlooked role of African American males' hypermasculinity in the epidemic of unintended pregnancies and HIV/AIDS cases with young African American women. *Journal of the National Medical Association*, *95*, 846-852.

Wright, K. (2001, June 6). The great down low debate: A new black sexual identity may be an incubator for AIDS. *Village Voice*, 56.

Young, R.M., & Meyer, I.H. (2005). The trouble with "MSM" and "WSW": Erasure of the sexual-minority person in public health discourse. *American Journal of Public Health*, *95*, 1144–1149.

Zierler, S., Krieger, N., Tang, Y., Coady, W., Siegfried, E., DeMaria, A., & Auerbach, J. (2000). Economic deprivation and AIDS incidence in Massachusetts. *American Journal of Public Health*, *90*(7), 1064–1073.

Chapter 10

Social Determinants of Substance Abuse among Older African-American Men

Robert Pope

Learning Objectives

- Analyze the historical effects of slavery and the resultant racial residential segregation as factors for targeted marketing of commodities in African-American communities.
- Locate the intersection of age, race, and illicit drugs in African-American communities.
- Develop insight into why an individual begins illicit drug use.
- Describe a theoretical framework for understanding illicit drug use in older African-American men.

• • •

By the year 2020, there will be approximately 5 million older Americans with substance abuse disorders (Gfroefer, Penne, Pemberton, & Folsom, 2003). A disproportionate number of these older Americans, almost half a million, will be males of African descent. One early, unexpected outcome from the AIDS epidemic was the discovery of the high percentage of older African-American males infected with the AIDS virus, a large number of whom had been intravenous (IV) drugs abusers (Centers for Disease Control and Prevention [CDC], 2003). In 2003, African-Americans constituted 37 percent of persons 50 years and over who had been diagnosed with HIV/AIDS, which was a strong indicator of illicit drug use in this population. The relationship between these issues lies in transmission; IV drug use (primarily of heroin) caused 30 percent of the cases of HIV/AIDS in African-American males 65 and older (CDC). Age-related changes, such as a decrease of reserve and efficiency, from the cellular level to the system level when responding to stress, when superimposed on this phenomenon, will predispose this vulnerable population of older African-American males to a myriad of undesirable social, psychological, and health outcomes such as homelessness, mental illness, HIV, and hepatitis C. These potential outcomes can lead to health disparities—that is, differential patterns of morbidity or mortality and life expectancies (Smedley, Stith, & Nelson, 2003)—in this vulnerable population. Health disparities experienced by vulnerable populations are differential patterns of morbidity or mortality, and life expectancies (Smedley et al., 2003).

Because most research indicates that drug use is initiated at a young age (Willengbring, 2006), drug use across the lifespan will be examined. Therefore, the questions that direct this inquiry into substance abuse in older African-American males are: Why do African-American males begin illicit drug use and why do some African-American males continue this illicit drug use into old age? The purpose of this chapter is to explore the social determinants of substance abuse in older African-American men. Pope, Wallhagen, and Davis (2010) studied the effects of family, media images, and environment on illicit drug use in African-American men. Pope, the principal investigator, used grounded theory methodology to explore the social processes involved in the use of illicit drugs in older African-American men as an underpinning to the development of approaches to care and treatment. Interviews were conducted with 23 older African-American illicit substance users (20 male, 3 female) who were currently in drug treatment programs. Responses to the questions were recorded, transcribed, and analyzed using constant comparative methods. Three core themes emerged: (1) family, (2) media images, and (3) environment.

Throughout this chapter, the Pope et al. (2010) study will be referenced, and the responses of the male participants will be used to illustrate possible determinants of substance abuse in older African-American men. This chapter explores the conditions into which older African-American men were born, grew up, lived, worked, and aged. These social determinants contributed to, but are not solely responsible for, the higher trends of illicit drug use in older African-American males; these trends must also be considered in the context of historical and contemporary social and economic inequality. These types of inequality provide evidence of persistent racial disparities in America (Smedley et al., 2003) and serve as the rationale for making racial distinctions when exploring substance abuse among older persons. In order to locate the intersection of age, race, and illicit drug use in older African-American male substance abusers today, an understanding of the history of illicit drugs in black America is essential.[1]

History of Illicit Drug Use in African-American Communities

Drug abuse among the older population is not a new phenomenon. As early as 1910, there were reports of white contractors supplying black stevedores with cocaine to increase their work productivity (Courtwright, 1983). Although cocaine use occurred in both the black and white communities, cocaine increasingly became negatively associated with blacks in much the same way that opium was negatively associated with the Chinese (Musto, 1989b) and marijuana with Mexicans (Himmelstein, 1983). Musto called it the linkage of a feared group to an illegal substance; such a linkage helps to stigmatize and further marginalize that group from mainstream society (Musto, 1991).

In 1914, the *New York Times* printed an article "Negro Cocaine Fiends: New Southern Menace" (Williams, 1914). Within the body of this opinion editorial, the author underscores the perceived threat that African-American men who used cocaine presented to southern society. Articles like this one, although accepted as truth by some, were generally dismissed by academia, and Musto called them "fantasies fueled by white fear" (Musto, 1992). Ironically, in its summation, this diatribe against African-American males who used cocaine during the early part of the 1900s poignantly observed that their cocaine use was "a new and terrible form of slavery upon thousands of colored men; a hideous bondage from which they cannot escape by mere proclamation or civil war" (Williams, 1914). In the United States, the legal sale and use of cocaine and morphine was uncontrolled until federal regulation occurred following the passage of the Dangerous Drugs Act in 1920 (Teff, 1972).

The black struggle for equal rights in America saw small gains in times of America's armed engagement in the great wars. During the Civil War, for example, black males gained the rather dubious honor of fighting on the battlefield and the possibility of dying for the country. During this period, morphine began to be used as a battlefield drug for dulling pain following serious injury. It was first used orally and later, after the invention of the syringe by Dr. Charles Wood between 1840 and 1850 (Berridge & Mars, 2004), it was used intravenously. In 1874, German manufacturers (quite erroneously) marketed heroin as a nonaddictive alternative to the highly addictive morphine (Modell, 1957). The prevalent practice of treating war-related injuries from the Civil War, both World Wars, and the Vietnam War with the analgesic morphine led to rising numbers of morphine- and heroin-addicted veterans, both black and white (McCormack, 1988; Stanton, 1976).

Prior to 1961, illicit drug use was recognized by health care providers as a problem among older people, and persons over the age of 50 were the largest group of users (Barton, 2003). However, following World War II, there was an increased use of illicit drugs by younger adults, which was partly related to the counterculture that began developing in the 1950s with the beatniks and that continued into the 1960s with the hippies. This counterculture engulfed the large cohort of people born between 1946 and 1964 (baby boomers) and signaled a large-scale experimentation with illicit substances.

During the 1960s and early 1970s, many in the white baby boom cohort experimented with hallucinogenics such as marijuana and lysergic acid diethylamide (LSD). However, due to historical factors such as slavery, which was followed by exploitative labor practices on freed slaves (Williams, 1914), and the resultant institutional practice of **racial residential segregation** (Williams & Collins, 2001), the commercial activity and use of illegal drugs such as heroin and cocaine took root in black neighborhoods before it became widespread elsewhere (Johnson, Williams, Dei, & Sanabria, 1990).

Racial Residential Segregation

Racial residential segregation did not happen by chance; rather, it was the result of institutional practices, segregationist zoning ordinances, and racially restrictive covenants between private individuals (Williams & Collins, 2001). Jonnes (1996) notes that, as far back as 1950, there were reports of the resurgence of illicit drug use, but little mention was made of the fact that the new users were disproportionately black. Institutional racism and racial residential segregation resulted in little being done about the epidemic until heroin use spread to white youth of suburban America, college students, and American military personnel in Vietnam (Agar, 1994). As a result, this social choice to ignore inconvenient facts that did not impact white America led to the creation of the urban ghetto. The consequences included a lack of capital in inner-city communities and a lack of opportunity in segregated minority neighborhoods. This is consistent with the extant Chicago studies in which illegal drug use and trafficking activities were also linked to the socially disorganized sections of the city (Dai, 1935).

Targeted Marketing of Commodities

The environment consists of the physical and social settings in which we live. Researchers reason that the social environment is associated with disease and mortality risks beyond individual proximate risk factors; is a fundamental cause of racial disparities in health; and is influential in disease processes (Krieger, 2003; Lambert, Brown, Phillips, & Ialongo, 2004; Smedley et al., 2003; Storr, Chen, & Anthony, 2004; Williams & Latkin, 2007; Xanthos, Treadwell, & Holden, 2010). One of Krieger's (2003) five key pathways through which racism becomes an eco-social factor is through "**targeted marketing of commodities**" such as malt liquor (Bluthenthal et al., 2008) in African-

American communities. This targeted marketing of commodities also includes psychoactive substances, which includes illicit drugs (Krieger, 2003).

Storr and co-authors (2004) labeled the likelihood of contact with drug dealers as an unequal opportunity when they examined subgroups of people living in disadvantaged neighborhoods compared with persons living in more advantaged areas. The researchers collected data from a cross-sectional ($n = 25,000$) survey of the 1998 United States National Household Survey on Drug Abuse (NHSDA, 2009). The NHDSA used a nationally representative sample of persons age 12 or older (excluding those institutionalized). Determination of a recent drug purchase opportunity was confirmed by asking respondents: "In the past 30 days, has anyone approached you to sell an illegal drug?" They found that residents of the most disadvantaged neighborhoods had an estimated 2.2 times greater opportunity to obtain drugs than residents living in more advantaged neighborhoods and that African-Americans were at a 4.2 percent greater risk of such an interaction than were whites. The authors posit that a drug purchase opportunity can be located within the larger macrosocial context associated with disadvantage.

Media Images

In the Pope et al. study on older African-Americans and illicit drug use (2010), respondents identified several dimensions of **media images** that portrayed African-American culture and influenced African-American baby boomers: harmful, one-dimensional characterizations surrounding criminal culture/drug culture; negative characterizations; and comedic renderings. The media of film and television were the primary sources of influential one-dimensional characterization, but literature and comedic renderings also played a part.

This exposure to **negative one-dimensional characterization** led many in this cohort to think of their illicit substance abuse as the activity of a successful outlaw (Bourgois et al., 2006). Bourgois et al.'s (2006) study informs us as to how the differences in race and culture help frame the ways in which older substance abusers perceive themselves and how they are viewed by others. This cohort was inundated with negative images from both external and internal sources that influenced how drug use was perceived. External influences refer to influences from outside the community (e.g., filmmakers, television producers, and news organizations), whereas internal influences refer to influences from within the community (e.g., literature and comedic renderings from black authors and black comedians). The following excerpt from the Pope et al. (2010) study illustrates media influences on this cohort of older African-American men.

One-Dimensional Characterizations: Film

Respondent 4 from the study on older African-Americans and illicit drug use (Pope et al., 2010) expressed his views on media influence:

> *Superfly*, the movie, was, well, what they did was popularize drugs. Any time you look up a black movie, it's always about drugs, you know?

From 1963 to 1975, when this cohort was between 16 and 24 years of age, its members were exposed to more than a dozen black exploitation films. Black exploitation films had largely black casts and catered to black audiences. Many of these films had a central theme surrounding drug use/criminal lifestyles and were widely viewed by African-American baby boomers. Chief among them was *Superfly*.

Television

Respondent 6 from the study on older African-Americans and illicit drug use (Pope et al., 2010) expressed his views on media influence:

> Basically, back then there wasn't too many—I would say that was positive back then. Huh. That was black. Back in the Sixties, there wasn't many black people on TV to look at. Every time you turned on the TV, you know, it was somebody white doing something. They didn't have—the only black person on TV back then, let me see who that was, Amos and Andy. Well, they had Flip Wilson back then, but . . . you know, I didn't take him very seriously, you know? Couldn't take what he was talking about very seriously, a black man wearing a dress on TV.

During this time period, television produced stereotypical images of African-American men as buffoons (*Amos and Andy*) and cross-dressers (*The Flip Wilson Show*). The images produced on these two television programs were perhaps even more harmful than movies in their one-dimensional depictions of African-American men delivered weekly to the nation. Although few outside the African-American community saw African-American exploitation films or read popular African-American literature, many outside the African-American community watched negative depictions on television without the benefit of fact-based interactions and accepted these depictions at face value.

The media plays a substantial role in developing an individual's perception of the world and then attempts to influence the individual's thoughts, feelings, and opinions about that image. A large proportion of what we know about the world comes to us from movies, television, newspapers, and the Internet. Substance abuse is a significant problem in the African-American community, and the media serves as a gatekeeper in the social construction of racialized others (Nairn, 2006). If the media functions in this way, one can reason that framing an event or issue in terms of race increases the likelihood that the event will be understood in terms of race by the audience (Haider-Markel, Delehanty, & Beverlin, 2007; Nelson, Oxley, & Clawson, 2007). The image of African-American behavior as deviant in the newspapers, on television, and in movies is socially constructed and detrimental. Granted, these two television shows were in no way associated with drug activity in older African-American men; however, they were instrumental in negatively depicting and stigmatizing this cohort as being capable of deviant acts.

But not all of the harmful images of African-American male baby boomers were external depictions; some were generated from within the community, which made such depictions appear less exploitive. African-American author Beck produced two widely read accounts of African-American life that were negative characterizations. In *Pimp: The Story of My Life* (Beck, 1969), Beck glamorized cocaine use and the associated lifestyle. This work was followed by *Trickbaby* (Beck, 1971), which chronicled and glamorized the choices of the son of a prostitute as he led a life characterized by criminal activity and drug abuse.

Comedic Renderings

During the young adulthood of the baby boom generation, the cultural mores surrounding drug use and drug experimentation had evolved into a more accepted norm (Leary, 1965). Despite his history of drug abuse, Richard Pryor was a popular comedian who was revered by many in this cohort. Pryor's use of humor simultaneously critiqued and reinforced negative images [or stereotypes] related to illicit drug use and other issues in the African-American community.

Respondent 4 from the study on older African-Americans and illicit drug use (Pope et al., 2010) expressed his opinion on this form of media influence by noting:

> I really blame, what's the comedian's name? Richard Pryor! Richard Pryor had the media, the African American, and the white audiences listening to him. He made it like it was fun and a joke. And people went behind it.

News: Television and Print

African-American men are seen all too often on the evening news as criminals; this portrayal is sometimes justifiable, sometimes not. The "looting versus finding" phenomenon witnessed during the aftermath of Hurricane Katrina is an interesting example of media influence (Haider-Markel et al., 2007). In this scenario, African-Americans were described as criminals and whites as scavengers when securing food by any means necessary during the hurricane and flood. Respondent 5 was a Katrina survivor who tells a story related to the negative media images of African-American men that were witnessed nightly by the nation and the consequences of this depiction.

Respondent 5 from the study on older African-Americans and illicit drug use (Pope et al., 2010) expressed his opinion on negative media images:

Respondent: A black man was running from some other black dudes that was jumping on him, and beating him up. He's running and this was when they told us to stop there and wait for the buses to come. And he ran toward the police car. Before he got to the police car, police shot him.

I: How do you feel about that?

Respondent: Oh, it ain't a good feeling, but I'm looking at it, man, and I talked to police. They were protecting themselves, 'cause we done tried to kill them, and they were scared, and so at that time that might have been justifiable. It's not a good feeling, you know, but him running to the car, the police not giving him a chance. I mean it was wrong, 'cause they, you know, they coulda gave him a chance to see what was happening, but then by him running to the car, they just opened fire on him. And that's it. He dropped right there and they threw something over his head. That don't feel good to see, they just put a blanket over him and kept going up and down the street.

One can only wonder what the response of the police would have been if the man in question had not been African American. This is a case of negative media portrayal in the daily news influencing judgment. The officer was shooting at a criminal as described by the television and print news media.

Family

The theme of family and the possible loss of family because of continued use of illicit substances is an often-mentioned motivation for voluntary admission into a drug rehabilitation program. The patterned microsocial adaptations (Cicchetti & Cohen, 2006) or behaviors learned through emulation, which foster perceptions of control (Wallhagen & Lacson, 1999) to these older African-American men, are influenced by larger societal forces such as family, media images, and the environment. Merton (1968) believed that deviant behavior rather than conformist conduct sometimes manifests societal forces. Influenced by the mainstream lens but unable to engage society in the mainstream fashion, these individuals develop other avenues to reach desired goals; this often translates into participation in illicit drug activity, which conflicts with the "American Dream" and leads to a dual consciousness (Du Bois, 1903). This leads to the marginality expressed by Park (1928) and the various adaptations to external pressures by these older, substance-abusing African-American baby boomers. The data from the Pope et al. (2010) study suggest that close relationships and the context of those relationships are factors for continuing substance abuse into old age and, in some cases, beginning substance abuse in old age.

There have been numerous studies examining children of alcoholics (Heuyer, Mises, & Dereux, 1957; Rodney, 1996; Ullman & Orenstein, 1994), beginning with Heuyer et al.'s classical study in 1957. All of the cited studies suggest a relationship between family history of alcohol use and the entrance of offspring of these users into alcoholism themselves as adults. Rodney (1996) examined the literature for inconsistencies related to African Americans, and Ullman and Orenstein (1994) looked at emulation as a factor. Although less has been done in relationship to heroin abusers and their children (Bucknall & Robertson, 1985; Nichtern, 1973; Suwanwela, Kanchanahuta, & Onthuam, 1979) and even less for the relationship between cocaine users and their children (O'Brien & Anthony, 2005), the published literature suggests a relationship between family history of illicit drug use and the entrance of offspring of these users into illicit drug use themselves as adults. Below are excerpts from the Pope et al. study (2010) that illustrate the influence of family on this cohort of older African-American men.

Respondent 8 from the dissertation study on older African Americans and illicit drug use (Pope, Wallhagen, & Davis, 2010) commented about his influence on his siblings:

I: Did . . . Are you the only sibling that used drugs?

R: No, everyone except my baby brother.

I: And who was the first to use?

R: On a continuous basis, I believe I was.

I: Did you introduce them to drugs?

R: No, but by example probably.

Respondent 15 from the dissertation study on older African Americans and illicit drug use (Pope et al., 2010) noted how his family influenced his choices yet were unaware of the consequences:

I: Okay. And any of your brothers and sisters use drugs?

R: Yeah, we all were using drugs.

I: Hard street drugs?

R: Yeah, yeah, because nobody knew the gun was loaded [the impact of cocaine].

And then everybody was getting, you know, here's something new, try this, you know. Nobody knew. You didn't need to know. If we knew smoking cocaine would get you hooked 30 years later, I don't think people would do it.

Emulation of an Admired Person or Lifestyle

The two themes above—media images and family—can be viewed as significant components of a larger core category called "emulation of an admired person or lifestyle." This core category captures all aspects of emulation, including family and media images as well as those involving other, less well-defined symbolic interactions. **Emulation** is defined here as identification and imitation of a model with resources desired by the emulator (Ullman & Orenstein, 1994). It is the development of a pattern of thinking and behaviors based on an emotional attachment to that model (Ullman & Orenstein, 1994): in this case, admiration of a drug lifestyle.

The initiation of drug use is a function of symbolic interaction with other people that produces a motivation to imitate admired others. Clearly, there are elements of role modeling; yet, for the purposes of this phenomenon, it is not role modeling because such a relationship would necessitate the role model's awareness of occupying this role and purposefully influencing the individual. Emulation is an emic desire and the result of the emulator's proactive attempts to model a given role, which often goes without input from, in this case, the admired person. Further, adolescents rarely attempt to emulate lifestyles associated with economically poor resources, and this idea adds another level of understanding to emulation versus role modeling. Additionally, in families in which the substance-abusing father is held in low esteem by the non–substance-abusing mother, the rate of emulation by male teenage offspring is only 38 percent. Conversely, when the substance-abusing father is held in high esteem by the non–substance-abusing mother, the rate of emulation by male teenage offspring is 73 percent (McCord, 1988). Below are excerpts from the Pope et al. study (2010) on the emulation of admired persons, such as family members, and admired lifestyles.

Respondent 15 from the dissertation study on older African Americans and illicit drug use (Pope, 2010) mentioned an admired person and lifestyle adding further depth to the idea of emulation versus role modeling:

I: Okay. And did any of your schoolteachers make an impression on you? It's okay if they didn't.

R: Yeah, I probably had one that was a coach. I thought he was a player [i.e., a male who is skilled at manipulating or "playing" others, especially women].

I: A coach?

R: Yeah.

I: So you admired him because he had game [i.e., the ability to seduce another].

R: Yeah. He thought he had game.

I: Thought he was slick [i.e., A smooth operator]?

R: Yeah.

In the following example, the same respondent expressed admiration for certain people and their lifestyles:

> **R:** I was in the county jail. Me and about one or two cats [men] on our tier—we were the youngest guys up there—everybody up there was all hardcore dope fiends and stuff. And they used to talk about it all the time—the Puerto Ricans and the blacks that was up there. Everybody'd talk about it and stuff. I thought it was the coolest thing going—all these cats been in the penitentiary, living this lifestyle, you know, kinda attracted my attention because I wanted a part of that lifestyle. Cause I'd been on the streets for I don't know how long, doing my little old stuff. So that part of it appealed to me and I'm looking at all these musicians—jazz musicians that I knew that were getting high—Miles Davis and all them cats and stuff, you know, getting high and shit and you see 'em in they little nods [to doze off when high on opiates] and looked so cool [laid back and relaxed] and shit. You know, I'm like, yeah that's hip [trendy] there, yeah, and I want to be this little hip cat.

Emulation has been suggested here as a point of initiation and provides insight into the question of why an individual might begin illicit drug use at a young age. It does not, however, fully address the reasons why one would continue this use into old age nor why a person 55 years of age or older might begin illicit drug use. Several of the respondents made explicit remarks concerning targeted marketing of commodities in their communities and suggested that the environment was a factor in their continued drug use after initiation and into old age.

Environment

As was stated earlier, the environment consists of the physical and social settings in which we live and may be instrumental in one's decision to participate in commercial drug activity.

Commercial Drug Activity

Disadvantaged, largely black communities in America have been inundated with **commercial drug activity**. The supply and demand of commercial drugs in these communities has taken on an open-air-market quality through corner drug sales, largely unabated by law enforcement, and a fast-food approach to delivering the product. Although financial status dictates the likelihood that one will partake in fine dining, fast-food restaurants offer a product that is cheap and can be consumed daily if an individual chose to do so. One fast-food franchise boasted "over one million" served, and this appropriately reflects the higher trends of illicit drug use in disadvantaged black neighborhoods. Many in the mainstream will dismiss the findings from the discourse on how drugs became pervasive in this community as conspiratorial in tone, but historical factors such as the Tuskegee experiment and the CIA Contra Crack controversy are powerful reasons for African-American mistrust of researchers and government entities. It has been well documented that, in the Tuskegee experiment, the government knowingly withheld treatment from African-American patients infected with syphilis to advance scientific research (Gray, 1998; Jones, 1981; Reverby, 2000; Washington, 2007). It has also been reported that, for the better part of a decade, a San Francisco Bay area drug ring sold huge amounts of cocaine to the Crips and Bloods (street gangs of Los Angeles) and funneled millions in drug profits to a Latin American guerrilla army run by the U.S. Central Intelligence Agency (Bewley-Taylor, 2001), further fueling this dual consciousness felt by many in the African-American community. Seemingly, furthering research and waging a war in Latin America at the expense of lives within the African-American community appeared acceptable to some within the U.S. government.

Several respondents in the Pope et al. study (2010) made tacit references to government conspiracies to "confine drugs" or target marketing of such commodities in African-American neighborhoods. Combine these findings with the recently televised response to the plight of African-American victims of Hurricane Katrina in New Orleans by the government, and it is understandable how a dual consciousness has developed in this community. The government's less-than-enthusiastic response to Hurricane Katrina's primarily African-American victims is a powerful example of malfeasance for those within this community to combat the notion that victimization and oppression are imagined.

The discourse on the pervasiveness of drugs in the African-American community became apparent while considering the reasons why contemporary African Americans are reluctant to participate in research. The Tuskegee experiment and its consequences and the Rodney King incident must also have seemed unthinkable to the mainstream when first uncovered, and yet both are points of fact. This thinking also led to the discourse of African Americans as an oppressed people who live in an area that has easy access to and casual attitudes toward drugs in their neighborhoods as acceptable as narrated by the perceived oppressors. Clearly, there is a need to refine the field's theoretical understanding of the social determinants associated with substance abuse among African-American male baby boomers and the consequences of substance abuse.

Respondent 2 from the study on older African Americans and illicit drug use (Pope et al., 2010) commented:

> I: Okay. You know, after you started using street drugs, what things kept you using them?
>
> R: Uh . . .
>
> I: Why do you think you—was it just addiction, or was it . . .
>
> R: It, it was being accepted into a certain environment. You know what I'm saying? It's, it's like even if I go away for one or two or three years, and I can come back and go right back to the corner of the drug use . . .

When discussing environmental influences, Respondent 2 from the study on older African Americans and illicit drug use (Pope et al., 2010) said:

> R: Yeah, see your environment is really a large portion of your makeup.
>
> I: Now when you say environment, what do you mean?
>
> R: I'm talking about the people in your community.
>
> I: Elaborate on that, there are people in every community. What do you mean about that?
>
> R: I say, in the community in which I was the environment is infested with people that are using drugs.

Respondent 12 from the dissertation study on older African Americans and illicit drug use (Pope et al., 2010) had the following observations about environmental influences:

> I: And when you came back out [of jail] did you use again? Talk to me in general.
>
> R: When I was in jail and then I come out, I stayed clean for awhile but I got back into the same crowd. I was hanging out with that same crowd of users and sellers.
>
> I: I guess by being back into that environment, the temptation was too great not to indulge back into the drugs.

Respondent 16 from the dissertation study on older African Americans and illicit drug use (Pope et al., 2010) expressed environmental influence as follows:

> R: Let me finish with this. I rebuilt that house—11 years—on that corner in West Oakland but the environment was too polluted. They throw

cocaine in the yard. I picked it up. I hid it. . . . The next thing I know I'm back in the nest [den of iniquity]. I talked to my brother in Hayward and he said: "Look, you know, it's better to let the house go if you can't handle it." I sold the house and moved over here in 2000. Because I know me, that girl [heroin] and me just don't get along. I can't be around anybody doing it.

I: So, [it's] environmental.

R: I call it environment pollutant, so it was better for me to leave the house.

Respondent 13 from the dissertation study on older African-Americans and illicit drug use (Pope et al., 2010) expressed environmental influence in this way:

> **I:** Okay, so tell me what your thoughts are on the environment and drug use.
>
> **R:** Well, it's simple as this, man. As far as if you say you want to quit using drugs, you can't be around a drug dealer when he's selling drugs. You can't be upstairs if somebody's selling drugs downstairs, something you love, something you like. That's like saying I don't like a girl, but she keeps coming in front of me. You understand me? Now you tell me, okay, I'm trying to stay in a drug-free environment. Now how are you going to quit using drugs if your buddy's sticking himself, and you know you want it. . . . So now you're thinking about all the excuses in your head. Man, should I do this? I'm just going to shoot a little bit. I'm just going to shoot a few ccs, right? And you plum well get caught up. You get caught up every time, man. . . .

Not all illicit drug use in older African-American males begins in adolescence, however, as this next exemplar evidences. Only Respondent 7 out of the 20 male respondents discussed late-onset addiction. He was a 51-year-old non-user until the death of his wife, which would suggest that he was responding to late-life stressors; however, he still credits environmental influences with the development of his late-life addiction to drugs.

Respondent 7 from the dissertation study on older African Americans and illicit drug use (Pope et al., 2010) discussed his late-onset drug use:

> **R:** My immediate environment. The guys around me where I used to live. I lived in the Ingleview district, the Lakeside district, and, after that, I started using drugs.
>
> **I:** So, that was in '89? How old were you in 1989?
>
> **R:** Let's see . . .
>
> **I:** This is 2008, huh, let's make it 2009, that was about 20 years ago. So you were like 51 years old?

R: Yeah, something like that.

I: You began after the death of your wife?

R: Yeah, after the . . .

I: You hadn't used before that?

R: No, I hadn't.

This latter quotation suggests that, although environment plays a role in drug use across the life span, the determinants of drug use in later life may be distinct from those involved in promoting drug use during adolescence or early adulthood. The unique experiences of older adults and specific stressors, such as the loss of a spouse or job, may be more pertinent to adopting a drug habit later in life. However, in the Pope et al. study (2010) there were insufficient data on which to make generalizations about late onset drug use. Differences in the possible triggers for entry into drug use, if confirmed by future studies, may suggest the need for different interventions for late versus early onset users.

Emulation

Emulation and role modeling are closely related concepts. However, in African-American culture, role modeling is most often framed as an etic account, "He serves as a civic role model for young men in his community," whereas emulation is most often framed as an emic account, "I want to be as popular as he is." Some will reason that role models are *emulated* and there will be no argument over that point within the confines of this discussion. The argument here, however, is that conceptually; the act of emulation and the act of role modeling are inversely related. They can occur simultaneously but are viewed from two different perspectives. Emulation is most often thought of in negative terms—a copying of undesired social characteristics or actions such as those that facilitate drug use. Conversely, role modeling is often positive, depicting socially desirable aspects and, therefore, can serve as a protective barrier against entry into substance abuse. Emulation of admired behavior of humans by other humans, unlike the emulation reproduced in the laboratory model by lab rats, occurs in no predictable temporal pattern (Panlilio, Thorndike, & Schindler, 2009), making it difficult to pinpoint an appropriate time for intervention to prevent unwanted social behaviors. Yet, numerous studies suggest the connection between emulation and illicit drug use by adolescents (Brook, Duan, & Brook, 2007; Hoffmann & Cerbone, 2002; Lam et al., 2004), and intervention studies of adolescents related to emulation are needed.

Theoretical Framework for Illicit Drug Use in Older African Americans

Policy Implications

Given our current limited understanding of drug use and abuse in this population, the appropriate function of any theoretical model is to stimulate new work in the area. Increasingly, health researchers have focused on the recognition that health outcomes emerge from both individual behaviors and complex interactions among a myriad of social and environmental factors. Differences in incidence and prevalence of illicit drug use exist across racial, ethnic, and socioeconomic groups. The well-documented research in health disparities suggests that factors beyond individual choices affect the health of individuals and lead to health disparities. With respect to illicit drug use in older African Americans, although health disparities across socioeconomic lines have been established in the literature, the underlying dynamics that contribute to these disparities are not fully understood. Predictive modeling methods could be applied to guide public policy in addressing the social determinants of health and to provide new insights for policy makers. The aim is to reframe the discussion of the social determinants of substance abuse by older African Americans. Such a model would serve as a useful tool for evaluating public health policies for their potential to reduce health disparities with respect to illicit drug use in older African Americans.

The belief that an individual is powerless to affect the environment and cope with stress plays a central role in illicit drug use, and internal thoughts and beliefs are factors in the development of maladaptive behavior. This supports the hypothesis that an individual's belief in the ability to control a situation strongly influences behavior.

The Organizing Concepts

Three assumptions underpin the conceptual framework designed to examine illicit drug use in older African Americans. These have been derived from the perspective that the concepts of both race and perceived control are situationally emergent (Brouillette & Turner, 1992; Lawton, 1982) constructs that can lead to role strain and role deprivation.

These concepts are: (1) race is significant to African Americans and is defined by existing race relations within a given historical period; (2) lower perceived environmental control contributes to drug activity and, as one ages, perceived control arises from contingencies based on learned experience; and (3) role strain and role deprivation lead to drug dependence. Omi and Winant's (1994) Racial Formation Theory helps locate race historically as the principal tenet of social

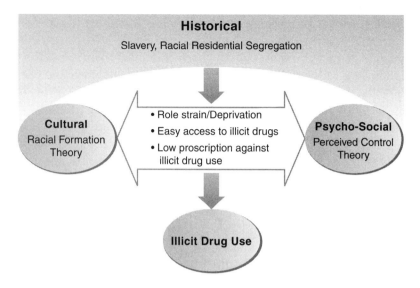

Figure 10.1. Historical–Cultural Psychosocial Model of Illicit Drug Use in Older African-Americans

order and organization in America, and Townsend and Belgrade (2000) recognize the significance of racial identity to African-Americans. Wallhagen's (1998) Perceived Control Theory examines the environment and offers a reframing of perceived control from a person–environment model that separates the sense of control from factors that may promote this experience. It has also been demonstrated that drug activity can result from lower perceived control and contingency (Lambert et al., 2004). Winick's (1974) Sociological Theory for the Genesis of Drug Dependence proposes that it is possible to locate within the social system the structural sources of role strain and deprivation that can lead to drug dependence. The organizing concepts in Figure 10.1 lay a foundation on which we may begin to seek information about the social determinants of substance abuse in older African-American men.

Summary

The questions that directed this inquiry into the social determinants of illicit drug use in older African Americans can now be expanded to explore the ways in which an analysis of empiricism and human science have contributed to an understanding of the phenomenon of substance abuse in older African Americans. Empiricists will insist that, if it exists, it can be measured, and there will be no argument over that point within the confines of this summary. However, constructionists would argue that such measurements offer little epistemological insight, only magnitude, and that essence is subjective and must be gained from an emic point of view. The older African-American male illicit drug users in the Pope et al. (2010) study offer insights unobtainable from any other source; they provide a view from within. For many, addiction begins as a way to deal with problems. However, unlike others in the same cohort, older African-American males often saw themselves as successful outlaws (Bourgois et al., 2006). Emulation (in adolescence) of an admired person or lifestyle was often mentioned as the catalyst for entry into illicit drug use and environment as the reason for continued abuse by these older African-American male illicit drug users. The need for an interdisciplinary approach to address this public health concern is clear because the social determinants of substance abuse, such as environment and larger societal forces, cannot be addressed by a single discipline or fulfilled by a mandate that clinicians move to an interdisciplinary approach. There must be a concerted effort from many disciplines to achieve a plan of care for this growing population.

Key Terms

commercial drug activity

emulation

media images

negative one-dimensional
characterization

racial residential segregation

targeted marketing of commodities

Discussion Questions

1. What was one of the first clear health indicators of illicit drug use among older African-American males? What physical and psychosocial health problems are these older African-American male illicit drug users at risk for?

2. The advertisement and marketing of malt liquor in African-American communities is an example of what social determinant? Relate the slogan "over one million sold" and a fast-food approach to illicit drug use in African-American communities.

3. Why is adolescent illicit drug use a concern for illicit drug use in older African-American males?

4. What are black exploitation films and what role did they play in influencing illicit drug use in this cohort of older African-American males? What is emulation and how does it relate to family and admired lifestyles?

Note

1. This chapter draws largely from R. Pope, M. Wallhagen, and H. Davis. (2010). The social determinants of substance abuse in African American baby boomers: Effects of family, media images, and environment. *Journal of Transcultural Nursing, 21*(3), 246–256. Copyright Sage (2010).

References

Agar, M. (1994, April–June). A heroin epidemic at the intersection of histories: The 1960s epidemic among African-Americans in Baltimore. *Medical Anthropology, 21*(2), 115–156.

Barton, A. (2003). *Illicit drugs*. New York, NY: Routledge.

Beck, R. (1969). *Pimp: The story of my life*. Los Angeles, CA: Holoway House.

Beck, R. (1971). *Trickbaby*. Los Angeles, CA: Holoway House.

Berridge, V., & Mars, S. (2004). History of addictions. *Journal of Epidemiology and Community, 58*, 747–750.

Bewley-Taylor, D. (2001). Cracks in the conspiracy: The CIA and the cocaine trade in south central Los Angeles. *International Journal of Drug Policy, 12*, 167–180.

Bluthenthal, R., Cohen, D., Farley, T., Scribner, R., Beighley, C., Schonlau, M., & Robinson, P. (2008, March). Alcohol availability and neighborhood characteristics in Los Angeles, California and Southern Louisiana. *Journal of Urban Health, 85*(2), 191–205.

Bourgois, P., Martinez, A., Kral, A., Edlin, B. R., Schonberg, J., & Ciccarone, D. (2006). Reinterpreting ethnic patterns among white and African American men who inject heroin: A social science of medicine approach. *PLoS Medicine, 3*(10), e452.

Brook, J., Duan, T., & Brook, D. (2007). Fathers who abuse drugs and their adolescent children: Longitudinal predictors of adolescent aggression. *American Journal on Addictions, 16, 5*, 410–417.

Brouillette, J., & Turner, R. (1992). Creating the sociological imagination on the first day of class: The social construction of deviance teaching sociology. *Teaching Sociology, 20*(4), 276–279).

Bucknall, A., & Robertson, J. (1985). Heroin misuse and family medicine. *Family Practice, 2*(4), 244–251.

Centers for Disease Control and Prevention. (2003). *Statistics and trends: Basic statistics, surveillance reports, populations at risk, trends*. Retrieved from http://www.cdc.gov/hiv/topics/aa/index.htm

Cicchetti, D., & Cohen, D. (2006). *Developmental psychopathology: Developmental neuroscience*. Hoboken, NJ: Wiley.

Courtwright, D. (1983). The hidden epidemic: Opiate addiction and cocaine use in the south. *Journal of Southern History, 49*(1), 57–72.

Dai, B., (1935). *Opiate addiction in Chicago*. Unknown binding.

Du Bois, W. (1903). *The souls of black folks*. Chicago, IL: McClurg.

Gfroefer, J., Penne, M., Pemberton, M., & Folsom, R. (2003). Substance abuse treatment need among older adults in 2020: The impact of the aging baby boom cohort. *Drug and Alcohol Dependence, 69*, 127–135.

Gray, F. (1998). *The Tuskegee syphilis study: The real story and beyond.* Montgomery, AL: New South Books.

Haider-Markel, D., Delehanty, W., & Beverlin, M. (2007). Media framing and racial attitudes in the aftermath of Katrina. *Policy Studies Journal, 35,* 587–605.

Heuyer, G., Mises, R., & Dereux, J. (1957). Off-spring of alcoholics. *Presse Medicine, 65*(29), 657–658.

Himmelstein, J. (1983). From killer weed to drop-out drug: The changing ideology of marihuana. *Crime, Law and Social Change, 7*(1), 13–38.

Hoffmann, J., & Cerbone, F. (2002). Parental substance use disorder and the risk of adolescent drug abuse: An event history analysis. *Drug and Alcohol Dependency, 66,* 255–264.

Johnson, B., Williams, T., Dei, K., & Sanabria, H. (1990). Drug abuse in the inner city: Impact on hard-drug users and the community. *Crime and Justice, 13,* 9–67.

Jones, J. H. (1981). *Bad blood: The Tuskegee syphilis experiment.* New York, NY: Free Press.

Jonnes, J. *1996 hep-cats, narcs, and pipe dreams: A history of America's romance with illegal drugs.* New York, NY: Scribner.

Krieger, N. (2003). Does racism harm health? Did child abuse exist before 1962? On explicit questions, critical science, and current controversies: An ecosocial perspective. *American Journal of Public Health, 93*(2), 194–199.

Lam, W., Wechsberg, J., & Zule, W. (2004). African-American women who use crack cocaine: A comparison of mothers who live with and have been separated from their children. *Child Abuse & Neglect Journal, 28*(11), 229–247.

Lambert, S., Brown, T., Phillips, C., & Ialongo, N. (2004). The relationship between perceptions of neighborhood characteristics and substance use among urban African American adolescents. *American Journal of Community Psychology, 34*(3–4), 205–218.

Lawton, M. (1982). Competence, environmental press, and the adaptation of older people. In M. P. Lawton, P. G. Windley, & T. O. Byerts (Eds.), *Aging and the environment: Theoretical approaches* (pp. 33–59). New York: Springer.

Leary, T. (1965). *Turn on, tune in, drop out.* Oakland, CA: Ronin.

McCord, J. (1988). Identifying developmental paradigms leading to alcoholism. *Journal of Studies on Alcohol, 49,* 357–362.

McCormack, N. A. (1988). Substance abuse among Vietnam veterans: A view from the cap control perspective. *International Journal of Addiction, 23*(12), 1311–1316.

Merton, R. (1968). *Social theory and social structure.* New York, NY: Free Press.

Modell, W. (1957). The search for a morphine substitute. *American Journal of Nursing, 57*(12), 1565–1567.

Musto, D. (1989b). Evolution of American attitudes toward substance abuse. *Annual of NY Academy of Science, 562,* 3–7.

Musto, D. (1991). Opium, cocaine and marijuana in American history. *Science America, 265*(1), 40–47.

Musto, D. (1992). Cocaine's history, especially the American experience. *Ciba Funded Symposium, 166,* 7–14; discussion 14–19.

Nairn, R. (2006). Media, racism and public health psychology. *Journal of Health Psychology, 11*(2), 183–196.

National Household Survey on Drug Abuse (NHSDA). (1999). Washington, DC: U.S. Government Printing Office.

Nelson, T., Oxley, Z., & Clawson, R. (1997). Toward a psychology of framing effects. *Political Behavior*, *19*, 221–246.

Nichtern, S. (1973). The children of drug users. *Journal of American Academy of Childhood Psychiatry*, *12*, 24–31.

O'Brien, M., & Anthony, J. (2005). Risk of becoming cocaine dependent: Epidemiological estimates for the United States, 2000–2001. *Neuropsychopharmacology*, *30*, 1006–1018.

Omi, M., & Winant, H. (1994) *Racial formation in the United States: From the 1960s to the 1990s*. New York, NY: Rutledge.

Panlilio, L., Thorndike, E., & Schindler, C. (2009). A stimulus-control account of dysregulated drug intake. *Pharmacology, Biochemistry and Behavior*, *92*, 439–447.

Park, R. (1928). Human migration and the marginal man. *American Journal of Sociology*, *33*, 881–893.

Pope, R., Wallhagen, M., & Davis, H. (2010). Social determinants of substance abuse in African American baby boomers: The effects of family, media images, and environment. *Journal of Transcultural Nursing*, *21*(2).

Reverby, S. (2000). *Tuskegee's truths: Rethinking the Tuskegee syphilis study*. Chapel Hill: University of North Carolina Press.

Rodney, H. (1996). Inconsistencies in the literature on collegiate adult children of alcoholics: Factors to consider for African Americans. *Journal of American Collegiate Health*, *45*(1), 19–25.

Smedley, B., Stith, A., & Nelson, A. (2003). *Unequal treatment: Confronting racial and ethnic disparities in health care*. Washington, DC: National Academies Press.

Stanton, M. D. (1976). Drugs, Vietnam, and the Vietnam veteran: An overview. *American Journal of Drug and Alcohol Abuse*, *3*, 557–570.

Storr, C., Chen, C., & Anthony, J. (2004). "Unequal opportunity": Neighborhood disadvantage and the chance to buy illegal drugs. *Journal of Epidemiology and Community Health*, *58*, 231–237.

Suwanwela, C., Kanchanahuta, S., & Onthuam, Y. (1979). Hill tribe opium addicts: A retrospective study of 1,382 patients. *Bulletin of Narcotics*, *31*(1), 23–40.

Teff, H. (1972). Drugs and the law: The development of control. *Modern Law Review*, *35*(3), 225–241.

Townsend, T., & Belgrade, F. (2000). The impact of personal identity and racial identity on drug attitudes and use among African American children. *Journal of Black Psychology*, *26*(4), 421–436.

Ullman, A., & Orenstein, A. (1994). Why some children of alcoholics become alcoholics: Emulation of the drinker. *Adolescence*, *2*(113), 1–11.

Wallhagen, M. (1998). Perceived control theory: A recontextualized perspective. *Journal of Clinical Geropsychology*, *4*(2), 119–140.

Wallhagen, M., & Lacson, M. (1999). Perceived control and psychosocial/physiological functioning in African American elders with type 2 diabetes. *Diabetes Educator*, *25*, 568–575.

Washington, H. (2007). *Medical apartheid: The dark history of medical experimentation on black Americans from colonial times to the present.* New York, NY: Random House.

Willengbring, M. (Writer) (2006). *Understanding relapse, addiction.* United States: HBO.

Williams, C., & Latkin, C. (2007). Neighborhood socioeconomic status, personal network attributes, and use of heroin and cocaine. *American Journal of Preventive Medicine, 32*(6, Suppl.), S203–S210.

Williams, D., & Collins, C. (2001). Racial residential segregation: A fundamental cause of racial disparities in health. *Public Health Reports, 116,* 404–416.

Williams, E. (1914, February 8). Negro cocaine "fiends" are a new southern menace. *New York Times,* p. 1.

Winick, C. (1974). *Sociological aspects of drug dependence.* New York, NY: CRC Press.

Xanthos, C., Treadwell, H., & Holden, K. (2010). Social determinants of health among African-American men. *Journal of Men's Health, 7,* 11–19.

Part Three

Social Determinants
of Health Care

Chapter 11

Prejudiced Providers

Unequal Treatment as a Determinant of African-American Men's Health

Clare Xanthos

Learning Objectives

- Appreciate the role of **unequal treatment** as a determinant of **African-American men**'s health.
- Acquire an overview of **health care inequities** affecting African-American men.
- Understand the role of **provider-level factors** (**health care interactions**) in health care inequities affecting African-American men.
- Understand the role of provider-level factors (**health care decisions**) in health care inequities affecting African-American men.
- Gain an awareness of potential strategies for addressing provider-level health care inequities affecting African-American men.

• • •

African-American ("African American" and "black" are used interchangeably throughout this chapter) men face well-documented, staggering health care inequities, which are associated with appreciably higher rates of morbidity and mortality as compared with their white counterparts. A full understanding of the social determinants of health among African-American men must include an account of these health care inequities. Although the better-known **social determinants of health** include low income, poor housing, poor neighborhood conditions, environmental hazards, and poor educational opportunities, unequal treatment is an often overlooked **health care risk factor** and **social risk factor** that determines health. As with other social risk factors, health care risk factors are to be distinguished from behavioral risk factors as being beyond the individual's control. In other words, these risk factors are not linked to the individual's behavior; rather, they are caused by societal stereotypes and biases that impact health providers' behavior, which leads to health care inequities.

Much of the existing public health literature on the topic of **health care disparities** affecting African-American men does not take a "social determinants of health approach"; more exactly, it reflects the predominant public health perspective on African-American men, which frequently focuses on behavioral risk factors or "**patient-level factors**" as significant causes of the health care disparities affecting them. Thus, existing literature often characterizes this population as "hard to reach" with "poor **help-seeking attitudes and behaviors**" (e.g., mistrust of the health care system, poor health literacy, negative attitudes toward screening services, inadequate utilization of health services). The role of "provider-level factors" (**stereotyping** and **bias** among health care providers) in health care disparities affecting African-American men has been virtually ignored in public health literature, yet there has been emerging evidence, which points to the significance of provider-level factors in racial health care disparities. Although a body of literature on this topic is slowly developing, there is nothing that specifically addresses this issue in relation to the health care of African-American men. The goal of this chapter is to take the first steps toward filling this gap, and lay the foundation for considering unequal treatment in health care as a determinant of African-American men's health. African-American men's health care is impacted by other social risk factors (e.g., insurance status, residential segregation), but the scope of this chapter is to review what has not been covered elsewhere, that is, the role of provider-level factors in the health care inequities affecting this population.

First, this chapter presents an *overview of inequities in health care affecting African-American men* (e.g., health care inequities in cancer, cardiovascular disease, kidney disease, HIV/AIDs, mental health). Second, it critically assesses *the role of provider-level factors in health care inequities affecting African-American men*, including a definition of provider-level factors, and the key ways in which provider-level factors manifest themselves (through health care interactions and health care decisions among health care providers and African-American men). Third, the author *offers suggestions for reducing provider-level health care inequities affecting African-American men.* These include:

- Conducting interventions that reduce racial bias among health care providers
- New legislation to reduce health care discrimination
- Increasing the number of African-American physicians
- Increasing research on provider-level health care inequities

Health Care Inequities Affecting African-American Men: An Overview

In discussing social determinants of health care inequities affecting African-American men, the first step is to provide an overview of the health care inequities affecting this population. The lower quality health care provided to African Americans, as compared with the majority population, is well documented in the public health research literature. African-American men are impacted by lower quality health care across a wide range of disease areas and medical services. A variety of examples are cited below with reference to the health care inequities between African-American men and their white counterparts.

Cancer

- Black men are less likely to receive "definitive therapy" (the most effective therapies for prostate cancer) (Underwood et al., 2004).
- African-American men's prostate cancer is more likely to be handled initially through "watchful waiting" (i.e., defer immediate prostate cancer treatment). This cannot be adequately explained by racial differences in the characteristics of the disease or life expectancy (Shavers et al., 2004a).
- African-American men on a watchful waiting protocol receive disproportionately low medical monitoring visits and procedures. These disparities cannot be explained by the characteristics of the disease or socio-demographic characteristics (Shavers et al., 2004b).
- African-American men who have been diagnosed with prostate cancer are less likely to receive treatment with "curative intent" (TCI) (the goal of the treatment is to cure the patient). These differences cannot be explained by characteristics of the disease or sociodemographic characteristics (Richert-Boe et al., 2008).

Cardiovascular Disease

- Black men are less likely to be recommended for "coronary artery bypass grafting" (CABG) (a surgery that improves blood flow to the heart) than either white men or black women (van Ryn, Burgess, Malat, & Griffin, 2006). In the study conducted by van Ryn et al. (2006), 21 percent of black men received a recommendation for CABG, as compared with 40 percent of white men, and 40 percent of black women.

- Black men are less likely to receive "reperfusion therapy" (a potentially life-saving therapy which restores blood flow to tissues and organs) than white men (Canto et al., 2000).

Cerebrovascular Disease (Leading to Stroke)

- African-American men are less likely to be prescribed a life-saving medication for ischemic stroke (Courtenay, 2002).

Kidney Disease

- Black men with end-stage-renal-disease (ESRD) frequently receive inferior care as compared with their white counterparts (Felix-Aaron et al., 2005).

- African-American men and women with ESRD are less likely to receive a kidney transplant than other racial/ethnic groups (Navaneethan & Singh, 2006). Further, African-American men are less likely than white men to be referred for evaluation at a transplantation center (53.9 percent versus 76.2 percent) (Ayanian, Cleary, Weissman, & Epstein, 1999). These disparities could not be accounted for by patients' preferences and attitudes about transplantation, socio-demographic characteristics, dialysis facilities, perceptions about care, health status, or the characteristics of the disease (Ayanian et al., 1999).

HIV/AIDs

- HIV-positive black men who have sex with men (MSM) are less likely than HIV-positive white MSM to be on "antiretroviral therapy" (ART) (a drug that suppresses the progression of HIV) (Millett, Flores, Peterson, & Bakeman, 2007).

Mental Health

- Black men are overdiagnosed with schizophrenia at five times the rate of other racial/ethnic and gender groups (Metzl, 2009).

- Recent studies suggest that in primary care settings, depressed African Americans are often underdiagnosed and ineffectively treated (Das, Olfson, McCurtis, & Weissman, 2006). For example, black Medicaid patients diagnosed with depression are less likely to be treated with newer antidepressant medications (which have fewer side effects than the older antidepressant medications) (Sambamoorthi, Olfson, Wei, & Crystal, 2006). Waldman et al. (2009) found depression-care disparities to be particularly marked among African-American men, with only 22 percent of moderately-to-severely depressed African-American men receiving treatment with antidepressant medication as compared with 43 percent of white men.

Hospital Services

- African-American men are more likely to experience difficulties obtaining insurance authorization when accessing emergency care than their white counterparts (Courtenay, 2002).

Although racial inequities in health care are disconcerting in and of themselves, they are associated with worse health outcomes, making them even more troubling (Smedley, Stith, & Nelson, 2002). Indeed, a study conducted by Peterson et al. (1997) indicated that the lower levels of coronary artery bypass surgery among African Americans was a key factor in the racial disparity in five-year survival rates among heart disease patients. Thus, racial inequities in medical care affecting African-American men have important implications for their health outcomes in the respective disease areas.

Finally, it is important to note that the above examples of health care inequities affecting this population are not meant to be exhaustive; rather, they are intended to provide a snapshot of the types of inequities faced by African-American men when they access health services.

The Role of Provider-Level Factors in Health Care Inequities Affecting African-American Men

In studying the social risk factors that contribute to health care inequities affecting African-American men, this chapter focuses on a major set of health care risk factors known as "provider-level factors" (see Smedley et al., 2002). Provider-level factors refer to biases, stereotypes, and clinical uncertainty among health care providers (Smedley et al., 2002). There are two key ways in which provider-level factors manifest themselves—*health care interactions* and *health care decisions* (Penner, Albrecht, Coleman, & Norton, 2007). Health care interactions refer to in-person patient–provider communication, which can lead to health care inequities, while health care decisions refer to health care providers' diagnosis and treatment decisions, which similarly can result in health care inequities (Penner et al., 2007). In short, provider-level factors are significant health care risk factors and social risk factors that can contribute to unequal treatment in health care and, as such, constitute an important social determinant of health (see McGibbon, Etowa, & McPherson, 2008).

Provider-level factors should be distinguished from the other identified causes of health care disparities—"**health system-level factors**" and "patient-level factors" (Penner et al., 2007). Health system-level factors are associated with socioeconomic variables (e.g., low incomes, medically underserved neighborhoods) that affect access to quality health care (e.g., quality health insurance plans, quality primary care practices, and hospitals). Although health system-level factors clearly affect access to health care, health care inequities persist among populations with the same health insurance plans and medical facilities (Penner et al., 2007).

Patient-level factors consist of patients' attitudes and behaviors, which can have an effect on their health care outcomes (Penner et al., 2007; Smedley et al., 2002). As indicated in the introduction, much of the existing literature discussing health care disparities affecting African-American men focuses on these patient-level factors, which are associated with poor help-seeking attitudes and behaviors. Examples of work with this perspective include studies of African-American men's mistrust of the health care system (Blocker et al., 2006), poor health literacy (see Friedman, Corwin, Dominick, & Rose, 2009), negative attitudes toward screening services (Blocker et al., 2006), inadequate utilization of health services (Richardson, Webster, & Fields, 2004), and interventions that have focused on improving African-American men's health behavior (see, for example, Taylor et al., 2006). Although patient-level factors obviously play a role in health care inequities, they do not adequately account for these inequities (see Ayanian et al., 1999).

Provider-level factors are often overlooked in the literature pertaining to African-American health, especially *the effect of provider-level factors on patient-level factors.* Diala et al. (2000) found that, before using mental health services, African Americans' mental health help-seeking attitudes were similar to or more positive than whites': however, following the receipt of mental health services, African Americans held more negative attitudes towards mental health services, and were not as likely to seek help again as compared with their white counterparts. As such, provider behavior may have a significant impact on help-seeking behavior among African Americans. (This issue is further explored later in this section.)

Provider-level factors are considered in depth in the following section in relation to health care interactions and health care decisions affecting African-American men.

The Social Determinants of Health Care Interactions and Health Care Decisions in Health Care Encounters with African-American Men

An emerging literature indicates that health care interactions and health care decisions are often influenced by the social stereotypes and biases that health care providers have about their patients (see, for example, Penner et al., 2010;

van Ryn et al., 2006). Certainly, in wider society, African-American men are often subjected to significant stereotyping. Woods, Montgomery, Belliard, Ramírez-Johnson, and Wilson (2004, p. 394) note that "the dominant stereotypic perception of black men in American society as a 'bad guy' (e.g., thug, drug dealer) often limits the opportunity for a positive patient–physician relationship and black male engagement." In a similar vein, in the health care setting, Malebranche (2004, p. 223) observes the frequency with which black men are labeled as "'aggressive,' 'threatening,' 'difficult,' or . . . 'noncompliant'" when they ask questions, also pointing out that "the same physicians refer to white male patients who ask similar questions as 'well-read,' 'inquisitive,' or 'knowledgeable.'"

The above-mentioned observations are consistent with the theory that physicians are more likely to hold negative stereotypes of black patients than white patients (Penner et al., 2007). This also corresponds with research. In a study that measured physicians' **implicit and explicit attitudes** about race, Sabin, Nosek, Greenwald, and Rivara (2009) found that physicians showed implicit preferences for whites over blacks. In another study (van Ryn & Burke, 2000) physicians generally had more negative stereotypes regarding African Americans as compared to whites. For example, physicians were more likely to view black patients as being potentially noncompliant, would-be substance abusers, and were less likely to perceive black patients as intelligent or to feel positive about black patients.

Health Care Interactions   Perhaps not surprisingly, a significant number of African-American men have experienced negative interactions with health care providers. In a study conducted by Woods et al. (2004), 62.8 percent of black men considered that their race/ethnicity was the reason for the poor treatment that they received, and 58.6 percent believed that their race/ethnicity affected the quality of care that they received. Respondents were discouraged by their verbal and nonverbal communications with health care providers, describing a lack of respectful interaction, as well as generally limited interaction with health care providers (Woods et al., 2004). This is consistent with the findings of other studies documenting negative health care experiences among black men (Malebranche, Peterson, Fullilove, & Stackhouse, 2004; Ravenell, Whitaker, & Johnson, 2008). Interestingly, these studies (Malebranche et al., 2004; Ravenell et al., 2008) indicate that the stereotyping of African-American men, lack of respect, and lack of interaction may be as significant among foreign-born physicians (often non-white) as it is among their white American counterparts. Drawing on their study of barriers to health care among African-American men, Ravenell et al. (2008, p. 1157) quote the following remark from one participant: "Every time I go to the hospital . . . I'm getting a foreign doctor who barely speaks English and they treat me like a young black hoodlum so you know it's like, why even go." In a similar vein, in a study that explored perceptions of health care among black men who have sex with men, Malebranche et al. (2004, p. 103) cite a number of respondents' comments on this issue, including "[I've] seen some [foreign doctors] interact with white patients in a more personable, more sociable [*sic*] . . . but when it comes to black patients, some of them are like, 'whatever,' and they'll just do this and do that."

Negative health care interactions can lead to *negative help-seeking behavior and the underutilization of health services*, which is well documented among African-American men. Malebranche (2004) considers that the negative stereotyping of black men is a significant factor in men losing an interest in their own health care (e.g., reluctance to seek medical help, refusal of tests, noncompliance with medication regimens). This is consistent with Woods et al.'s (2004) study, which indicated that negative health care interactions had a significant impact on preventive health behavior among black men. In short, contemporary negative health care interactions can lead to "cultural mistrust" in the health care system (see Whaley, 2004) and "negative help-seeking behavior" among this population. It is worth noting the distinction between *cultural mistrust based on ongoing discrimination* as opposed to *historical mistrust* of health services. This is pointed out because public health literature often focuses on African American mistrust of the health care system in terms of historical mistrust of health services, emanating particularly from the Tuskegee experiments, which were conducted on African-American men between 1932 and 1972. The Tuskegee experiments are certainly a good reason for ongoing mistrust, but it is important not to overlook mistrust that is generated from contemporary health care experiences. If today, in twenty-first century America, African-American men have reason to believe they will be discriminated against by health service providers at a time when they are unwell and vulnerable, is it surprising that they delay or avoid seeking care? In short, contemporary negative health care interactions play a potentially important role in the underutilization of health services among African-American men, which has important implications for their health outcomes. As such, health care interactions are significant determinants of health among this population.

Health Care Decisions   The stereotyping of African-American men can result in disparities in health care decisions concerning African-American men as compared with their white counterparts. In other words, stereotyping can result in discriminatory behavior in the health care setting. In a study conducted by Bogart, Catz, Kelly, and Benotsch (2001), findings indicate that physicians' stereotypes of African-American men resulted in physicians' assumptions that African-American men would be less likely to comply with highly active antiretroviral therapy (HAART) treatment. These kinds of predictions have serious implications as they are likely to have an effect on treatment decisions (Bogart et al., 2001).

It is important to note that in contemporary health care settings, discriminatory decision making is likely to be subtle and unconscious as opposed to overt or intentional (Penner et al., 2007). Penner et al. (2007) propose that the **aversive racism** theory developed by Gaertner and Dovidio (1986) is particularly applicable to discriminatory decision making in the health care setting (see Penner et al., 2007). Aversive racism theory holds that while "aversive racists" consciously support racially egalitarian values, concurrently they have unconscious negative emotions and stereotypes about specific racial/ethnic groups (Dovidio et al., 2008). Thus, there is an inherent contradiction between their "explicit egalitarian attitudes" and their "implicit negative racial attitudes" (Dovidio et al., 2008, p. 479). Further, automatic and unconscious negative attitudes and stereotypes are particularly likely to lead to discriminatory behavior when health care providers are coping with time constraints or tasks that require extensive thought and deliberation (Dovidio et al., 2008). Drawing on Geiger's work (2001), Dovidio et al. (2008) note that racial disparities in medical treatment appear to be greater when physicians are dealing with "high-discretion" procedures (e.g., making a referral for a procedure or drug) than when they undertake "low-discretion" procedures (e.g., emergency surgery) (Geiger, 2001). For example, in a study that explored race disparities in treatment recommendations for men with coronary artery disease, black men were less likely to be recommended for coronary artery bypass grafting (CABG) than either their white male or black female counterparts. Concurrently the physicians in this study also exhibited negative stereotypes about the black male patients as compared with their white counterparts with regard to a number of factors, including medical compliance, substance abuse, and intelligence (van Ryn et al., 2006). High-discretion decision making is particularly pertinent in the mental health setting. Drawing on a number of scholars' work (Abreu, 1999; Loring & Powell, 1988; Rosenfield, 1984), Whaley (2004) argues that the unconscious stereotype that black men are violent plays a significant role in the misdiagnosis of paranoid schizophrenia in black men.

In summary, the literature suggests that discriminatory decision making contributes to health care inequities affecting African-American men. This has important implications for health outcomes among this population. As such, health care decision making is an important determinant of health among African-American men.

Reducing Provider-Level Health Care Inequities Affecting African-American Men

To date, the public health community (funding bodies, researchers, program developers, policy makers) has often overlooked social determinants of health care inequities affecting African-American men, frequently focusing on African-American men themselves, as the chief "cause" of their health care inequities. The earlier part of this chapter has demonstrated that this is not the case, that in fact, health care provider-level factors play a critical role in health care inequities affecting African-American men. To this end, the following section sets out some key areas that stakeholders should consider in reducing the health care inequities affecting this population.

Conduct Interventions That Reduce Racial Bias

African-American men are a population group that is particularly vulnerable to racial bias in health care, facing special challenges with stereotyping from health care providers. As such, it is imperative that strategies are developed that address this issue head-on. Although significant funds have been dedicated to programs that improve health care providers' communication with patients from diverse cultures (Burgess, van Ryn, Dovidio, & Saha, 2007) these programs tend to neglect issues of racial bias (Gregg & Saha, 2006) and thus are limited in their potential to adequately address unconscious stereotyping (Burgess et al., 2007). Accordingly, the author recommends interventions that draw on a social cognitive psychology framework developed by Burgess et al. (2007), which outlines evidence-based strategies and skills, and addresses the shortcomings of cultural competency curricula. The aim is to teach strategies and skills to medical trainees and practicing physicians, which will address the unconscious racial attitudes and stereotypes that negatively impact health care interactions and health care decisions. Burgess et al. (2007) emphasize the need for interventions to be implemented in a safe space, where new skills can be practiced, and that intervention implementers should be careful not to make providers feel ashamed of having stereotypes. The proposed strategies and skills (Burgess et al., 2007) are intended to:

- Develop providers' personal motivation to reduce bias
- Develop providers' psychological understanding of bias
- Develop providers' confidence in interacting with patients from different racial/ethnic groups
- Increase providers' ability to regulate their emotions

- Increase providers' ability to understand patients' perspectives and be empathetic
- Improve providers' ability to effectively partner with patients

New Legislation to Address Health Care Discrimination

Research indicates that discrimination in health care is likely to be a frequent reality among African-American men. While intervention strategies to reduce racial bias in health care are vital as outlined in the last section, it is also imperative to provide for legislation that better protects African-American men and other vulnerable populations from discriminatory health care. Current civil rights legislation has significant shortcomings in that it was originally designed to address overt forms of discrimination, and does not address subtle discrimination that is a feature of contemporary health care settings (Randall, 2006). In view of that, Randall (2006) argues for legislation that expands the law to deal with more than overt or intentional discrimination. In other words, the law should allow for the more subtle kinds of discrimination (e.g., aversive racism) that is experienced by African-American men in the twenty-first-century health care setting. Randall (2006) proposes a Health Care Anti-Discrimination Act designed to:

- Acknowledge a variety of forms of discrimination (e.g., "intentional discrimination"; "subtle discrimination"; and "unthinking discrimination").
- Approve and finance the use of individuals appointed as "medical testers" to provide evidence of discrimination.
- Provide individuals (including testers) and organizations (e.g., civil rights organizations) the right to bring a case before a court.
- Require health care organizations to collect disaggregated race-based health care data to make discrimination in health care more detectable.
- Require a health report card for health agencies, providers, or facilities to encourage accountability in health care discrimination issues.
- Establish an equality health care council as a key agency for antidiscrimination work in health care.
- Set adequate fines for antidiscrimination law violations.
- Pay the attorney fees of individuals and organizations who win lawsuits.
- Permit the punitive damages awarded to be used to fund health care equity programs.

Increase the Number of African-American Physicians

Increasing the number of African-American physicians is another strategy that can be used to improve the health care experiences of African-American men (see Cooper et al., 2003). Research indicates that patients with physicians of the same race have longer physician visits, are more satisfied, and regard their physicians as more participatory than those who do not (Cooper et al., 2003). In a study conducted by Malebranche et al. (2004, p. 103), several of the black male interviewees indicated a preference for black physicians because they considered that they could "relate on a more personal level" as compared with non-black physicians. Moreover, individuals who have been subject to discrimination in health care frequently prefer same-race health care providers (Malat & van Ryn, 2005). At present, the lack of African-American physicians (only 4 percent of physicians are African American) has meant that this preference cannot be easily exercised among African-American men (African Americans make up 13 percent of the population in the United States) (see Rao & Flores, 2007).

The following recommendations are an adaptation of the Institute of Medicine's proposed strategy to increase diversity in the health care workforce (Smedley, Butler, & Bristow, 2004) with an emphasis on increasing the numbers of African-American physicians, an underrepresented group of minority physicians:

- Health education institutions should have African Americans represented on admission committees, and they should consider the race of applicants in admission decisions.
- Congress should increase funding for initiatives to increase the number of African-American physicians.
- Health profession accreditation groups should encourage medical schools to recruit African-American students, and include African Americans on their boards.

Increase Research on Provider-Level Health Care Inequities

Public health research relating to African-American men has focused largely on their health behavior (patient-level factors) as a cause of health care disparities; interventions have frequently sought to address poor health-seeking attitudes and behaviors. Although these efforts are worthy in and of themselves, focusing on African-American men's health behavior in isolation is not enough. As this chapter has argued, provider behavior plays a key role in health care inequities affecting African-American men. There is also a need to contextualize health behavior by exploring the impact of provider-level factors on health behavior/patient-level factors. Suggestions for addressing this research gap are discussed in the following sections.

The effect of racial bias and stereotypes on health care interactions and health care decisions.

There is a need for research that examines stereotypes and attitudes of providers toward African-American men, and how these might have an impact on physician recommendations, physician referrals, and receipt of the optimum treatments (see National Institutes of Health [NIH], 2010). This should include experimental studies on the effect of providers' stereotypes and attitudes on health care decisions, as well as health care interactions (Penner et al., 2007). Future researchers might consider using aversive racism theory (e.g., consider implicit attitudes and stereotypes among providers). As stated earlier, health care provider implicit attitudes and stereotypes are particularly appropriate for studying discrimination in contemporary health care settings (Penner et al., 2007).

The effect of health care interactions and health care decisions on health care disparities.

Although there is a great deal of indirect evidence that points to the association between provider-level factors and racial health care disparities, there is a need for research that directly addresses this issue (Smedley et al., 2003). Further, since African-American men are impacted by specific forms of stereotyping, there is a particular need for gender-specific research on this topic.

The effect of provider behavior on help-seeking behavior.

The predominant focus within the public health literature concerning African-American men is on their help-seeking and health behavior. To the author's knowledge, there is currently no work that has explored the *impact of racialized health care interactions on help-seeking and health behavior among African-American men.* To be sure, the need for research on this issue has been emphasized by the National Institutes of Health (NIH) in a 2011 funding opportunity announcement (http://grants.nih.gov/grants/guide/pa-files/PA-11-162.html), which identifies the need for research that explores patients' experiences of discrimination in health care and its association with future help-seeking behavior and health behavior. Moreover, Penner et al. (2009) argue that future research must consider that the sources of racial health care disparities may emanate from patients' *experiences of discrimination in health care* rather than from patients per se. This is consistent with Ford and Airhihenbuwa's (2010) assertion that currently, public health literature is overly colorblind, and in many instances does not deal adequately with issues pertaining to race and racism. In this vein, future researchers may wish to consider utilizing Critical Race Theory (CRT) to study the effect of racialized provider behavior on patients' help-seeking behavior, as well as other aspects of provider-level health care inequities.

CRT places race at the forefront of inquiry, and is a useful theory for studying the causes of health disparities; since it critiques colorblindness, it is particularly helpful in keeping the discussion focused on the principles of equity and social justice (Ford & Airhihenbuwa, 2010).

Summary

This chapter has shown that African-American men face health care inequities across a wide range of disease areas and medical services, and has focused on *provider-level factors* as important determinants of these inequities. To be sure, these unique health care risk factors have significant implications for health care experiences, health care quality, and health outcomes among African-American men. In exploring the role of provider-level factors in health care inequities, this chapter has emphasized the need to seriously consider the impact of negative health care interactions (e.g., lack of respect, lack of interaction) on African-American men's health care experiences, and particularly their future utilization of health services. It has also underlined the significance of discriminatory health decision making (e.g., questionable prostate cancer decision making, biased cardiovascular referral decisions) in contemporary health care settings, and its association with health care inequities. Together, negative health care interactions and discriminatory health decision making not only reduce health care quality, they also have obvious implications for the worsening of health conditions, which may have been previously manageable, and thus implications for increased morbidity and mortality among African-American men.

Finally, this chapter has drawn from multidisciplinary sources to propose a number of recommendations for tackling the social determinants of health care inequities affecting African-American men. This includes interventions that reduce racial bias among health care providers, new legislation to address health care discrimination, increasing the number of African-American physicians, and developing the research base on provider-level health care inequities.

Unequal treatment in health care has huge implications. Health care (or the lack of it) tends to impact individuals when they are ill, a time when they are at their most vulnerable. Moreover, poor health care is a basic denial of an individual's human rights. As Martin Luther King Jr. (1966) argued, "Of all the forms of inequality, injustice in health care is the most shocking and inhumane." It is imperative that policy makers place the issue of health care equity for African-American men, and other vulnerable minorities higher up the policy agenda than is currently the case. There is also a need to move beyond patient-level factors in understanding and addressing these inequities.

Key Terms

African-American men

aversive racism

bias

health care decisions

health care disparities

health care inequities

health care interactions

health care risk factor

health system–level factors

help-seeking attitudes and behaviors

implicit and explicit attitudes

patient-level factors

provider-level factors

social determinants of health

social risk factor

stereotyping

unequal treatment

Discussion Questions

1. Unequal treatment is presented in this chapter as being a significant determinant of African-American men's health. Do you agree with this assessment? Why/Why not?

2. Were you surprised to learn the extent of health care inequities affecting African-American men? Why/Why not?

3. How important are negative health care interactions versus discriminatory health care decisions as determinants of health among African-American men? In other words, are health care interactions and health care decisions equally important in terms of their potential to affect African-American men's health outcomes? Why/Why not?

4. Discuss the advantages and potential barriers to implementing the strategies suggested in this chapter for tackling health care inequities affecting African-American men. Can you think of any additional strategies?

References

Abreu, J. M. (1999). Conscious and nonconscious black stereotypes: Impact on first impression and diagnostic ratings by therapists. *Journal of Consulting and Clinical Psychology*, *67*, 387–393.

Ayanian, J. Z., Cleary, P. D., Weissman, J. S., & Epstein, A. M. (1999). The effect of patients' preferences on racial differences in access to renal transplantation. *New England Journal of Medicine*, *341*, 1661–1669.

Blocker, D. E., Romocki, L. S., Thomas, K. B., Jones, B. L., Jackson, E. J., Reid, L., & Campbell, M. K. (2006). Knowledge, beliefs and barriers associated with prostate cancer prevention and screening behaviors among African-American men. *Journal of the National Medical Association, 98*(8), 1286–1295.

Bogart, L. M., Catz, S. L., Kelly, J. A., & Benotsch, E. G. (2001). Factors influencing physicians' judgments of adherence and treatment decisions for patients with HIV disease. *Medical Decision Making, 21*, 28–36.

Burgess, D., van Ryn, R., Dovidio, J., & Saha, S. (2007). Reducing racial bias among health care providers: Lessons from social-cognitive psychology. *Society of General Internal Medicine, 22*(6), 882–887.

Canto, J. G., Allison, J. J., Kiefe, C. I., Fincher, C., Farmer, R., Sekar, P., . . . Weissman, N. W. (2000). Relation of race and sex to the use of reperfusion therapy in Medicare beneficiaries with acute myocardial infarction. *New England Journal of Medicine, 342*, 1094–1100.

Cooper, L. A., Roter, D. L., Johnson, R. L., Ford, D. E., Steinwachs, D. M., & Powe, N. R. (2003). Patient-centered communication, ratings of care, and concordance of patient and physician race. *Annals of Internal Medicine, 139*, 907–915.

Courtenay, W. H. (2002). A global perspective on the field of men's health. *International Journal of Men's Health, 1*, 1–13.

Das, A. K., Olfson, M., McCurtis, H. L., & Weissman, M. M. (2006). Depression in African Americans: Breaking barriers to detection and treatment. *Journal of Family Practice, 55*, 30–39.

Diala, C., Muntaner, C., Walrath, C., Nickerson, K. J., LaVeist, T. A., & Leaf, P. J. (2000). Racial differences in attitudes toward professional mental health care and in the use of services. *American Journal of Orthopsychiatry, 70*(4), 455–464.

Dovidio, J. F., Penner, L. A., Albrecht, T. L., Norton, W. E., Gaertner, S. L., & Shelton, J. N. (2008). Disparities and distrust: The implications of psychological processes for understanding racial disparities in health and health care. *Social Science & Medicine, 67*(3), 478–486.

Felix-Aaron, K., Moy, E., Kang, M., Patel, M., Chesley, F. D., & Clancy, C. (2005). Variation in quality of men's health care by race/ethnicity and social class. *Medical Care, 43*, 172–181.

Ford, C. L., & Airhihenbuwa, C. O. (2010) Critical race theory, race equity, and public health: Toward antiracism praxis. *American Journal of Public Health, 100*, 30–35.

Friedman, D. B., Corwin, S. J., Dominick, G. M., & Rose, I. D. (2009). African American men's understanding and perceptions about prostate cancer: Why multiple dimensions of health literacy are important in cancer communication. *Journal of Community Health, 34*(5), 449–460.

Gaertner, S. L., & Dovidio, J. F. (1986). The aversive form of racism. In J. F. Dovidio & S. L. Gaertner (Eds.), *Prejudice, discrimination, and racism: Theory and research* (pp. 61–89). Orlando, FL: Academic Press.

Geiger, H. J. (2001). Racial stereotyping and medicine: The need for cultural competence. *Canadian Medical Association Journal, 164*, 1699–1700.

Gregg, J., & Saha, S. (2006). Losing culture on the way to competence: The use and misuse of culture in medical education. *Academic Medicine, 81*(6), 542–547.

King, M. L. Jr. (1966). Presentation at the Second National Convention of the Medical Committee for Human Rights. Chicago, March 25, 1966.

Loring, M., & Powell, B. (1988). Gender, race, and DSM-III: A study of the objectivity of psychiatric diagnostic behavior. *Journal of Health and Social Behavior*, *29*, 1–22.

Malat, J., & van Ryn, M. (2005). African American preference for same-race doctors: the role of discrimination. *Ethnicity & Disease*, *15*(4), 739–747.

Malebranche, D. J. (2004). Learning about medicine and race. *Health Affairs*, *23*(2), 220–224.

Malebranche, D. J., Peterson, J. L., Fullilove, R. E., & Stackhouse, R. W. (2004). Race and sexual identity: Perceptions about medical culture and healthcare among black men who have sex with men. *Journal of the National Medical Association*, *96*(1), 97–107.

McGibbon, E., Etowa, J., & McPherson, C. (2008). Health care access as a social determinant of health. *Canadian Nurse*, *104*(7), 22–27.

Metzl, J. M. (2009). *The protest psychosis: How schizophrenia became a black disease*. Boston, MA: Beacon Press.

Millett, G. A., Flores, S. A., Peterson, J. L., & Bakeman, R. (2007). Explaining disparities in HIV infection among black and white men who have sex with men: A meta-analysis of HIV risk behaviors. *AIDS*, *21*(15), 2083–2091.

National Institutes of Health. (2011). *The effect of racial and ethnic discrimination/bias on health care delivery*. Funding opportunity announcement. Retrieved from http://grants.nih.gov/grants/guide/pa-files/PA-11-162.html

Navaneethan, S., & Singh, S. A. (2006). A systematic review of barriers in access to renal transplantation among African Americans in the United States. *Clinical Transplantation*, *20*(6), 769–775.

Penner, L. A., Albrecht, T. L., Coleman, D., & Norton, W. E. (2007). Interpersonal perspectives on black-white health disparities: Social policy implications. *Social Issues & Policy Review*, *1*, 63–98.

Penner, L. A., Dovidio, J. F., Edmondson, D., Dailey, R. K., Markova, T., Albrecht, T. L., & Gaertner, S. L. (2009). The experience of discrimination and black-white health disparities in medical care. *Journal of Black Psychology*, *35*, 180–203.

Penner, L. A., Dovidio, J. F., West, T. V., Gaertner, S. L., Albrecht, T. L., Daily, R. K., & Markova, T. (2010). Aversive racism and medical interactions with black patients: A field study. *Journal of Experimental Social Psychology*, *46*(2), 436–440.

Peterson, E. D., Shaw, L. K., DeLong, E. R., Pryor, D. B., Califf, R. M., & Mark, D. B. (1997). Racial variation in the use of coronary-vascularization procedures: Are the differences real? Do they matter? *New England Journal of Medicine*, *336*, 480–486.

Randall, V. (2006). *Dying while black*. Dayton, Ohio: Seven Principles Press.

Rao, V., & Flores, G. (2007). Why aren't there more African-American physicians? A qualitative study and exploratory inquiry of African-American students' perspectives on careers in medicine. *Journal of the National Medical Association*, *99*, 986–993.

Ravenell, J. E., Whitaker, E. E., & Johnson, W. E. (2008). According to him: Barriers to healthcare among African American men. *Journal of the National Medical Association*, *100*(10), 1153–1160.

Richardson, J. T., Webster, J. D., & Fields, N. J. (2004). Uncovering myths and transforming realities among low-SES African American men: Implications for reducing prostate cancer disparities. *Journal of the National Medical Association*, *96*(10), 1295–1302.

Richert-Boe, K. E., Weinmann, S., Shapiro, J. A., Rybicki, B. A., Enger, S. M., Van Den Eeden, S. K., & Weiss, N. S. (2008). Racial differences in treatment of early-stage prostate cancer. *Urology*, *71*(6), 1172–1176.

Rosenfield, S. (1984). Race differences in involuntary hospitalization: Psychiatric vs. labeling perspectives. *Journal of Health and Social Behavior*, *25*(1), 14–23.

Sabin, J., Nosek, B. A., Greenwald, A., & Rivara, F. P. (2009). Physicians' implicit and explicit attitudes about race by MD race, ethnicity, and gender. *Journal of Health Care for the Poor and Underserved*, *20*(3), 896–913.

Sambamoorthi, U., Olfson, M., Wei, W., & Crystal, S. (2006). Diabetes and depression care among Medicaid beneficiaries. *Journal of Health Care for the Poor and Underserved*, *17*(1), 141–161.

Shavers, V. L., Brown, M., Klabunde, C. N., Potosky, A. L., Davis, W., Moul, J.W., & Fahy, A. (2004b). Race/ethnicity and the intensity of medical monitoring under "watchful waiting" for prostate cancer. *Medical Care*, *42*, 239–250.

Shavers, V. L., Brown, M. L., Potosky, A. L., Klabunde, C. N., Davis, W.W., Moul, J.W., & Fahy, A. (2004a). Race/ethnicity and the receipt of watchful waiting for the initial management of prostate cancer. *Journal of General Internal Medicine*, *19*, 146–155.

Smedley, B. D., Butler, A. S., & Bristow, L. R. (2004). (Eds.). *In the nation's compelling interest: Ensuring diversity in the health-care workforce.* Washington, DC: National Academies Press.

Smedley, B. D., Stith, A. Y., & Nelson, A. R. (Eds.). (2002). *Unequal treatment: Confronting racial and ethnic disparities in health care.* Washington, DC: National Academies Press.

Taylor, K. L., Davis, J. L. III, Turner, R. O., Johnson, L., Schwartz, M. D., Kerner, J. F., & Leak, C. (2006). Educating African American men about the prostate cancer screening dilemma: A randomized intervention. *Cancer Epidemiology, Biomarkers & Prevention*, *15*(11), 2179–2188.

Underwood, W., DeMonner, S., Ubel, P., Fagerlin, A., Sanda, M. G., & Wei, J. T. (2004). Racial/ethnic disparities in the treatment of localized/regional prostate cancer. *Journal of Urology*, *171*, 1504–1507.

van Ryn, M., Burgess, D., Malat, J., & Griffin, J. (2006). Physicians' perceptions of patients' social and behavioral characteristics and race disparities in treatment recommendations for men with coronary artery disease. *American Journal of Public Health*, *96*(2), 351–357.

van Ryn, M., & Burke, J. (2000). The effect of patient race and socio-economic status on physicians' perceptions of patients. *Social Science & Medicine*, *50*(6), 813–828.

Waldman, S. V., Blumenthal. J. A., Babyak, M. A., Sherwood, A., Sketch, M., Davidson, J., & Watkins, L.L. (2009). Ethnic differences in the treatment of depression in patients with ischemic heart disease. *American Heart Journal*, *157*, 77–83.

Whaley, A. L. (2004). Ethnicity/race, paranoia, and hospitalization for mental health problems among men. *American Journal of Public Health*, *94*(1), 78–81.

Woods, V. D., Montgomery, S., Belliard, J. C., Ramírez-Johnson, J., & Wilson, C. M. (2004). Culture, black males, and prostate cancer: What is reality? *Cancer Control*, *11*(6), 388–396.

Chapter 12

The Impact of the Correctional Health Care System on HIV/AIDS and the Health of African-American Men

Rhonda Conerly Holliday

Learning Objectives

- Enable the reader to understand that prison health promotion and health care has an impact on the community health environment to which the inmate returns.
- Highlight the major illnesses impacting the health of prisoners.
- Enable the reader to grasp the multidimensional nature of incarceration and the need for multiple community agencies to have a role in providing support services for inmates returning to the community.
- Enable the reader to internalize the observation that health disparities among AA inmates mirrors that of the community at large.

• • •

African Americans by far represent the largest percentage of persons under correctional supervision in the United States and are disproportionally represented. In 2008, African Americans constituted 38 percent of all imprisoned persons, with the vast majority being African-American males (Sabol, West, & Cooper, 2009). Comparatively, African Americans represented only 12.6 percent of the entire population (U.S. Census Bureau, 2010). Although the imprisonment rate for African-American males decreased between 2000 and 2008, the rate was six times higher than white males. The imprisonment rate for African-American males was 3,161 per 100,000 compared to 487 per 100,000 and 1,200 per 100,000 for white and Hispanic males, respectively (Sabol et al., 2009).

Educational and employment inequities among African-American men are correlated with incarceration rates. The unemployment rate for African-American men has consistently remained above the national average for decades. In 2009 the dropout rate for African-American males between the ages of 16 and 24 was 10.6 percent (Chapman, Laird, Ifill, & KewalRamani, 2010). Many persons who are incarcerated have received poor and/or limited education, thus directly impacting their ability to secure adequate and sustainable employment. This invariably leads to lack of health insurance and health care and thus inequities in health among this population.

Correctional Health Care

Prisoners are the only group in the United States with a constitutional right to health care. Following the *Estelle v. Gamble* court decision in 1976, prison systems in the United States were obligated to maintain the health and well-being of their inmates. Health is one of the universal and basic human rights; all people have the right to be absent of disease. The United Nations AIDS Office advances that "public health interests do not conflict with human rights. On the contrary, it has been recognized that when human rights are protected, fewer people become infected." (UNAIDS, 1998). Hence, public health and human rights are complementary and should not be regarded as independent policy initiatives. The application of basic human rights, particularly those concerning health among inmate communities, is a new advocacy movement, and policy makers have often ignored the concept of prison health. As a result of *Estelle v. Gamble*, three basic rights related to provision of health care in the prison system have emerged: (1) the right to access to care, (2) the right to care that is ordered, and (3) the right to a professional medical judgment.

The idea that inmates are entitled to the same level of health care provided in community settings is becoming more accepted in the United States. Many citizens, however, still hold to the belief that inmates do not deserve to be treated the same as the general population. They argue that inmates will take advantage of improved health care services while incarcerated at the expense of taxpayers. However, because not all inmates take advantage of improved health care, it seems inaccurate to label all incarcerated persons in this way and it is not a reason to deny adequate health care (Birmingham, 1997). As previously mentioned, health care in prisons is a necessity and a right, not just for the inmates themselves but also for the many communities at large (where many of these inmates return).

Many persons enter correctional facilities with a compromised health status or having received inadequate access to health care. Incarcerated persons are faced with a multiplicity of health-related issues ranging from all to a combination of the following: drug dependence and withdrawal, infectious disease problems, and psychiatric and traumatic emergencies (Challoner, 1999). These conditions are associated with poverty, homelessness, lack of formal education, and chronic unemployment, all of which place a person at risk for incarceration and breed illness and disease.

The same social conditions that are present in the community are also present in correctional facilities. Prisons are the social petri dish and breeding grounds for infectious diseases. They encourage unhealthy behaviors and potentially have a negative impact on mental health (HIV InSite, 1998). Several factors associated with increased transmission of infectious diseases within correctional facilities include: overcrowding, poor ventilation, lack of education, lack of medical care, sharing of drug injecting equipment, tattooing or skin piercing, and unprotected sex (UNAIDS, 1997). Due to the transient nature of inmates, as well as visitation of family, friends and commercial sex workers, adverse prison conditions can exacerbate the spread of infection and risk the health of inmates, visitors, and prison health and human services staff (Duncan, 1999).

Although inmates are subject to many adverse health effects associated with prison conditions, they often lack proper care and health education. This exacerbates the risks inherently present in the prison environment that lead to poor health outcomes. "Prisons serve as a social determinant of health by mediating the vicious cycle of concentration, amplification, deterioration, dissemination or overburdening, and post-release morbidity and mortality. . . . Prisons amplify adverse health conditions through a culture that normalizes behaviors that are deleterious to health." (Awofeso, 2010).

Prison health has an impact on the general population and must be viewed in the larger context of community public health concerns. Since the majority of inmates return to community settings, prison health affects not only inmates but also members of the general community at large (Braithwaite, Hammett, & Mayberry, 1996; Health in Prisons Project, 1998). There should be little debate about the question of whether or not inmates have the right to adequate care.

The sheer volume of prisoners who leave prison each year is astounding. During the year 2000, 570,966 sentenced prisoners were released from state prisons, up from 526,905 in 1998. At the same time, total admissions to state prisons rose by 1.7 percent (from 572,779 in 1998 to 582,232 in 2000) (Beck, Karberg, & Harrison, 2002). In 2002 alone, more than 600,000 inmates were released back into local communities from public and private correctional institutions in the United States (U.S. Bureau of Justice Statistics, 2002). At the end of 2002, there were 753,141 adults on parole in the United States. In local jurisdictions, 70,804 detainees were supervised in their communities though electronic monitoring, home detention, day reporting, community services, weekender programs, other pretrial supervision, other work programs, and treatment programs (drug/alcohol, mental health, other medical treatment) (U.S. Bureau of Justice Statistics, 2002, p. 5). With more than 600,000 prisoners reentering their home communities each year, it is imperative that policy makers and other community-based organizations explore innovative and effective ways to improve the health status of incarcerated populations.

The "revolving door" phenomenon (the continuous flow of inmates into and out of correctional facilities) poses particular challenges for correctional health officials. The reentry of these prisoners back into local communities raises important questions about what correctional systems are doing to maintain the health and well-being of prisoners and the communities to which they ultimately return (National Commission on Correctional Health Care, 2003). Petersilia (2000) suggests that the volume of inmates released back into society creates "unfortunate collateral consequences" to include the spread of infectious disease. He writes:

> [I]nmates have always been released from prison, and officials have long struggled with helping them succeed. But the current situation is different. The numbers of returning offenders dwarf anything known before, the needs of released inmates are greater, and corrections system has retained few rehabilitation programs. A number of unfortunate collateral consequences are likely, including increases in child abuse, family violence, the spread of infectious diseases, homelessness, and community disorganization. (p. 1)

When a prisoner returns to the community, they are returning to the same social conditions that impacted their lives prior to incarceration, including poverty, lack of education, lack of job opportunities, and access to adequate health care. Incarceration also leads to disenfranchisement. Formerly incarcerated individuals with felony convictions have been denied voting rights in many states either for a defined period of time or indefinitely. Recent reports suggest that 4.6 million felons are disenfranchised, while 1.7 million ex-felons (those who have completed their sentences) are disenfranchised (ACLU, 2005). Among African Americans, 1.4 million are disenfranchised. This leads to a lack of political power for a large segment of the population and a lack of means for the formerly incarcerated to advocate for themselves politically. In essence, their voices are silenced. Further exasperating the plight of formerly incarcerated persons is the stigma of being labeled a convict, which limits many opportunities for self-improvement. Once released from a correctional facility, the health care received during incarceration is often not continued in the community.

A Public Health Approach to Correctional Health Care

Periods of incarceration and community supervision represent important opportunities for intervening to prevent and treat disease and promote health among populations with generally high rates of morbidity and historically poor access to health care and prevention services.

Once incarcerated, prisoners continue to face barriers to adequate health services. In a survey conducted on prison health care managers, it was found that despite the prevalence of HIV in prison (the rate of HIV in male prisoners is 15 times higher than that of men not imprisoned), more than half of prisons have no sexual health policy (BBC News, 2005). The lack of sexual health policy suggests that the needs of a significant proportion of the inmate population are not being adequately addressed. This may lead to increased morbidity and mortality due to lack of information and services, because one cannot do what he/she does not know. Similarly, correctional health officials struggle to balance high demand for services, stressful work conditions, and their mandate to provide adequate health care. Short stays and high inmate turnover rates intensify health care challenges, especially in city and county jails settings.

Jails and prisons are faced with different health care challenges and they have different intervention opportunities. This is due to the variation in lengths of stay between these two types of confinement facilities. Health promotion programs that might work well within short-term facilities may not be as effective or even appropriate in long-term facilities and vice versa. Systems struggle to make improvements in suicide prevention, accessibility of substance abuse treatment programs, more intensive mental health support services (e.g., individual and group counseling), dental health services, chronic disease management, and gerontological services for a rapidly aging inmate population.

The high percentages of black and Latino male prisoners complicate concerns about cultural sensitivity in health care delivery and HIV/AIDS education. Forms of racial discrimination serve as a barrier to health care, not only in the community but also in correctional facilities. Reports from several institutions indicate that white inmates receive more favorable responses to "sick call" requests than do African-American inmates and that white inmates tend to receive less strenuous prison work details. The lack of consistent, effective HIV prevention education targeting male prisoners of color is merely a symptom of the larger problem of incarcerated men of color having relatively poor health status. Thus, the period of incarceration offers a unique opportunity, particularly for men of color, to access medical services that may have been otherwise difficult to obtain when they were in the community.

Correctional facilities provide a unique opportunity to provide health care and to relay prevention messages that focus on high-risk behaviors outside the secured setting, given the constant flow of convicted persons into the prison system and the release of inmates back into the general population. A public health approach to correctional health care is essential to the prisoners and the entire community (Gaiter & Doll, 1996; MacDougall, 1998; Travis 2002). A public health approach involves working not only to prevent the spread of these conditions, but also to reduce the burden of chronic disease and mental health illness. A public health approach to correctional health "involves bringing together correctional systems, public health agencies, and community-based organizations to design an array of prevention and support services for inmates and ex-offenders" (Gaiter & Doll, 1996, p. 1202). One central tenet of the public health approach is to encourage collaboration across community-based organizations, universities, federal, state, and local correctional systems and private prisons across the nation to work together using best practices to improve public health.

Evaluating correctional health care with a public health approach addresses the needs of prisoners and the communities to which they eventually return. The rapid increase in the number of prisons, jails, and bureaucratic structures required to incarcerate and monitor these millions of people, combined with high rates of disease and incarceration, push the limits of the correctional health communities' ability to meet prisoners' health needs.

In the United States, prisoners have significantly higher rates of infectious and chronic disease than the general population. Other issues with prison health care include apathetic health care workers and prison employees, as well as the subculture of a hierarchical power structure typically formed by inmates in most prison systems (Veeken, 2000). Correctional health officials struggle to meet the need for proper inmate health, but are plagued by high turnover and burnout rates, understaffing, and difficult working conditions.

For correctional health care providers, a struggle exists among security concerns, the quality of inmate health care—and perhaps most importantly—how to promote future behavioral change from within the confines of a secured facility. Physicians faced with the care of inmates should be aware of the spectrum of problems as well as the high-risk nature of their care (Challoner, 1999). The most common infectious diseases in prison populations are HIV and sexually transmitted infections, tuberculosis, hepatitis, meningitis and other infections. Presently, the largest cause of mortality in this population is due to AIDS (Challoner, 1999).

HIV and AIDS in Correctional Institutions

The prevalence of individuals with HIV infections in correctional institutions is higher than age-adjusted rates in surrounding communities (Altice et al., 1998). However, it should be noted that the majority of HIV infection in the United States occurs prior to incarceration (Braithwaite et al., 1996). By the end of

1999, the rate of confirmed AIDS cases in United States prisons was five times higher than in the total United States population (Maruschak, 2001). The *2000 Census of State and Federal Adult Correctional Facilities* surveyed 84 federal facilities, 1,295 state facilities, 22 facilities under state and local authority, 3 facilities operated by the District of Columbia, and 264 privately operated facilities (Maruschak, 2000). This census collects data on HIV/AIDS testing policies and prisoner statistics. The *1999 Census of Jails* included 3,365 locally administered correctional facilities (e.g., city and county correctional facilities) that held inmates beyond arraignment and were staffed by municipal or county employees (U.S. Bureau of Justice Statistics, 1999). Data from this survey indicate that significant numbers of local jail inmates were infected with HIV/AIDS.

By the end of 2008, there were an estimated 8,733 state and federal inmates with AIDS and 16,254 known to be HIV-positive. The 1999 U.S. Census of Jails indicates that there were 8,615 jail inmates known to be positive for HIV (Marusck, 2010). Among state prisoners between 1991 and 1996, the number of males infected with HIV increased 35 percent and the number of females infected increased 84 percent (Hammett, Harmon, & Maruschak, 1999). In 2000, AIDS was the third leading cause of death among all U.S. inmates, following natural causes and suicide, accounting for 174 state inmate deaths and 21 federal inmate deaths. AIDS-related deaths in state prisons peaked in 1995 and have since declined; from 2005 to 2007 the number of deaths per 100,000 decreased from 11 to 9 (Maruscak, 2010). Maruscak (2000) also reports that nearly a third of inmates with AIDS in state and federal prisons were housed in 25 facilities, most of which are concentrated in the southeastern United States. Although the number of confirmed AIDS cases in state systems dropped in 2000 for the first time since 1991, state correctional systems such as New York and Florida, still hold a disproportionate percentage of HIV-positive inmates. Nearly half of all jail inmates known to be HIV-positive were housed in 43 of the 50 largest local jurisdictions, most of which are clustered, again, in the southeastern United States. The five jurisdictions with the highest rates of HIV/AIDS cases as a percentage of the total jail population were Palm Beach County, Florida (10.6 percent); New York City, New York (7.1 percent); King County, Washington (5.8 percent); San Francisco City/County, California (4.9 percent); and Fulton County, Georgia (4.8 percent) (U.S. Bureau of Justice Statistics, 1999). These statistics represent only correctional systems and facilities that reported their HIV prevalence data. It is possible that nonreporting systems and facilities have higher or lower rates of HIV-infected inmates. With the concentration and distribution of confirmed AIDS cases and HIV-positive inmates as they are, it is reasonable to believe that effective disease prevention efforts should be targeted at those populations in greatest need (Nicholson-Crotty & Nicholson-Crotty, 2004).

HIV infection upon prison admission has been found to be associated with being black or Hispanic, 40 years or older, and an intravenous drug user (Macalino et al., 2004). Older black males are the most likely segment of the inmate population to contract HIV while incarcerated as compared to whites, Hispanics, and Native Americans (Krebs & Simmons, 2002). Further, inmates with HIV and AIDS are likely to be poor, less educated, black, have had an STD in the past 10 years, and engage in an assortment of HIV risk behaviors, including IV drug use, crack cocaine use, and sex with multiple partners. Additional research has identified characteristics that are associated with seroconversion in prison including male–male sex in prison, older age, ≥ five years served on current sentence, tattooing in prison, black race, and having a BMI upon entering prison of ≤ 25.4 kg/m (Taussig et al., 2006). Age may be an important factor in intraprison HIV transmission, especially as sentence lengths increase.

The HIV/AIDS epidemic has attacked prisons with severity (Human Rights Watch, 2003). Two main factors can be held accountable for the increasing incidence of AIDS in prison populations: (1) the tendency of people entering prison to have a high incidence of HIV, and (2) prison conditions that provide an ideal environment for the growth and transmission of the virus (Human Rights Watch, 2003). Due to the characteristics of incarcerated persons, prison populations contain a disproportionate number of people who are likely to be at risk of HIV infection (Semelamela & Mugabem, 1996). Drug use with needle sharing and unprotected sex make HIV a "time bomb for the prison population" (Veeken, 2000). As the prevalence of HIV infection among new prison entrants increases, so does the risk of transmission to other inmates within prison and to sexual partners upon release (Gama Vaz, Gloyd, & Trindade, 1996).

Unlike tuberculosis, HIV/AIDS is not an airborne disease, and people living with HIV/AIDS do not have to be isolated from others during treatment, as do people that have active pulmonary tuberculosis. The World Health Organization (WHO) *Guidelines on HIV Infection and AIDS in Prisons* advances that: "Since segregation, isolation and restrictions on occupational activities, sports and recreation are not considered useful or relevant in the case of HIV-infected people in the community; the same attitude should be adopted towards HIV-infected prisoners" (WHO, 1993). However, this policy guideline is not often practiced, especially in prisons in developing countries. Though isolation of HIV-positive inmates may not be necessary for the same reason as tuberculosis isolation, there may be positive consequences in some situations. However, situations involving mandatory isolation cross into the realm of the health versus human rights debate.

The issue of ethics and human rights is important because inmates living with HIV should be treated the same as the general HIV-negative population. There also exist public health reasons, in relation to the general public, for the humane treatment and proper care of inmates infected with HIV. Prison conditions, as noted earlier, are conducive to the spread of HIV. As with the tuberculosis scenario, without proper treatment and acknowledgment, transmission of the virus within the prison population increases as well as the risk of spreading the virus to the general community upon release.

Intravenous Drug Use

Despite the strict laws and controls against drugs, random drug testing of inmates in the United States typically finds 3 to 10 percent positive for illicit substances (Purdy, 1995). Drugs enter the prisons in a variety of ways, including staff, visitors, and personal mail. In the general population, injection drug use is the second most common means of HIV exposure (Gaiter, Jurgens, Mayer, & Hollibaugh, 2000). For inmates with HIV, injection drug use is the primary vector of exposure before their incarceration (Gaiter et al., 2000). There are more intravenous drug users in correctional facilities than in drug treatment centers (Dixon et al., 1993). High-risk behaviors do not simply stop when the prison doors close. In fact, during focus groups with prisoners, one participant stated, "[J]ust because I was locked up didn't mean I was going to stop getting high" (Mahon, 1996). Syringes are relatively difficult to find in jails or prisons and are therefore almost always shared. Inmates will pick out dirty syringes from medical garbage, or use basketball pump needles, pieces of light bulbs, and pens as their injecting equipment (Mahon, 1996). According to unpublished data from the Nevada Department of Corrections, 12 inmates who seroconverted while incarcerated reported using a hypodermic needle at least once during their incarceration, but denied engaging in any sexual activity (May & Williams, 2002).

Tuberculosis, Hepatitis, and Other STIs in Correctional Institutions

Tuberculosis (TB) rates among inmates represented approximately 35 percent of all TB cases in the United States in 1999 (Adams & Leath, 2002). Conditions such as overcrowding, demoralized and underfunded (and therefore poorly motivated) prison health services, and the unofficial power structure or hierarchy that forms in all prisons create an environment in which it is difficult to treat tuberculosis (Reyes & Coninx, 1997).

The conditions in prisons encourage the development and spread of multidrug-resistant tuberculosis because of the highly intensive treatment method for the disease. Directly Observed Treatment Short-Course (DOTS) is the only tuberculosis control strategy to produce consistently an 85 percent cure rate (WHO, 2000). The DOTS is a comprehensive strategy in which health workers (in this case prison health workers) counsel and observe their patient swallowing each dose of a combination of medicines, and then monitor the patient's progress until each is cured (WHO, 2000). The DOTS strategy has been implemented worldwide in order to effectively combat tuberculosis.

In the late 1980s and early 1990s and through to the present day, correctional facilities encountered a resurgence of tuberculosis (Davis, 2002). In 1997, it was estimated that 7.4 percent of prisoners had TB infection, .04 percent had tuberculosis disease, and between 17 and 18.6 percent had hepatitis C (Davis, 2002). Correctional facilities have improved efforts to control tuberculosis, but outbreaks continue. In addition, transmission from former inmates to members of the community has been amply documented in the communicable disease literature. Lobato (1999) discovered that in 1997, correctional facilities reported 729 cases, representing almost 4 percent of national cases reported to the CDC. Selwyn et al. (1989) found that the incidence of TB in correctional institutions and urban communities have since risen drastically because of reactivation due to HIV and secondary spreading. A survey of 29 state departments conducted by Anno (1991) revealed that during 1984 and 1985, the incidence of tuberculosis among inmates was more than three times higher than that for nonincarcerated adults 15 to 64 years of age. The CDC Surveillance Summaries (1991) reported that since 1985, the national case rate for tuberculosis has increased alarmingly. Although more inmates are now receiving either treatment or prophylaxis for tuberculosis, containment of tuberculosis reactivation, subsequent intramural spread, and postrelease transmission cannot be addressed solely by prophylaxis. Vlahov et al. (1991) mentions that previous efforts have suggested that control of TB outbreaks in correctional facilities may result in diminution of subsequent community spread.

The most important prevention strategy in the treatment and prevention of tuberculosis is prompt drug treatment. All of the drugs used in the treatment must be taken in order to completely destroy the infectious agent as well as to prevent an outbreak of drug-resistant tuberculosis (WHO, 1998). Education may still play a key role; everyone involved has to realize the serious health risks to everyone of contracting and not treating, or incomplete treatment of, this disease. Signs and symptoms need to be recognized to determine when physician care is necessary.

Hepatitis B and C are also rapidly becoming health problems within correctional facilities. Decker, Vaughn, Brodie, Hutcheson, and Schaffner (1984) found that inmates have a high prevalence rate of hepatitis B virus (HBV) serologic markers. The rate of positive markers among male prison inmates was 19 percent in Wisconsin, 29 percent in Tennessee, and 47 percent in New Mexico. Hull et al. (1985) reported that, although small subgroups such as inmates serving unusually long sentences or those using injectables while incarcerated are at risk for new infection, the overall incidence of new HBV infection during incarceration is low. Chisolm (1988) reports that infection control programs must be aggressively promoted to ensure appropriate utilization of respiratory isolation, restrictions on transfer of ill inmates, rigorous surveillance, and contact tracing. Neaigus et al. (1990) suggest that the continuity of care after release, especially for tuberculosis infection control, will help improve compliance with preventative therapy and treatment of active disease, thereby reducing the emergence of drug resistance and secondary transmission in the community.

The prevention of hepatitis B and C virus (HBV, HCV) infections is also of major public health concern due to the fact that infected individuals carry a substantial risk of chronic liver disease and (especially with HBV) may transmit the virus to their sexual partners (and in the case of women to their children) (Stark, Bienzle, Vonk, & Guggenmoos-Holzmann, 1997). The main risk factor for HBV and HCV is injection drug use.

HBV and HCV are more easily transmitted by needle-stick injection than HIV (Stark et al., 1997). Due to the nature of the prison system and lack of acknowledgment concerning use and sharing of needles between inmates, the high rates of infection with the hepatitis viruses has remained a prison health problem.

Stark et al. (1997) reported that intravenous drug users who had shared syringes and had been imprisoned, and particularly those who had shared syringes while in prison, were more likely to be seropositive for HBV, HCV, and HIV. This was especially pronounced in inmates who had shared syringes in prisons more than 50 times. Again, this shows that the risk of syringe contamination by hepatitis and HIV viruses is much higher in prison than outside, where syringes are usually shared with only one or two other people.

The overall failure to apply a pragmatic and effective response to the HIV/AIDS epidemic and other health issues in prisons is due to preexisting inadequacies in prison health care; the lack of independence in prison medical services, and the adoption of policies that serve the needs of institutions rather than those of inmates.

Conclusion

The studies cited throughout this chapter present evidence to support the need for improved health care in prisons. However, it is important to realize that it is not just the health of those who are incarcerated that is jeopardized, but also that of the general public. Adequate health care for inmates is not a privilege; it is a basic necessity (Birmingham, 1997).

An anonymous editorial appearing in *The Lancet* (Anonymous, 1998) outlined one of the major obstacles to improved prison health care—the challenges faced by prison health doctors. Prison physicians have to work within the constraints of a "triangular doctor, patient, and prison/judicial-service relationship." Confusion concerning whether the medical or prison officer is in charge of health care, and a population more difficult and manipulative than usual, are further challenges encountered by prison health care workers. Ironically, the rapid spread of diseases such as HIV, tuberculosis, and hepatitis within prisons may have stimulated interest and attracted physicians to prison health care (Anonymous, 1998). Now it is vital that programs promoting prison health are supported in order to better equip physicians to work with prison communities.

Prison health care is good public health (Levy, 1997). In terms of communicable diseases, the relationship between prisoners' health, their families' health, and the health of the general community needs to be recognized by prison and health authorities, inmates, and the community at large as a complex constellation of interrelationships. Limiting the spread of diseases in prison benefits both the prisoner and the general population (HIV InSite, 1998). Thus, it is important to provide adequate health care and to arm inmates with health education information and skills while they are captive and incarcerated. The practice of healthy behaviors on release will further the general health and well-being among family and community residents. Moreover, providing inmates with such health education has the potential of creating strong ambassadors and champions for disseminating health education messages to others they encounter while incarcerated and on release.

Another basic, yet a difficult, strategy to improve health care is education of inmates, staff, and health care providers. It is important that education occur at all levels of the prison system. Inmates need to be educated to know the facts and risks, as well as how to prevent or protect themselves from exposure to any of the many diseases that threaten their health. Prison officials also need to be educated, in part to realize that inmates are people and deserve to be treated as such, as well as to learn that they increase their chances of exposure (thus exposing their families and community) by the act of denying health care to inmates. The guards in many prison systems are important in conveying the inmates' concerns to the prison administration, so it is essential for them to realize that their actions affect them as well as the inmates. Prison doctors also need to be well informed for the same reasons as the guards and other officials. Prison health does not stop at the prison entrance. Health care providers have ethical responsibilities to the prisoners as well as to the general public.

Inmates are the only segment of the U.S. population with a constitutional right to adequate medical care (Heckman, Kelly, Bogart, Kalichman, & Rompa, 1991). Health care in correctional settings should *promote* the health of prisoners, identify prisoners with health problems, assess their needs and deliver treatment, or refer them to other specialist services as appropriate. An important factor in the improvement of prevention and treatment services in correctional and criminal justice settings is expanding and strengthening collaborations among public health departments, correctional and criminal justice agencies, and community-based organizations. These health entities must cooperate with one another to find ways to quantify and offer standardized indicators to measure outcomes for public health programs. This can be achieved through the use of partnerships with schools of public health or medical schools.

There exists a need to heed the call for action issued by researchers and practitioners alike for the delivery of effective health care and infectious disease prevention education behind prison walls. Prison systems have an obligation not only to execute measures aimed to prevent the spread of these infectious diseases among inmates in prisons but also to care for prisoners living with infectious diseases. It is common knowledge that high-risk activities, likely to transmit infectious diseases, are prevalent in prisons; refusing to approve adequate prevention measures could even be interpreted as facilitating the spread of infectious diseases among prisoners and within the community after their release.

In essence, correctional facilities must enhance the development of comprehensive and collaborative health promotion and disease interventions to effectively deal with the challenges that are present in the system. This would involve developing new programs, modifying some existing strategies, and providing consistent input to evaluate the effectiveness of the implemented interventions. The success of the programs will be contingent on the involvement of prison administrators, correctional officers, educators, counselors, researchers, as well as the inmates themselves.

Bold and progressive risk reduction policy action is required by correctional policy makers to advance the health and well-being of incarcerated populations and ultimately the community at large. Recent political developments in Los Angeles, New York, Florida, and nations around the world indicate that politicians and correctional administrators are heeding the call to augment infectious disease prevention strategies behind prison walls to demand condom availability for inmates. Incarcerated populations represent high-risk groups in need of effective health care and health prevention programs and services, particularly relative to infectious diseases such as HIV/AIDS.

Recommendations

To conclude, we would like to suggest specific policy initiatives that may further these aims and improve the health of the citizenry.

- Adoption of mandatory HIV testing by state prison systems is highly recommended, although it is acknowledged that this position runs counter to the WHO position supporting voluntary testing. It is paramount that this testing only be offered in a nonprejudicial setting by health personnel who can ensure medical confidentiality. Currently only 24 states and the federal prison system have such mandatory testing. Mandatory testing will surface numerous undiagnosed cases and facilitate case finding and subsequent treatment. The surfacing of new cases will, however, have budgetary implications as it relates to the provision of treatment. Many state departments of corrections have external health care providers servicing the prison population. These providers often have a capitation formula for health care services provided, and fear that the identification of new cases will have a negative financial impact on their "bottom line." The state legislatures must be educated to see the bigger picture of "paying now or paying later"; or that prevention is more cost-effective than intervention. The legislatures must increase the funding support to state departments of corrections to accommodate the new HIV cases that will result from a mandatory testing policy.

- Support for an increase in initiatives that reinforce the "continuity of care" for inmates returning to community settings. Continuity of care for African-American and Latino offenders is especially daunting, given their low representation among the health insured. As it relates to connecting these offenders to health care providers in the community, deliberate policy action is needed to extend the responsibility for medical treatment from the prison to community settings. Most state correctional systems are divorced of this responsibility, once the inmate is released; and parole departments typically do not have strong articulation agreements with local and county health departments. Interagency collaboration between corrections and municipal health providers will need to be legislated to ensure such articulation.

- Improved opportunities for community-based organizations and AIDS service organizations to gain access to incarcerated populations for delivery of education and prevention programs. Many state departments of corrections and local jails allow these organizations to offer prevention programs, but it is not without grief. These prevention specialists are frequently humiliated and negatively stereotyped by correctional officers for the positive services they provide. Herein lies an apparent need for increased staff training and education designed to modify attitudes about infectious diseases among correctional personnel. Such in-service training should be a requirement of all correctional staff and administrators as a certification for employment.

- Conduct epidemiological and ethnographic research on the sexually transmitted infection risks faced by prisoners during the period of time from incarceration through their transition back into the community. This research would include assessing risk behaviors, attitudes, and personal histories, while respecting the sensitive nature of discussing sexuality with men in same-sex institutions. Our research reveals that these social psychological factors are underappreciated in corrections research. In the absence of hard epidemiological evidence regarding the transmission of sexually transmitted infections, it is critical to understand the social contexts in which sexual contact occurs in prison and jail and link these circumstances to prisoners' perceptions of their choices and interactions with others.

- The concerns raised in this chapter ought to be placed in a larger public health context that includes not only specific diseases and the means of preventing their spread, but also a wide range of other important health issues, such as access to care and health disparities. Our correctional institutions must work, either collaboratively or independently, to help prisoners transition back into the community with their health intact and the support systems and programming necessary to ensure their emotional and physical well-being.

Summary

This chapter has outlined some of the major health issues faced by prison populations. Risks, modes of transmission and infection, and general health concerns to the prison as well as the general community have been discussed. We outlined recommendations on how to improve health of inmates, decrease risk behavior, and increase knowledge and awareness of both inmates and prison staff. Correctional institutions need to take advantage of their access to the prison population, as a period of imprisonment may be the only opportunity for people incarcerated to benefit from screening and treatment programs (Ford, 2000). Innovative, coordinated, and collaborative health interventions will benefit the health of inmates and their families (a historically underserved population), as well as the health of the community at large (Hammett et al., 1999). This is an important field of public health research that should no longer be ignored.

Key Terms

African-American men	HIV/AIDS
correctional health care	incarceration

Discussion Questions

1. How did the *Estelle v. Gamble* court decision in 1976 affect prison health care? What has this court decision meant for prison systems nationwide?

2. How do social determinants of health influence the health status and health care of incarcerated persons?

3. What is the relationship between health care for prisoners and the communities to which they return?

References

ACLU. (2005, September). *Voting while incarcerated: A toolkit for advocates seeking to register and facilitate voting by eligible people in jail*. Retrieved from http://www. aclu.org/pdfs/votingrights/votingwhileincarc_20051123.pdf

Adams, D. L., & Leath, B. A. (2002). Correctional health care: Implications for public health policy. *Journal of the National Medical Association*, 94, 294–298.

Altice, F. L., Mostashari, F., Selwyn, P. A., Checko, P. J., Singh, R., Tanguay, S., & Blanchette, E. A. (1998). Predictors of HIV infection among newly sentenced male prisoners. *Journal of Acquired Immune Deficiency Syndromes & Human Retrovirology*, 18, 444–453.

Anno, B. (1991). *Prison health care: Guidelines for the management of an adequate delivery system*. Washington, DC: U.S. Department of Justice, National Institute of Corrections.

Anonymous. (1998). Correction of attitudes to prison medicine. Editorial. *Lancet*, 351 (9113), 1371.

Awofeso, N. (2010). Prisons as social determinants of hepatitis C virus and turberculosis infections. *Public Health Reports*, 125(Suppl. 4), 25–33.

Beck, A. J., Karburg, J. C., & Harrison, P. M. (2002). *Prison and jail inmates at midyear 2001*. U.S. Bureau of Justice Statistics, Department of Justice. NCJ 191702.

BBC News. (2005). Call for free condoms in prisons. Retrieved from http://news.bbc.co. uk/2/hi/uk_news/4434136.stm

Birmingham, L. (1997). Should prisoners have a say in prison health care? *British Medical Journal*, 315(7099), 65–66.

Braithwaite, R. L., Hammett, T., & Mayberry, R. (1996). Prisons and AIDS: A public health challenge. San Francisco, CA: Jossey-Bass.

CDC Surveillance Summaries. (1991, December). *Morbidity & Mortality Weekly Report*, 40(33-3), 23–27.

Challoner, K. (1999). Correctional medicine. *Top Emergency Medicine*, 21(3), 49–54.

Chapman, C., Laird, J., Ifill, N., & KewalRamani, A. (2010). *Trends in high school dropout and completion rates in the United States: 1972–2009*. U.S. Department of Education. NCES 2012-006. Retrieved from http://nces.ed.gov/pubs2012/2012006.pdf

Chisolm, S. A. (1988). Infection control in correctional facilities: A new challenge. *American Journal of Infectious Control*, 16, 107–113.

Davis, L. (2002, December). Health profile of the prison population. Paper presented at the National Reentry Rountable: Public health dimensions of prisoner reentry addressing the health needs and risks of returning prisoners and their families, Los Angeles, California.

Decker, M., Vaughn, W., Brodie, J., Hutcheson, R., & Schaffner, W. (1984). Seroepidemiology of hepatitis B in Tennessee prisoners. *Journal of Infectious Disease*, *150*, 450–459.

Dixon, P., Flanigan, T. P., DeBuono, B. A., DeCiantis, M. L., Hoy, J., & Stein, M. (1993). Infection with the human immunodeficiency virus in prisoners: Meeting the health care challenge. *American Journal of Medicine*, *95*(6), 629.

Duncan, N. (1999, October). WMA to tackle adverse health conditions in prisons. *British Medical Journal*, *319*(7217), 1090.

Ford, P. W. (2000). Health care problems in prisons. *Journal of the American Medical College*, *162*(5), 664–665.

Gaiter, J., & Doll, L. S. (1996). Improving HIV/AIDS prevention in prisons is good public health policy. *American Journal of Public Health*, *86*(9): 1201–1203.

Gaiter, J., Jurgens, R., Mayer, K., & Hollibaugh, A. (2000). Harm reduction inside and out: Controlling HIV in and out of correctional institutions. *AIDS Reader*, *10*(1), 45–53.

Gama Vaz, R., Gloyd, S., & Trindade, R. (1996). The effects of peer education on STD and AIDS knowledge among prisoners in Mozambique. *International Journal of STD & AIDS*, *7*, 51–4.

Hammett, T. M., Harmon, P., & Marushcak, L. M. (1999, July). *1996–1997 update: HIV/AIDS, STDS, and TB in correctional facilities*. Washington, DC: U.S. Department of Justice, National Institute of Justice.

Health in Prisons Project. (1998). Consensus statement on mental health promotion in prisons. Available at http://www.hipp-europe.org/events/hague/0040.htm

Heckman, T. G., Kelly, J. A., Bogart, L. M., Kalichman, S. C., & Rompa, D. J. (1991). HIV risk differences between African-American and white men who have sex with men. *Journal of the National Medical Association*, *91*(2), 92–100.

HIV InSite. (1998). *WHO guidelines on HIV infection and AIDS in prisons*. Available at http://HIVInSite.ucsf.edu/topics/prisons/2098.3842.htm

Hull, H. F., Lyons, L. H., Mann, J. M., Hadler, S. C., Steece, R., and Skeels, M. R. (1985). Incidence of hepatitis B in the penitentiary of New Mexico. *American Journal of Public Health*, *75*, 1134–1135.

Human Rights Watch. (2003). *HIV/AIDS in prisons*. Human Rights Watch prison project. Retrieved from http://www.hrw.org/advocacy/prisons/hiv-aids.htm

Krebs, C. P., & Simmons, M. (2002). Intraprison HIV transmission: An assessment of whether it occurs, how it occurs, and who is at risk. *AIDS Education and Prevention*, *14* (Suppl. B), 53–64.

Levy, M. (1997). Prison health services: Should be as good as those for the general community. *British Medical Journal*, *315*(7120), 1394–1395.

Lobato, M. (1999). Tuberculosis in United States correctional facilities. *HIV Education Prison Project News*, *2*, 3.

Macalino, M. E., Vlahov, D., Sanford-Colby, S., Patel, S., Sabin, K., Salas, C., & Rich, J. D. (2004). Prevalence and incidence of HIV, hepatitis B virus, and hepatitis C virus infections among males in Rhode Island prisons. *American Journal of Public Health*, *94*(7), 1218–1223.

MacDougall, D. S. (1998, April). HIV/AIDS behind bars: Incarceration provides a valuable opportunity to implement HIV/AIDS treatment and prevention strategies in a high-risk population. *Journal of IAPAC (International Association of Physicians in AIDS Care)*. http://www.thebody.com/iapac/prisons.html

Mahon, N. (1996). New York inmates' HIV risk behaviors: The implications for prevention policy and programs. *American Journal of Public Health 86*(9), 1211–1216.

Maruschak, L. M. (2001, July). *HIV in prisons and jails, 1999*. Washington, DC: U.S. Bureau of Justice Statistics, Office of Justice Programs. Report No.: NCJ 187456.

Maruschak, L. M. (2002, October). *HIV in prisons, 2000*. Washington, DC: U.S. Bureau of Justice Statistics, Office of Justice Programs. Report No.: NCJ 196023.

Maruschak, L. M. (2010, January), *HIV in prisons, 2007–08*. Washington, DC: U.S. Bureau of Justice Statistics, Office of Justice Programs. Report No.: NCJ 228307.

May, J. P., & Williams, E. L. (2002). Acceptability of condom availability in a U.S. jail. *AIDS Education and Prevention*, *14* (Suppl. B), 85–91.

National Commission on Correctional Health Care. (2003). *The health status of soon-to-be-released inmates*. A report to Congress.

Neaigus, A., Sufian, M., Friedman, S., Goldsmith, D., Stephenson, B., Douglas, S., & Mota, P. (1990). Effects of outreach intervention on risk reduction among intravenous drug users. *AIDS Education Prevention*, *2*, 253–271.

Nicholson-Crotty, J., & Nicholson-Crotty, S. (2004). Social construction and policy implementation: Inmate health as a public health issue. *Social Science Quarterly*, *85*, 240–256.

Petersilia, J. (2000). *When prisoners return to the community: political, economic, and social consequences. Research in brief: Executive sessions on sentencing and corrections.* Department of Justice, Office of Justice Programs, National Institute of Justice.

Purdy, M. (1995, December 17). Officials ponder expansion of drug searches in prison. *New York Times*, *145*(50278), p. 54.

Reyes, H., & Coninx, R. (1997). Pitfalls of tuberculosis programmes in prisons. *British Medical Journal*, *315*(7120), 1447–1450.

Sabol, W. J., West, H. C., & Cooper, M. (2009). *Prisoners in 2008*. Washington, DC: U.S. Bureau of Justice Statistics, Office of Justice Programs; December Report No. NCJ 228417.

Selwyn, P., Hartel, D., Lewis, V., Schoenbaum, E., Vermund, S., Klein, R., . . . Friedland, G. H. (1989). A prospective study of the risk of tuberculosis among intravenous drug users with human immunodeficiency virus infection. *New England Journal of Medicine*, *320*, 545–550.

Semelamela, L., & Mugabem, M. (1996). Knowledge, attitudes, beliefs and practices about HIV/AIDS/STDs among male prison inmates in Botswana. *International Medical Journal*, *3*(1), 31–34.

Stark, K., Bienzle, U., Vonk, R., & Guggenmoos-Holzmann, I. (1997). History of syringe sharing in prison and risk of hepatitis B virus, hepatitis C virus, and human immunodeficiency virus among injecting drug users in Berlin. *International Journal of Epidemiology*, *26*(6), 1359–1365.

Taussig, J., Shouse, R. L., LaMarre, M., Fitzpatrick, L., McElroy, P., Borkowf, C.B., . . . Jafa, K. (2006). HIV transmission among male inmates in a state prison system—Georgia, 1992–2005. *Morbidity and Mortality Weekly Report, 55*, 421–426.

Travis, J. 2000. Research brief No 7: But they all come back: Rethinking prisoner reentry. *Sentencing and corrections: Issues for the 21st century*. U.S. Department of Justice.

Veeken, H. (2000). Lurigancho prison: Lima's "high school" for criminality. *British Medical Journal, 320*(7228), 173–175.

Vlahov, D., Brewer, F., Castro, K., Narkunas, J., Salive, M., Ullrich, J., & Munoz, A. (1991). Prevalence of antibody to HIV-1 among entrants to U.S. correctional facilities. *Journal of American Medical Association, 265*, 1129–1132.

UNAIDS. (1997). Prisons and AIDS: UNAIDS point of view. Retrieved from http://www .unaids.org/html/pub/Publications/IRC-pub05/Prisons-PoV_en_pdf.htm

UNAIDS. (1998). HIV/AIDS and human rights: International guidelines. Retrieved 2003, http://www.unaids.org.HR/PUB/98/1

U.S. Bureau of Justice Statistics. (2002). *Sourcebook of criminal justice statistics, 2002*. [NCJ 203301]. Washington, DC: Bureau of Justice Statistics, U.S. Department of Justice.

U.S. Bureau of Justice Statistics (Stephan, J. J.). (1999). *Census of jails*. Department of Justice, Office of Justice Programs.

U.S. Census Bureau. (2010). *State and Country Quickfacts*. Retrieved from http:// quickfacts.census.gov/qfd/states/00000.html

World Health Organization [WHO]. (1993). *WHO guidelines on HIV infection and AIDS in prisons*. Retrieved from http://www.unaids.org/htm.pub/publications.htm

World Health Organization (WHO). (1998). *Guidelines for the control of tuberculosis in prisons*.

World Health Organization. (2000). *WHO tuberculosis site*. Available at http://www .who.int/gtb/dots/index.htm

Part Four

Addressing Social Determinants of Health Inequities

Chapter 13

Building Communities of Opportunity

Pathways to Health for African-American Men

Angela Glover Blackwell

Learning Objectives

- Learn how neighborhood environments impact the health of African-American men.
- Recognize that interventions beyond the health sector are needed to eliminate health disparities.
- Understand the basic principles of community-change strategies to improve the health of African-American men.
- Recognize the importance of policy change in achieving health equity.

• • •

To help readers understand why building communities of opportunity is essential for improving the health of African-American men, this chapter begins with a review of the social and economic roots of health disparities. The chapter then explains how distressed neighborhood environments, particularly lack of access to opportunity, contribute to high rates of illness and premature death. The chapter presents four principles for equitable community transformation that can eliminate health disparities and improve the health of African-American men. Policy solutions are discussed and promising programs are spotlighted.

The Roots of Health Disparities

African-American men cannot be healthy if their communities are ailing. No doctor can undo the ill effects of living in communities without the essentials for healthy living: affordable fresh foods, clean air, safe streets, parks and other green spaces that invite exercise or an afternoon's relaxation. No medication can reverse the damaging consequences of living in neighborhoods with sweeping, systemic obstacles to wellness: poverty, dilapidated housing, abysmal schools, high unemployment, gangs, violence, crime, and despair.

African-American men need better **access** to health care, but the ability to obtain health services, alone, will not eliminate health disparities or put African-American boys and men on a life course of health and prosperity. To improve the health of African-American men and boys, we must intentionally change the conditions in which they live, work, learn, and play.

Health is more than the absence of disease or injury. According to the World Health Organization, health is "a state of physical, mental, and social well-being" (World Health Organization, 2003). Local environments either nourish or undermine well-being. A deep body of research shows all too clearly which way it cuts in communities of color, and for African-American men and boys especially. Policies, programs, and strategies well beyond the health sector are needed to address the health crisis in communities of color. We must transform ailing, disinvested communities into healthy **communities of opportunity**—places that support all residents to make healthy choices, achieve educational success, obtain living-wage jobs, engage in social and cultural networks, and connect to robust business environments. For African-American men, investments aimed at building healthy communities are literally a matter of life and death.

By almost any measure, the health status of African-American males is a national disgrace. Compared with white men, African-American men are 30 percent more likely to die from heart disease, the nation's number-one killer (Kung, Hoyert, Xu, & Murphy, 2008). They are twice as likely to die from prostate cancer (Centers for Disease Control and Prevention, 2009a), 7.4 times more likely to develop AIDS, and 9 times more likely to die from it (Centers for Disease Control and Prevention, 2009b). They suffer disproportionately from asthma (Moorman et al., 2007), diabetes (Centers for Disease Control and Prevention, 2008), poor oral health (Office of Minority Health, n.d.), and stroke (Pleis & Lucas, 2009). They are less likely to drive or own cars, yet they die at higher rates in motor vehicle crashes (Cohen Mikkelsen, & Srikantharajah, 2009). African-American men and boys are disproportionately victimized by violence and crime and vulnerable to drug and alcohol addiction (Lee, 2008). Although **health disparities** persist regardless of income (House & Williams, 2000), entrenched poverty in communities of color, coupled with the persistent segregation of so many neighborhoods along the lines of race and income, demand that we view this health crisis through overlapping lenses of race, socioeconomic status, and place.

Poor access to health care exacerbates the health disparities. African-American men are far more likely than white men to have no regular source of medical care and no health care coverage (Doty & Holmgren, 2006). In poor communities of color, residents are in dire need of practitioners who understand their culture, speak their language, counsel healthy habits, diagnose diseases early, prescribe the right treatments, and follow up on care. Affordable high-quality care must be made available immediately, and equitably.

The health reform legislation passed by Congress and signed by President Obama in 2010 marked a tremendous step forward. The law, upheld by the Supreme Court in June 2012, addressed core concerns that many people of color have had about the status quo. It expanded coverage to upwards of 30 million people. It ended the most egregious abuses of the insurance industry and helped low-income Americans afford coverage with subsidies. One of the most promising provisions was the creation of a prevention and public health trust fund to invest billions of dollars in proven **prevention**, wellness, and public health activities such as increasing bicycle paths, playgrounds, sidewalks, and hiking trails. As public health prevention and expanded coverage become a reality, African-American men stand to benefit at least as much as the rest of the population.

Yet critical as it is, an insurance overhaul represents only one of the many changes needed to eliminate health disparities and achieve **health equity**. Lack of access to health care is one of a multitude of factors contributing to disease risk and mortality in the United States (Ford et al., 2007). Local conditions—the physical environment, the economic landscape, the presence (or absence) of strong social networks and community services—play a major role. Simply put, where you live affects your health. In fact, a person's address is an astonishingly good predictor of his risk of disease, injury, early death, and, indeed, many of the risk factors that physicians track in their patients, such as excess weight, high blood pressure, high cholesterol, and elevated blood sugar (Bell & Rubin, 2007). With millions of African-American men and boys trapped in disadvantaged neighborhoods, is it any mystery why their health is suffering, or why the risks are accumulating and worsening over time?

Neighborhood conditions affect air quality, physical activity levels, and the availability of the necessities for healthy living, such as fresh, nutritious foods. Local conditions also impact health by providing access—or throwing up barriers—to economic and social opportunities, including jobs, education, and social networks. Access to opportunity, to resources for healthy living, and to health care are inextricably linked. Gaps in all three areas feed on one another in complex ways.

Deteriorated housing and schools, which are the norm in many poor inner-city neighborhoods, are frequent and hazardous sources of mold, lead, and vermin. Bus depots and other facilities that spew pollutants are disproportionately located in low-income communities of color, and truck-choked highways often run through them. These foul the air of already vulnerable communities, contributing to high rates of asthma and other respiratory diseases. For example, just a few miles from my office, the predominantly African-American community of West Oakland, California, abuts a busy freeway, a major port, and an airport. A 2003 study found the air inside some homes to be five times more toxic than in other parts of the city (Lee, 2003).

Poor communities on average have half as many supermarkets as wealthy communities, and predominantly African-American neighborhoods have especially limited access to supermarkets, farmers' markets, and grocery stores (Flournoy & Treuhaft, 2005). In Albany, New York, for example, 80 percent of residents of color live in neighborhoods where one cannot find low-fat milk or high-fiber bread, staples in any middle-class community (Hosler, Varadarajulu, Rosani, Fredrick, & Fisher, 2006). Predominantly white areas of Los Angeles have 3.2 times as many supermarkets as predominantly African-American areas and 1.7 times as many as predominantly Latino areas (Flournoy & Treuhaft, 2010). The absence of supermarkets in many low-income urban and rural communities, combined with inequitable transportation resources, often leaves residents with no convenient access to fresh, healthy foods—and all too reliant on fast-food outlets and convenience stores stocked with high-fat snacks and processed foods. These same communities also generally offer few, if any, options for physical activity: no parks, ball fields, recreation centers, or bicycle lanes; no well-maintained sidewalks or community bustle to encourage walking; and crime rates that keep residents indoors (Powell, Slater, Chaloupka, & Harper, 2006). In low-income, predominantly African-American neighborhoods, residents are often inundated with advertising for tobacco and alcohol, further stacking the deck against positive health choices.

Obesity, heart disease, diabetes, liver disease, and lung cancer are often viewed as "lifestyle" ailments attributable to an individual's behavior. In reality, they are the consequences of inequitable resources for healthy living. These both reflect and contribute to the economic and social inequities that lie at the heart of the health crisis facing African-American men.

Race, Poverty, Geography

Although the fanciful idea of a "postracial" America gained currency in the media in the wake of the 2008 election of President Obama, racial and economic segregation remain pernicious facts of life in many inner cities, inner-ring suburbs, and rural communities. On every major economic indicator—

income, wages, employment levels—African Americans are worse off today than a decade ago (Austin, 2008a). The reversal began long before the financial meltdown of 2008, leaving African-American men all the more vulnerable when the nation's economy tumbled.

African-American men led the unemployment surge that would become one of the harshest hallmarks of the recession, and they were the hardest hit. In April 2009, the official jobless rate among African-American men was 15.4 percent, double the rate for white men. The reality was much bleaker, because the statistics do not include men who are incarcerated, who are under-employed, or who have given up on finding work (Wessler, 2009). More than one-third of African-American men ages 16 to 19 in the labor force were out of work—a higher unemployment rate than the United States suffered during the Great Depression. African-American families with a hard-earned toehold in the middle class disproportionately felt the fallout of the massive loss of union jobs, especially in the automobile industry, and the subprime mortgage fiasco—the other hallmark of the recession.

Nationally, African-American homebuyers were two to nine times more likely than white buyers to receive subprime mortgages and other exotic home loans. In Bakersfield, California, for example, 55.5 percent of African-American home owners had high-risk mortgages. By the end of 2009, the city had one of the highest foreclosure rates in the state (which itself had one of the highest rates in the nation), with one of every 16 owner-occupied homes on the foreclosure market (Ojeda, 2009). By mid-2009, the African-American middle class was shrinking, and nearly half of all African Americans were living in poverty or severe financial distress. With the loss of jobs, homes, and assets accumulated over years, the impact on the African-American middle class may turn out to be one of the most lasting, disastrous effects of the recession and a significant threat to health in the African-American community for years to come.

Income is an important determinant of health (Braveman & Egerter, 2008), and the association between poverty and poor health is well documented. This is more than a matter of an individual's income. The economic environment of a community has a significant impact on the physical and psychological health of residents (Bell & Rubin, 2007). A study in Alameda County, California, found that residents of a high-poverty neighborhood had an increased risk of death over a nine-year period, regardless of individual income, age, gender, education, and other personal factors. This is explained in large part by the geography of poverty: Poor people in the United States tend to live in communities with many other poor people, and low-income African Americans often live in the poorest places of all. African Americans are nearly twice as likely as whites to live in high-poverty neighborhoods (Rivera, Huezo, Kasica, & Muhammad, 2009).

The combination of **residential segregation** and **concentrated poverty** leaves millions of African Americans cut off from the essential services and opportunity structures that form the ladder to the American dream. It also disadvantages African Americans from generation to generation. A study by the Economic Mobility Project, a nonpartisan collaborative effort of the Pew Charitable Trusts, found that 42 percent of children born to low-income families (the bottom 20 percent) will remain there, and another 42 percent will make it out just barely (Isaac, 2008). Race is a key factor in determining economic mobility, and African Americans are far less likely than whites to advance beyond the income level of their parents.

Many African-American males struggle to overcome the odds of an uphill, even Sisyphean, battle from birth, or even earlier. Low-income African-American women are less likely to receive high-quality prenatal care and have disproportionate rates of infant mortality and low birth weight. The effects of poverty and limited opportunity snowball from there:

- Disinvested communities with less access to high-quality preschools that provide the foundation for academic success and self-esteem
- Underfunded elementary, middle, and high schools with inexperienced teachers and inadequate materials
- Overcrowded, outdated, ill-equipped school facilities
- A frayed (and in some places dysfunctional) foster care system that often fails its charge to provide a safe haven for youth
- A job market with fewer and fewer sustainable opportunities for less-educated workers and often insurmountable barriers for ex-offenders
- Neighborhoods that often lack amenities such as transportation to connect to jobs around the region, yet that are saturated with gangs, violence, and illegal drugs
- Police who are quick to detain and harass African-American boys and men
- A criminal justice system far more willing to incarcerate them than to reintegrate them into society after their release

African-American boys have a one-in-three chance of going to prison in their lifetimes, and African-American youth are four times as likely as white youth to be incarcerated (Austin, 2008b). In California, African Americans accounted for 8 percent of the youth population but 25 percent of incarcerated juveniles in 2003—an overrepresentation echoed in many states (Chura, 2010). United States incarceration rates are by far the highest documented in the world. Yet as the prison and incarcerated youth population has swelled, support for rehabilitation and reentry services has diminished. For example, Congress cut college aid for prisoners, known as Pell Grants, even though inmates who participate in such educational programs have significantly lower rates of recidivism (Marable, 2000). As a result of cuts in education and other critical services, a man has a slim chance of successfully reintegrating into mainstream society after his release from prison. In California, for example, more than 60 percent of formerly incarcerated men return to prison within three years (California Department of Corrections and Rehabilitation, 2009).

Although these patterns are devastating to incarcerated men, they are not the only people hurt by disproportionate imprisonment and the abject failure of rehabilitation. When so many men are marginalized economically and socially, in prison and after their release, their families and communities also suffer (Hyman, 2006). Just as African-American men cannot be healthy if their communities are ailing, communities cannot be healthy if their men are sick, jobless, poorly educated, or locked up.

Beyond the economic toll, poverty exacts enormous social costs. High-poverty communities often lack the tight civic bonds and sense of cohesion that are critical to physical and psychological health. Strong social networks are associated with lower rates of homicide, suicide, and alcohol and drug abuse (Centers for Disease Control and Prevention, 2009c). Research on HIV-related interventions aimed at adolescents suggests that membership in social organizations may be protective against involvement in risky sexual behavior; indeed, one study found that weak social bonds and networks (as measured by a concept known as **social capital**) are strong predictors of rates of four common sexually transmitted diseases: gonorrhea, syphilis, chlamydia, and AIDS (Holtgrave & Crosby, 2003). An analysis of deaths during a Chicago heat wave in 1995 found that mortality was linked to differences in individual relationships and supportive neighborhood institutions (Klinenberg, 2002). A neighborhood with low levels of social capital had a mortality rate 10 times higher than the rate in a neighborhood of similar income but with higher levels of social capital. Those who died from the heat were almost always alone and isolated.

Strong community networks promote health in two ways. First, they foster interpersonal connections. Neighbors look after neighbors, and communities build and sustain social and faith-based organizations. Not only do these organizations attend to the needs of local residents—they also provide life-affirming opportunities for volunteering and leadership development, which further nourishes the social lifeblood of a community. Second, strong networks enable residents to organize and advocate for new investment, government funding, policies, and programs. These are essential to improve opportunity and health for everyone, individually and collectively, today and for generations to come.

Cornerstones of Community Transformation

To effectively address the health crisis facing African-American men, we must focus on their needs at the beginning of political processes. We must ensure they participate in and benefit from decisions that shape the course of development in their neighborhoods and the systems that serve them. We must promote and secure funding for **multidisciplinary** approaches focused not only on expanding access to health care but also on improving the social, physical, and economic environments of underserved communities. We must deepen our collective understanding of the developmental stages for African-American males, from birth (or before) through adulthood. This **lifecycle** should illuminate the policies, programs, and services needed for success as well as the challenges and opportunities facing our boys and men at every pivotal stage.

Four interconnected approaches provide both the philosophical underpinnings of community transformation and the cornerstones of effective, sustainable, equitable action to improve health:

- *Community-driven* strategies must build on the wisdom, voice, and experience of African-American men and the reality of their communities. Health practitioners, advocates, program providers, neighborhood and business leaders, and residents should play instrumental roles in shaping and implementing efforts to effect change for African-American boys and men.

- *Focusing on people and places* grounds our work in the conditions that shape day-to-day life—and health—in a community. It capitalizes on the strengths of the neighborhood and its residents while acknowledging the challenges they face.

- *Comprehensive and interconnected* programs are critical to repair the systems and practices that alienate and exclude African-American boys and men from opportunity (e.g., early childhood education programs, K–12 schools, physical and mental health systems, workforce education, higher education, the regional labor market).

- *Research-based* initiatives must pinpoint areas of immediate need and opportunities for action. Data should be used to: (a) identify disparities by key social and economic indicators; (b) assess the performance of institutions responsible for serving African-American boys and men; and (c) determine the effectiveness of all policies in eliminating disparities and providing equitable opportunities to males of color.

Policy Implications

There are proven strategies to transform struggling communities into healthy places of opportunity. The Harlem Children's Zone (HCZ) is an inspiring example. Recognizing the myriad interconnected challenges that confront communities of color, HCZ offers families within a 100-block area of New York City a full range of services designed to tip the scales toward success: health clinics, parenting classes, cooking classes, schools, tutoring, job counseling, and more. The Obama administration has taken the HCZ concept as the model for its Promise Neighborhoods initiative, which supports the planning and implementation of communities of opportunity, centered around strong schools, across the country. As Obama said during the presidential campaign: "There's no reason this program should stop at the end of those blocks in Harlem. It's time to change the odds for neighborhoods all across America."

Community interventions achieve their greatest success when they are connected to **policy**. Policies establish the rules and parameters for factors that dramatically impact a person's health, for better or for worse—the types of housing, transportation, schools, and health and human services we invest in and where we provide them; the price and availability of food; the kinds of jobs we create and whom we hire; the quality of teachers, the standards of instruction, and the physical condition of school buildings. The list goes on, affecting virtually every aspect of our lives.

Our public policies must be aligned with the goal of changing the odds for neighborhoods all across America. Key elements of a policy agenda include the following.

Revitalize Disinvested Communities

More than 60 years of metropolitan sprawl have isolated the places where many African Americans live: first, inner-city neighborhoods and more recently, aging inner-ring suburbs. Development patterns have siphoned public investment and attention from these communities toward the affluent suburban edge. It is long past time to ensure that resources flow equitably. We must commit to and invest in the revitalization of long-neglected neighborhoods, through broad policies to promote economic and social development.

One good place to start: Fix physical conditions that are detrimental to health, and create neighborhoods that support active living and healthy eating.

Researchers have identified transportation, land use, parks, and the availability of green spaces as critical factors in the health of communities of color. Local, state, and federal governments all have roles to play in creating local environments that support active living. In many cases, this will not happen by itself—it will take pressure from broad-based groups of advocates, practitioners, officials, neighborhood leaders, and residents. The City Project of Los Angeles demonstrates what such pressure can achieve. Through coalition building, advocacy, and lawsuits when necessary, the group has worked to create a web of parks, playgrounds, high-quality school buildings, beaches, forests, and transportation that serves diverse low-income Los Angeles communities that for years have had little or no access to such amenities.

Grocery stores are also part of a thriving community. They draw foot traffic, create local jobs, and stimulate commerce. Further, access to fresh, nutritious food is critical to health. The Pennsylvania Fresh Food Financing Initiative has been a pioneer in bringing healthy food retailers to communities that have long struggled without. From 2004 to late 2010, the initiative helped to open 83 supermarkets and fresh-food outlets in underserved areas throughout the state, and the numbers continue to grow. A partnership among state and local officials, nonprofit groups, and the business sector, the initiative had also created or retained 5,000 jobs in communities, including the entry-level positions that allow young men to secure their first chance at employment. Like HCZ, the initiative has become a model for the Obama Administration. The President's FY 2012 budget includes more than $330 million in investments in a national Healthy Food Financing Initiative. By investing in new and expanded food retailers, the program would move the country a long way toward expanded access to healthy food while providing many communities with an important anchor for revitalization.

Expand Opportunities for Employment

As mentioned earlier, income is a key determinant of health. Study after study shows that being poor is bad for your health, and the more you earn, the healthier you are likely to be. The message in the research is clear: If we want African-American men to have better health, we must provide better opportunities for meaningful, well-paid employment.

The Bureau of Labor Statistics predicts that new jobs over the next decade will increasingly require a college degree or higher. This is worrisome for African-American and Latino communities, which have lower levels of educational attainment than white and Asian communities. Without new approaches that target education and training resources toward African-American men and boys, they will be left crowding the fewer and fewer positions that require no degrees. This will perpetuate racial inequity and thus health disparities, not to mention other problems such as gangs and violence that arise when the future offers no real chance for success.

Employment discrimination remains a concern. Despite antidiscrimination laws enacted decades ago, employers still make biased assumptions about the capacity of applicants of color (Moss & Tilly, 2001). Moreover, studies show that African Americans earn lower wages, even controlling for educational background and work experience. Enforcement of civil rights laws to secure fair employment is imperative. But it is also important to create pipelines for African-American youth and adults to move into jobs and ultimately careers.

This requires investments in education and vocational training, with an emphasis on skills that will meet the demands of high-growth sectors in regions.

A number of organizations, among them SCOPE (Strategic Concepts in Organizing and Policy Education) in Los Angeles, are doing exactly that. They are trying to connect disadvantaged groups to the emerging "green" industry. SCOPE has led a public policy campaign to ensure that low-income communities receive the benefits of the green economy, including the employment it will create. In 2009, the Los Angeles City Council adopted an ordinance to begin green retrofits in all municipal buildings and to connect low-income communities to the jobs created by the project. Like the most promising place-based workforce development strategies, SCOPE forcefully addresses the broad components that make a place healthy: economic development, by creating jobs with a career path; civic engagement, by enlisting residents in coalition building and advocacy to gain political support for their goals; the physical conditions, as green jobs will improve both the natural and built environments; and the social fabric, as public buildings will be upgraded to better serve city residents.

Invest in Human Development and Build a Skilled Workforce

The increasingly punitive environment in public schools, evidenced by zero-tolerance policies, has not only failed to make schools safer and more supportive of learning, but it has also been counterproductive (Skiba & Knesting, 2002). Zero-tolerance policies have been applied disproportionately against boys and young men of color, African Americans in particular, pushing more and more children out of school and often into the prison pipeline. Prevention and intervention strategies must be aimed at keeping African-American students in school, out of trouble, and on a path to success. We must ensure that at-risk students have access to counseling and other services to address mental health issues, emotional trauma, and other social and psychological problems that may underlie disruptive behavior.

But getting through school without expulsion is not enough. Young men need to see possibilities in the labor market and a way to grasp them. Acknowledging that youth in low-income neighborhoods sometimes cannot imagine themselves in college, the "multiple pathways" approach prepares students for higher education and careers, often by carving small, focused academic programs within large public high schools. An example is the Architecture, Construction, and Engineering (ACE) Academy at Locke High School in Los Angeles, opened in 2009. Developed by a partnership of community, business, and labor organizations, the school prepares a largely African-American and Latino student body for well-paid careers in the skilled and building trades.

In Oakland, the Cypress Mandela Construction Program prepares students for careers in construction through strong alliances with local organizations, including the county Building Trades Council, the Ella Baker Center for Human Rights, and the Oakland Green Job Corps, a job-placement program funded by the American Recovery and Reinvestment Act.

Community-based pipelines to employment such as these can be lifesavers, providing young men with self-confidence, marketable skills, and hope for the future. Promising practices can be strengthened by legislation that provides technical assistance and funding to education institutions that address local and regional industry needs while providing meaningful training for community youth.

Emphasize the Justice in the Juvenile and Criminal Justice Systems

In his book, *Punishment and Inequality in America* (2007), Harvard sociologist Bruce Western writes that punitive penal policies end up hurting the communities they were designed to protect. He argues that incarceration is not merely a symptom of social inequality but also a cause and fuel of inequality because it undermines families and further isolates them from the economic and social mainstreams.

McCullum Youth Court in Alameda County, California, represents an effort to change that picture. Working with police and probation departments throughout the county and with the Oakland Unified School District, Youth Court offers young nonviolent offenders a chance to avoid incarceration if they agree to a peer-led court process that includes case management, prosecuting and defense attorneys, jury deliberation, and sentencing. Defendants found guilty must accept responsibility, undergo needed treatment or counseling, and repay their victims, families, and communities for damage to property and relationships. According to Youth Court, nearly 80 percent of the young people who went through this alternative process did not recidivate, and almost 70 percent of those who were not in school when they came to the court eventually reenrolled.

Just as it is critical to help youthful ex-offenders stay out of jail, it is imperative to help ex-convicts reintegrate into their communities. The Getting Ready program in Arizona is working toward that goal by preparing prisoners for their eventual return home, almost from the day they are locked up. The program emphasizes job training for growth industries in the state, and it has reported great success in lowering prison violence, facilitating reentry, and reducing recidivism.

Keeping ex-offenders from returning to prison is good for them, but it's also good for everyone else. It means safer neighborhoods, more intact families, more dedicated workers, and more productive members of the community. In short, it means healthier places—and a healthier society—for all.

Summary

As we rightly push the health care system to respond more effectively to the urgent health needs of African-American men, we must acknowledge that better medical treatment and access to health care, alone, will not the solve the health crisis in our communities. We must advocate for policy reforms and investments aimed at improving the physical, economic, and social environments of struggling communities of color in cities, older suburbs, and rural areas. This requires public and political will as well as a new way of thinking about health and the means to achieve it.

This chapter argues that the health of African-American men is closely tied to the health of their communities. It explains how local environmental factors—including air-pollution levels; housing quality; and access to grocery stores, transportation, and jobs—negatively impact the health of African-American men. It describes the four underpinnings of community-change efforts that can improve the health of African-American men: These efforts should be locally driven, focused on people and places, comprehensive and interconnected, and based on research. Public policies must be aligned with the goal of creating healthy communities of opportunity. Key elements of a policy agenda include revitalizing distressed communities, expanding job opportunities, investing in workforce development, and reforming the justice system.

Key Terms

access	multidisciplinary
communities of opportunity	policy
concentrated poverty	prevention
health disparities	residential segregation
health equity	social capital
lifecycle	

Discussion Questions

1. What is the relationship between race and health? What is the relationship between place and health? Do you believe race or place is the primary driver of the health crisis facing African-American men?

2. How do environmental conditions contribute to poor diet and sedentary lifestyle? Describe how these elevate disease risk for African-American

men. How can interventions be aimed simultaneously and effectively at individuals and the conditions in which they live?

3. What policies currently catapult African-American boys and men into the criminal justice system and away from pathways to opportunity? How can these policies be mitigated? How can they be dismantled?

4. What inherent strengths in African-American communities can be tapped to organize for, effect, and sustain change?

5. What role should doctors, community clinics, and hospitals play in community transformation efforts? Do health and medical practitioners have a social responsibility to advocate for policy initiatives in land use, transportation, food access, workforce development, and other spheres that impact the health of their patients?

References

Austin, A. (2008a). *Reversal of fortune: Economic gains of the 1990s overturned for African Americans from 2000–02.* Briefing Paper No. 220 Washington, DC: Economic Policy Institute. http://www.epi.org/publications/entry/bp220/

Austin, A. (2008b). *What a recession means for black America.* Issue Brief No. 241 Washington, DC: Economic Policy Institute. http://www.epi.org/publications/entry/ib241/

Bell, J., & Rubin, V. (2007). *Why place matters: Building a movement for healthy communities.* Oakland, CA: PolicyLink. http://www.policylink.org/site/apps/nlnet/content2.aspx?c=lkIXLbMNJrE&b=5136581&ct=6997411

Braveman, P., & Egerter, S. (2008). *Overcoming obstacles to health.* Princeton, NJ: Robert Wood Johnson Foundation. http://www.rwjf.org/files/research/obstaclestohealth.pdf

California Department of Corrections and Rehabilitation. (2009). *Recidivism rate: Three year follow-up period by commitment offense.* Sacramento, CA: Adult Research Branch, California Department of Corrections and Rehabilitation. Retrieved from http://www.cdcr.ca.gov/Reports_Research/Offender_Information_Services_Branch/Annual/RECID3/Recid3d2005.pdf

Centers for Disease Control and Prevention. (2008). *Age-adjusted percentage of civilian, noninstitutionalized population with diagnosed diabetes, by race and sex, United States, 1980–2006.* Retrieved from http://www.cdc.gov/diabetes/statistics/prev/national/figraceethsex.htm

Centers for Disease Control and Prevention. (2009a). *Health, United States, 2008.* Hyattsville, MD: Centers for Disease Control and Prevention, National Center for Health Statistics. http://www.cdc.gov/nchs/data/hus/hus08.pdf

Centers for Disease Control and Prevention. (2009b). *HIV/AIDS surveillance report 2007.* Vol. 19. Atlanta, GA: Centers for Disease Control and Prevention, National Center for Health Statistics. http://www.cdc.gov/hiv/topics/surveillance/resources/reports/2007report/pdf/2007SurveillanceReport.pdf

Centers for Disease Control and Prevention. (2009c). *Report of the national expert panel on social determinants of health equity: Recommendations for advancing efforts to achieve health equity*. Atlanta, GA: Centers for Disease Control and Prevention. Retrieved from http://www.reversechildhoodobesity.org/sites/default/files/files-wfm/files/SDOH%20Expert%20Panel%20Report_0.pdf

Chura, D. (2010). *I don't wish nobody to have a life like mine: Tales of kids in adult lockup*. Boston, MA: Beacon Press.

Cohen, L., Mikkelsen, L., & Srikantharajah, J. (2009). Traffic injury prevention: A 21st century approach. In S. Malekafzali (Ed.), *Healthy, equitable transportation policy: Recommendations and research*. Oakland, CA: PolicyLink. http://www.ConvergencePartnership.org/atf/cf/{245a9b44–6ded-4abd-a392-ae583809e350}/HEALTHTRANS_FULLBOOK_FINAL.PDF

Dodakian, R. 2010. Promises to keep: The Obama poverty plan. *City Limits*. http://www.citylimits.org/news/article.cfm?article_id=3887

Doty, M. M., & Holmgren, A. L. (2006). *Health care disconnect: Gaps in coverage and care for minority adults* (Issue Brief, Vol. 21) New York, NY: Commonwealth Fund. http://www.commonwealthfund.org/Content/Publications/Issue-Briefs/2006/Aug/Health-Care-Disconnect—Gaps-in-Coverage-and-Care-for-Minority-Adults—Findings-from-the-Commonwealt.aspx

Flournoy, R., & Treuhaft, S. (2005). *Healthy food, healthy communities: Improving access and opportunities through food retailing*. Oakland, CA: PolicyLink. http://policylink.info/pdfs/HealthyFoodHealthyCommunities.pdf

Flournoy R., & Treuhaft, S. (2010). *Healthy food, healthy communities: Promising strategies to improve access to fresh, healthy food and transform communities*. Oakland, CA: PolicyLink. http://www.policylink.org/site/apps/nlnet/content2.aspx?c=lkIXLbMNJrE&b=5136581&ct=8020083

Ford, E. S., Ajani, U. A., Croft, J. B., Critchley, J. A., Labarthe, D. R., Kottke, T. E., & Capewell, S. (2007). Explaining decrease in U.S. deaths from coronary disease, 1980–2000. *New England Journal of Medicine*, 356, L2388–L2398.

Holtgrave, D. R., & Crosby, R. A. (2003). Social capital, poverty, and income inequality as predictors of gonorrhea, syphilis, chlamydia, and AIDS case rates in the United States. *Sexually Transmitted Infection*, 79, 62–64. Retrieved from http://www.hawaii.edu/hivandaids/Predictors_of_Gonorrhoea,_Syphilis,_Chlamydia_and_AIDS_Case_Rates_in_the_US.pdf

Hosler, A. S., Varadarajulu, D., Rosani, A. E., Fredrick, B. L., & Fisher, B. D. (2006). Low-fat milk and high-fiber bread availability in food stores in urban and rural communities. *Journal of Public Health Management Practice*, 12, 556–562.

House, J. S., & Williams, D. R. (2000). Understanding and reducing socioeconomic and racial/ethnic disparities in health. In B. D. Smedley & S. L. Syme (Eds.), *Promoting health: Intervention strategies from social and behavioral research*. Washington, DC: Institute of Medicine/National Academy Press.

Hyman, J. B. (2006). *Men and communities: African American males and the well-being of children, families, and neighborhoods*. Washington, DC: Joint Center for Political and Economic Studies. http://www.jamesbhyman.com/Publications/Men%20and%20Communities.pdf

Isaac, J. B. (2008). Economic mobility of black and white families. In *Getting ahead or losing ground: Economic mobility in America*. Washington, DC: Brookings Institution. http://www.economicmobility.org/assets/pdfs/PEW_EMP_GETTING_AHEAD_FULL.pdf

Klinenberg, E. (2002). *Heat wave: A social autopsy of disaster in Chicago*. Chicago, IL: University of Chicago Press.

Kung, H. C., Hoyert, D. L., Xu, J., & Murphy, S. L. (2008). *Deaths: Final data for 2005*. National Vital Statistics Report (Vol. 56, No. 10). Hyattsville, MD: Center for Disease Control and Prevention. http://www.cdc.gov/nchs/data/nvsr/nvsr56/nvsr56_10.pdf

Lee, H. K. (2003, November 26). Diesel exhaust poses health risks in West Oakland, study finds. *San Francisco Chronicle*. Retrieved from http://www.sfgate.com/cgi-bin/article.cgi?f=/c/a/2003/11/16/BAGQE334JL1.DTL

Lee, M. M. (2008). *The health challenge: Creating a policy agenda focused on place*. Working paper for the National Black Latino Summit. Oakland, CA: PolicyLink. http://www2.nationalblacklatinosummit.org/bls_health.pdf

Marable, M. (2000). Facing the demon head on: Institutional racism and the prison industrial complex. *Southern Changes*, *22*(3): 4–7.

Moorman, J. E., Rudd, R. A., Johnson, C. A., King, M., Minor, P., Bailey, C., & Akinbami L. J. (2007). *National surveillance for asthma—United States, 1980–2004*. Surveillance Summaries. Morbidity and Mortality Weekly Report (Vol. 56, SS-8). Atlanta, GA: Centers for Disease Control and Prevention, National Center for Health Statistics. http://www.cdc.gov/mmwr/PDF/ss/ss5608.pdf

Moss, P. & Tilly, C. (2001). Stories to tell: Race, skill, and hiring in America. New York, NY: Russell Sage Foundation.

Office of Minority Health, U.S. Department of Health and Human Services. (n.d.). *Oral health 101*. Retrieved from http://minorityhealth.hhs.gov/templates/browse.aspx?lvl=3&lvlid=246

Ojeda, R. H., (2009) *The continuing home foreclosure tsunami: Disproportionate impacts on black and Latino communities*. William C. Velasquez Institute White Paper. http://www.wcvi.org/data/pub/WCVI_Publication_Homeownership102309.pdf

Pleis, J. R., & Lucas, J. W. (2009). *Summary health statistics for U.S. adults: National health interview survey 2007*. Vital and Health Statistics, Series 10, No. 240. Hyattsville, MD: Centers for Disease Control and Prevention, National Center for Health Statistics. http://www.cdc.gov/nchs/data/series/sr_10/sr10_240.pdf

Powell, L. M., Slater, S., Chaloupka, F. J., & Harper, D. (2006). Availability of physical activity-related facilities and neighborhood demographic and socioeconomic characteristics: A national study. *American Journal of Public Health*, *96*(9), 1676–1680.

Rivera, A., Huezo, J., Kasica, C., & Muhammad, D. (2009). *The silent depression: State of the dream 2009*. Boston, MA: United For a Fair Economy. http://www.faireconomy.org/files/pdf/state_of_dream_2009.pdf

Skiba, R. J., & Knesting, K. (2002). Zero tolerance, zero evidence. An analysis of school disciplinary practice. In R. J. Skiba & G. G. Noam (Eds.), *New directions for youth development (No. 92: Zero tolerance: Can suspension and expulsion keep schools safe?)* (pp. 17–43). San Francisco, CA: Jossey-Bass.

Wessler, S. (2009). *Race and recession: How inequity rigged the economy and how to change the rules*. New York, NY: Applied Research Center. www.arc.org/recession

Western, B. (2007). *Punishment and inequality in America*. New York, NY: Russell Sage Foundation.

World Health Organization. (2003). *WHO definition of health.* Retrieved from http://www.who.int/about/definition/en/print.html

One City's Attempt at Treating the Effects of Social Inequities in African-American Men

Lessons Learned

Elizabeth M. Whitley
Jodi Drisko

Learning Objectives

- Understand how the social determinants of health influence African-American men's health status and behaviors.
- Identify how quantitative and qualitative data can be used to assess underlying need and inform program development.
- Recognize health policy implications that must be addressed to alleviate undue burden on disparate, underserved populations.

• • •

African-American men in Denver experience significant **disparities** compared to other men and women in terms of overall health status, insurance, health-seeking behaviors, mental health, risk of chronic disease(s), and health risk behaviors. The **social determinants of health** such as poverty, unemployment and underemployment, low educational attainment, and inadequate housing negatively affect health access and outcomes.

This chapter illustrates one community's experience working within a public health care system using an **outreach and navigation** model to address health, basic needs, and the social determinants of health for individual clients through direct service, partnering with community-based organizations, and influencing public policy.

Denver Community Context

The City and County of Denver is one geopolitical unit that covers 153 square miles at 5,280 feet above sea level. Denver is composed of 77 discrete neighborhoods, recognized by city government and residents alike. The population of Denver is 600,158 individuals, of which 52.2 percent are non-Hispanic white, 31.8 percent Hispanic, 10.2 percent black/African American, 3.4 percent Asian, 1.4 percent American Indian, and 1 percent other. Approximately 27.7 percent of individuals over the age of five speak a language other than English at home (U.S. Census Bureau, 2010).

Denver has 32 officially designated medically underserved neighborhoods with a population of 258,769 residents, of which 29.2 percent are non-Hispanic white, 51.4 percent Hispanic, 14.3 percent African American, and 5 percent others. When compared to the rest of Denver, the residents in these 32 neighborhoods are disproportionately minority, poor, and young.

Denver Health is the primary health care safety net institution for Denver. Denver Health serves one out of every four Denver residents, or approximately 150,000 unduplicated users each year, of which 52 percent are Hispanic, 14 percent African American, 27 percent Caucasian, 1 percent Native American, less than 1 percent Asian, and 5 percent of unknown race/ethnicity. More than 46 percent of Denver Health patients are uninsured and the system provided over $350 million of uncompensated care in 2009.

Understanding the Issue

Men and minorities often have a higher prevalence of poor health and risk factors and a lower prevalence of positive factors (Williams, 2003). Existing, readily available data, such as Behavioral Risk Factor Surveillance System (BRFSS) and Denver Health utilization data, were examined as a part of a needs assessment process to further understand the health status and issues of underserved men in Denver. Additionally, focus groups were conducted with uninsured Denver men to provide qualitative data about barriers to health care access.

The burden of chronic diseases and high-risk health behaviors among Denver's minority and male populations are well documented through the BRFSS as seen in Table 14.1.

Table 14.1. Health Status, Risk Behaviors, and Chronic Disease, Prevalence Estimates BRFSS 2006–2008 (Behavioral Risk Factor Surveillance System, 2006–2008)

Health Indicator	Denver Males				All Denver Adults			
	Black/African American	Hispanic	White/non-Hispanic	All Denver Males	Black/African American	Hispanic	White/non-Hispanic	Denver Total
Health status								
Fair to poor health status	14.5	35.7	9.5	18.4	15.1	34.3	9.8	16.5
Mental health not good 8+ days in last month	20.3	14.2	11.4	13.0	18.1	14.8	12.1	13.8
Physical health not good 8+ days in last month	12.1	12.9	9.1	13.3	14.8	14.3	10.6	11.7
Overweight or obese, BMI†=25.0 or higher	72.9	70.5	57.1	62.8	64.2	72.2	47.2	54.9
Obese, BMI†=30 or higher	28.1	28.7	12.3	19.1	24.0	31.0	13.6	18.8
No health insurance	18.9	51.5	9.5	25.3	20.4	50.6	9.1	21.6
Behavioral risk factors								
Binge drinking	17.0	27.6	25.8	26.3	13.6	16.9	20.6	19.4
Current smoker	25.6	31.0	16.7	23.7	24.3	23.5	17.0	19.9
No physical activity	9.9	29.9	10.3	17.7	20.0	32.7	13.3	19.6
Eat 5 or more servings of fruits/vegetables per day	*	13.8	25.0	19.8	7.5	16.5	31.4	25.9

(continued)

Table 14.1 (Continued)

Health Indicator	Denver Males				All Denver Adults			
	Black/African American	Hispanic	White/non-Hispanic	All Denver Males	Black/African American	Hispanic	White/non-Hispanic	Denver Total
Don't always wear seatbelt in car	33.1	16.2	17.4	18.1	18.7	18.9	15.0	16.5
Medical care and chronic disease								
Ever had colonoscopy (ages 50 and over)	*	*	64.0	57.1	59.1	37.0	60.4	55.5
Haven't had cholesterol checked in last 5 years	*	47.9	21.7	34.5	32.0	42.2	17.7	26.8
Diagnosed with diabetes	12.3	6.6	5.2	6.4	10.2	8.2	3.9	5.7
Have asthma	6.5	2.0	6.7	4.6	8.6	4.6	7.1	6.5
Been told have high cholesterol	*	27.6	36.6	36.0	48.5	26.9	32.2	31.8
Been told have high blood pressure	*	14.6	22.9	21.0	37.0	14.6	21.5	20.8

*small sample size unable to calculate estimate

†BMI = body mass index

Health Status

Nearly 19 percent of African-American men in Denver have no health insurance, private or public, compared to 10 percent of white/non-Hispanic men. About 15 percent of African-American men report that they have fair or poor health status, which is equivalent to all men in Denver. Almost 20 percent report that their mental health was not good eight or more days in the last month, which is 50 percent higher than that for all Denver men. Twelve percent report their physical health was not good eight or more days in the past month, similar to all men. Twenty-eight percent of African-American men are obese and another 45 percent are overweight, which means that almost three quarters (73 percent) are overweight or obese, putting them at great risk for diabetes and heart disease.

Certain behaviors are more likely to predict poor health and chronic disease. African-American men are just as likely to smoke (25.6 percent) as all men in Denver and are just as likely to participate in physical activity as white/non-Hispanic men. They are less likely to engage in binge drinking (having five or more alcoholic beverages in one sitting) than white/non-Hispanic or Hispanic men. However, about one third of African-American men do not always wear a seatbelt, compared to 18 percent of all Denver men. Data were not available for consumption of fruit and vegetables for African-American men, but African Americans in Denver consume five or more servings of fruits and vegetables at a much lower rate than all Denverites (7.5 percent compared to 25.9 percent).

In Denver, as in the rest of the United States, men are often less likely to seek medical care than women. Even though data are not available for some indicators, inferences can be made from the total rates for African Americans and other racial/ethnic groups. Almost 60 percent of African Americans over the age of 50 have had a colonoscopy. Thirty-two percent of African Americans have not had their cholesterol checked in the past five years, and men are less likely to report having their cholesterol checked than women, so probably more than one-third of African-American men have not had their cholesterol checked in five years. Of those who have had their cholesterol checked, almost half (48.5 percent) of African Americans report that their cholesterol was high and 37 percent report that their blood pressure was high. These rates are the highest of all racial/ethnic groups in Denver. Males, in general, are more likely to report having high cholesterol, but equally as likely as women to report having high blood pressure. More than 12 percent (12.3 percent) of African-American men report having been diagnosed with diabetes and 6.5 percent report currently having asthma. This diabetes rate is nearly double the rate for all men in Denver.

System Utilization

The fact that men access health care systems less than women is well documented in the literature (Brett & Burt, 2001; Sandman, Simantov, & An, 2000). The need to foster health promotion within all minority men was also demonstrated through an analysis of Denver Health utilization data from 1998 through 2001 that excluded visits with primary diagnoses related to administration, social services, and sex-specific conditions (fertility, prenatal, male and female genitourinary organs) (Day, 2003).

This analysis showed that within Denver Health patients, men constituted 7.8 percent fewer total unique outpatient users than women. This difference was even more salient within the Denver Health Hispanic population, where males constituted 13.8 percent fewer users than females. In the Denver population there are roughly equal proportions of males and females of all race–ethnicities, and these data show that more women are accessing the health care system than men. Overall, average visits per year were 33 percent lower for men than women. This trend was more pronounced for minority populations; average visits per year were 39 percent and 37 percent lower for African-American and Hispanic men than their female counterparts. Furthermore, this trend persisted for patients diagnosed with chronic conditions; the average visits per year for men were 25 percent less than women. Therefore, in comparison to females, male patients receive less outpatient care, routine care, or care for the management of chronic illnesses.

Men Identify Barriers to Health Care

Next, focus groups were conducted to identify barriers to accessing health care for uninsured African-American, Hispanic, and white men in Denver. Eight focus groups were conducted, stratified by ethnicity, age, and language preference (Whitley, Samuels, Wright, & Everhart, 2005). The results of the African-American men's focus groups are summarized briefly next.

Three African-American men's focus groups were conducted; one for adults ages 23 to 45, one for 45- to 61-year-olds, and one group of teenagers, between the ages of 14 and 17 years. The two adult men's groups had 10 and 9 participants, respectively, and 16 young men participated in the teenage focus group.

Questions were asked about attitudes related to health and health care, access to health care, the health care experience, ways to better deliver health care, and life priorities. Key findings for the African-American focus groups are described below.

1. **African-American men do not trust the health care system.** African-American men mentioned past mistreatment of African-Americans

within our country's health care system as a reason for continued skepticism and mistrust. One particular example cited by a couple of participants was the Tuskegee syphilis study and its negative impact on the African-American community.

2. **African-American men detect differences in health care based on race.** Some African-American men point to race as reasons that they are treated differently than those of another race, particularly white people. Several compelling examples of institutional racism experienced at the health care safety net institutions were shared.

3. **African-American men emphasize that lack of a good job (or no job) leads to lack of financial resources, lack of health insurance, and thus, lack of adequate access to health care.** African-American men commonly mentioned significant economic barriers to accessing health care.

4. **African-American men feel their community has been left out.** These men believed that proper health messages are not communicated to their community and that health care programs are not developed specifically for them, at least in part due to economic factors. Instances of racial discrimination were also pointed out by several participants.

5. **African-American men favor educational messages on health.** Men indicated educational messages on issues such as the importance of health and access to health care would be well-received.

6. **A genuine effort must be brought to the African-American community to be effective.** Men indicated that those in their community must see some genuine caring and some action in order to be accepting of any health care marketing efforts.

Although all the participants recognized the importance of health, they perceived substantial barriers to obtaining health care. These barriers include economic status, lack of insurance, lack of transportation, lack of information, mistrust, and fear.

The African-American participants were particularly concerned about men's diseases and disease that disproportionately affect African Americans such as prostate cancer, diabetes, and heart disease. They were also aware of the behaviors that affect their health, such as eating well, exercise, and stress reduction.

Several health care system issues were also identified, including long wait times, quality concerns, and distrust of the system. The participants also expressed the need for better, more respectful communication.

The teens described health as important for longevity and physical performance and discussed several health issues of concern, including STDs,

HIV/AIDs, diabetes, hypertension, and prostate cancer. The young men maintained their health through attention to diet, exercise, mental health, and sexual health. African-American teens pointed out the most unhealthful behaviors they have noticed include drug and alcohol use, violence, lack of attention to diet, and risky sexual behavior.

These findings are consistent with those in the literature (Institute of Medicine, 2002; Satcher & Rust, 2006). The results of the focus groups were used to inform organizational and public policy, and to guide the development of media messages and the program model for the Denver Health Men's Health Initiative.

Program Model

The goal for Denver Health's Men's Health Initiative (MHI) is to increase access and affordability, reduce disparity, and improve seamlessness of health care to underserved men in Denver. Two patient navigators conduct outreach and provide basic care management to men in the community and in the city and county jail. Examples of community settings include homeless shelters, work centers, and street outreach. The patient navigators have established formal partnerships with many community-based organizations where they hold office hours and/or the organization may call them to help a client.

The patient navigators meet with clients to assess their needs and insurance status. As most of the Men's Health Initiative clients do not have health insurance, the patient navigators take applications for the Colorado Indigent Care Program, the state adult discount program. They also make appointments with enrollment specialists for the few men that qualify for Medicaid, primarily due to disability. The patient navigators assist their clients in establishing a medical home and in scheduling and coordinating primary and specialty care visits. Bus tokens are provided to men as needed to reduce the barriers related to transportation. Additionally, co-payments for medical visits and medications are provided through the Patient Assistance Fund. The patient navigators also help their clients apply for grant funds to purchase prosthetics and other essential items. Through partnerships with many community-based organizations the patient navigators provide referrals to housing, employment programs, support groups, parole compliance, and other needed services.

Community Reentry from Jail

In Denver, as in the rest of the United States, a disproportionate percentage of African-American men are incarcerated (Colorado Department of Corrections, 2007; Justice Policy Institute, 2007). The Men's Health Initiative patient

---

A Client's Brief Story—Fred (as Told by the MHI Patient Navigator)

Fred is an African-American man a MHI patient navigator met at St. Frances Day Shelter. He had been homeless for just a couple of weeks after losing his job and his health insurance. Fred has a seizure disorder and is diabetic. He had just run out of medications and was worried about how he was going to maintain his health so that he could find a job and get off the streets. The MHI patient navigator was able to get him enrolled in the Colorado Indigent Care Program to help pay for medical care and also made him an appointment with a primary care provider. Then, Fred was able to get the medicine he needed. The patient navigator also helped him get some glasses and a bus pass.

Fred was able to get a job shortly thereafter. The patient navigator saw him a couple of Sundays ago at St. Frances—he was there to get his things out of storage as he had found an apartment. He thanked the patient navigator and said, "I could not have done this without you." The patient navigator told him that he was happy for him and that he was only doing his job. But we do wonder what would have happened to Fred if it were not for the Men's Health Initiative.

---

navigators visit the Denver city/county jail several times a week and meet with men who are due to be released in the near future. They assess the individual's needs and provide reentry planning. On release, the patient navigators meet with their clients to reduce barriers to health care access. In addition to returning to predominantly economically disadvantaged communities, ex-offenders face many obstacles, such as restricted access to housing and limited employment opportunities. The patient navigators also provide funds for individuals to obtain identification and driver's licenses as well as referrals to other community-based organizations that facilitate community reintegration. However, a quarter of people on parole in the Denver metro area end up in homeless shelters or other temporary housing (Piton Foundation, 2007).

Through a grant from Morehouse School of Medicine Center for Primary Care, Community Voices, the Patient Navigators are able to assist reentry clients with transportation and in accessing mental health services through a partner, the Mental Health Center of Denver. Mental health evaluations and limited therapy (up to six sessions) are provided for individuals referred by the patient navigators. Clients are selected for this program by the patient navigators based on their functionality, reliability, and interest in the program. A specific team at the Mental Health Center of Denver, including a licensed counselor and psychiatrist, work with the reentry clients.

Evaluation metrics include number of ex-offenders receiving services, types and number of services received, medication adherence, and recovery markers, measured via an instrument administered at intake and discharge. Although the number of clients receiving services is small, preliminary results are encouraging.

A Client's Story—Ed (as Told by the MHI Patient Navigator)

Ed is a 45-year-old African-American man who is severely mentally ill and is also a crack addict. He started coming around our office about a year and a half ago. He would not say much about himself except he just got out of prison; he was obviously desperate, looking for whatever he could get. He was always making up wild tales just so he could get bus tokens. Our relationship was not always smooth and I have to admit I did not look forward to him coming in. I once walked into the bathroom and found him smoking crack, he stole a charger cord from my office, and later a Palm Pilot.

At one point I asked him to just stay away from our office and that there was nothing more I could do for him for the time being. When I ran into him on the streets a few months later, I thought he might be angry or resentful. But he seemed very happy to see someone he knew and he told me that he had been back to jail.

Ed started to come back to the office although he would never make appointments. He was not interested or up to getting hooked into primary care and did not want drug treatment. But he kept coming in and slowly started trusting me and me him. He would come in just to talk almost every day and it became apparent that I was the only person in his life that he trusted and in fact, had any consistent contact with. He would often come in beat up, and was frightened most of the time.

After many months of him coming in every day he finally told me some of his life history. Ed had grown up in the south with his family, when he was 18 he went to prison for eight years, and when he got out his family had moved and no one knew where they were. So, this mentally ill man, with no family, job, income, or friends, ID, skills, or education, has been traveling around the country ever since he was 24 years old. He sleeps on the streets except when in jail, and he is too paranoid to go to shelters. He told me that at the age of 45, he has never had an ID, Social Security card, or a job.

The ending to this story, at least for now, is not very happy. I got him a psychological evaluation at Stout Street Clinic and into a program that serves homeless folks with dual diagnoses. But that same night Ed got arrested and I have not seen him since.

I have wondered what his life would have been like if he would have gotten just a little bit of support when he got out of jail (the first time), if someone would have checked to see that he had somewhere to go. Ed's life could have been totally different—he is very intelligent, and has a great smile and laugh. What a waste!

Marketing

A marketing campaign was created to increase awareness about men's health and the Men's Health Initiative among African-American and Hispanic men, as well as to encourage men to access preventive health care. The "It's not your time" campaign was created based on the results of the men's focus groups and focused on the communication of two messages: Men of color die younger than other men from preventable diseases and the Denver Men's Health Initiative offers affordable and accessible preventive health care for men in Denver.

The campaign included a press conference (resulting in six two-minute local news segments and several print articles), TV spots, bus benches, buses and print ads. Men's Health Initiative spokespeople included a senator, attorney, barber, and police commander. Fact sheets were also created and disseminated. During the quarter following the launch of the campaign, 1,500 new men accessed the Denver Health system.

Men's Health Initiative Results

As of December 31, 2009, 9,741 men had been enrolled into the program, including 2,737 African Americans. Demographics for all participants and African-American men in particular are summarized in Table 14.2. Men's Health Initiative participants' ethnicity remains evenly split between African-American, Hispanic, and white, although slightly more white men have enrolled in the program. Demographic characteristics for African-American men are similar to the characteristics of all men enrolled in the program. The majority of participants are either homeless or in jail and 43 percent of African-American men listed jail as their last source of health care. Approximately two thirds of program participants describe their general health status as fair or poor, in contrast to 18 percent of men in Denver as a whole. About three quarters of men in the program reported having no regular doctor upon enrollment. The average age of all participants is nearly 42 years.

Table 14.2. Demographic Characteristics of Men's Health Initiative Participants (2002–2009)

Characteristic	All MHI Participants ($n = 9,741$)		African-American MHI Participants ($n = 2,737$)	
Ethnicity	Number	%	Number	%
African-American	2,737	28	2,737	100
Asian	61	1		
Hispanic	2,892	30		
Native American	209	2		
White	3,695	38		
Other/missing	147	2		
Living arrangement				
Homeless	4,691	48	1,223	45
Jail	2,265	23	841	31
Independent	1,189	12	365	13
Other/missing	1,596	16	308	11
Health status				
Good	2,427	25	767	28
Fair or poor	6,761	69	1,822	67
Missing	553	6	148	5
Regular doctor				
Yes	1,736	18	532	19
No	7,604	78	2,105	77
Missing	401	4	100	4
Mean age at intake	41.7		42.7	

Table 14.3 displays the social and environmental determinants for African-American men enrolled in the Men's Health Initiative. The largest barriers to care were financial reasons (87 percent) and homelessness (81 percent), followed by lack of kin (44 percent), lack of knowledge (42 percent), and legal problems (36 percent). Transportation, unemployment, and substance abuse were other barriers experienced by at least 25 percent of participants. Eleven percent cited mental illness as a barrier to seeking care. Only about one third reported having a social support network that consisted of friends (35 percent) and family (31 percent). Social risks included drug abuse (25 percent), alcohol abuse (23 percent), and smoking (15 percent). The men reported the largest life stress as lack of housing (77 percent), poverty (77 percent), and unemployment (65 percent), followed by health issues (49 percent), and legal issues (41 percent). Educational attainment was also asked, but 88 percent of participants did not answer that question.

Table 14.3. Social and Environmental Determinants of Health for African-American Men's Health Initiative Participants, through 12/31/2009

Characteristic	African-American Men's Health Initiative Participants ($n = 2{,}737$)	
Barriers to care	Number	%
Financial problems	2,372	87
Homelessness	2,216	81
Lack of kin	1,206	44
Lack of knowledge	1,142	42
Legal problems	977	36
Mental illness	306	11
Substance abuse	693	25
Transportation	740	27
Unemployment	737	27
Social support		
Family	835	31
Friends	956	35
Other case management	347	13
Religion	39	1
Social risks		
Alcohol abuse	622	23
Drug abuse	680	25
Smoking	411	15
Life stressors		
Health issues	1,340	49
Lack of housing	2,095	77
Poverty	2,109	77
Unemployment	1,780	65
Mental illness	306	11
Legal issues	1,134	41

As stated previously, the main purpose of the Men's Health Initiative is to engage men and to assist them in connecting with the health care system, establish a medical home, and obtain needed services. Patient Navigators gave out 4,659 bus tokens, scheduled or coordinated 51 medical or enrollment specialist visits, and took 738 applications for the Colorado Indigent Care Program (CICP). The Men's Health Initiative paid for 91 copayments or fees associated with getting necessary identification for insurance enrollment.

Service utilization at Denver Health clinics was analyzed for all African-American MHI participants one year after their enrollment in the program. All visits after their enrollment date for a time period of one year were included in the analysis. However, of the 2,737 African-American men in the program, 233

Table 14.4. Health Care Service Utilization of African-American Men within One Year of Enrollment in Men's Health Initiative

Men's Health Initiative: African-American Utilization Data for One Year after Enrollment $N = 2,185$

Type of Visit	Number of Visits	Number of Patients	Percent Using Service
Medical specialty	2,586	600	27
Primary care	2,070	562	26
Urgent care	869	456	21
Emergent care	823	452	21
Ancillary services	414	238	11
Denver cares (detox)	1,423	229	10
Dental	398	217	10
Inpatient	361	212	10
Correctional care outpatient clinic	135	96	4
Denver public health	105	86	4
Behavioral health	146	85	4
Methadone clinic	2,268	39	2

did not have a valid medical record number and were eliminated from the utilization analysis. Additionally, all participants with an enrollment date after December 31, 2008 were eliminated from this analysis ($n - 319$) to ensure that all participants had one full year to utilize services from their date of enrollment. Thus, the number of African-American men matched with the Denver Health data was 2,185, with 1,347 or 61 percent actually having had a visit at Denver Health. In contrast, 71 percent of white men and 66 percent of Latino men registered in the Denver Health system had utilized services within one year of MHI program enrollment. Among all MHI participants enrolled in the program for at least one year (those with and without a medical record number at Denver Health), 55 percent of African-American men and 58 percent of white and Latino men utilized services at Denver Health.

Table 14.4 displays the number of visits by service type. These categories were created based on billing codes and similar services were grouped together. Approximately 27 percent of enrolled African-American men in the Men's Health Initiative had a medical specialty visit, with an average of almost four visits per patient. About 27 percent had at least one primary care visit, with an average of nearly four visits per patient. Emergency and urgent care visits were utilized by 21 percent of men and averaged almost two visits per patient in this category.

Although service utilization within one year of enrollment seems relatively low, more than 1,300 African-American men received health care services that they may not have had access to without the program and work of the patient navigators. Additionally, service utilization data could only be captured for those receiving services at Denver Health clinics. Many clients also utilized services at other low-income and homeless health clinics. Some also returned to jail and would not be able to access services. Many were uninsured, so they may not have sought services.

Sustainability

Denver Health has completed a return on investment analysis for the Men's Health Initiative, which is described in great detail in a previous article (Whitley, Everhart, & Wright, 2006). Briefly, the Men's Health Initiative has increased access to primary and specialty care for underserved men, while also helping men use safety net services more appropriately. Inpatient, urgent care, and behavioral health visits decreased for men participating in the program compared with previous utilization of services prior to contact with the patient navigator. However, most of the Men's Health Initiative participants were uninsured, or perhaps only eligible for adult discount programs.

The favorable return on investment analysis resulted in stable funding for the Men's Health Initiative. Staff salaries are paid from the operational budget of Denver Health Community Health Services, primary care support. Other program costs, such as copays and bus tokens, are supported by the Denver Health Foundation Patient Assistance Fund.

Denver Health has also leveraged funds to provide outreach, education, and referral services to vulnerable men. For example, a grant from the Colorado Department of Public Health and Environment currently provides screening, referrals, and follow-up to African-American men in Denver barbershops. Additionally, new funds have been made available through the Denver Department of Corrections to pay for drug copayments for individuals released from jail.

Policy Implications

The Men's Health Initiative has increased awareness about men's health on several levels: throughout the Denver Health system, locally, statewide, and nationally. However, little progress has been made to address the barriers to care for underserved men through health care reform.

One of the most acute barriers is the exclusion of low-income adult men (without dependent children or disability) from publicly funded health insurance combined with work in jobs without employer-sponsored health insurance and insufficient resources to purchase coverage (Meyer, 2003). Additionally, access to Colorado Indigent Care Program (adult discount program) is not available to men in transition between incarceration and release. To date, there seems to be little political will at the state and federal levels to expand health coverage to vulnerable men.

Summary

This chapter has provided the reader with a description of how one community addressed the health effects of the social determinants of health for African-American clients of the Men's Health Initiative. The ill effects of poverty, unemployment, low educational attainment, and inadequate housing are evident beginning with the review of available data on the health status of Denver's African-American men, their health-seeking behavior, and the use of the safety net health system and barriers to health care. The Men's Health Initiative effectively increased access, affordability, and continuity for underserved African-American men in Denver. Policy reform is necessary to eradicate the negative effects of the social determinants of health and eliminate health disparities.

Key Terms

disparities

outreach and navigation

social determinants of health

Discussion Questions

1. Discuss what components of the program worked well to serve the African-American clients.

2. What changes would need to be made for the program to better serve the African-American clients?

3. What are some ways to address the root causes of poor health in African-American men in a more proactive fashion?

4. How can African-American men play a role in developing solutions to overcome the detrimental effects of the social determinants of health?

References

American Community Survey. (2008, July 1). *County characteristics resident population estimates file*. U.S. Census Bureau. Retrieved from http://www.census.gov/popest/counties/asrh/CC-EST2008-alldata.html

Behavioral Risk Factor Surveillance System. (2006–2008). Colorado Health Information Dataset. Colorado Department of Public Health and Environment. Retrieved from http://www.cdphe.state.co.us/cohid

Brett, K. M., & Burt, C. W. (2001). Utilization of ambulatory medical care by women: United States, 1997–1998. *Vital and Health Statistics*, *13*(149), 1–46.

Bureau of Justice Statistics. (2008). *Prison statistics*. Washington, DC. Retrieved from http://bjs.ojp.usdoj.gov/index.cfm?ty=pbdetail&iid=1763

Colorado Department of Corrections. (2007). *General statistics*. Retrieved from http://www.doc.state.co.us/Statistics/7GeneralStatistics.htm

Day A. D. (2003). *A quantitative analysis of utilization patterns for male patients in a safety-net health care system*. MPH Thesis. University of North Carolina at Chapel Hill.

Institute of Medicine. (2002). *Unequal treatment: Confronting racial and ethnic disparities in health care*. Washington, DC: National Academy Press.

Justice Policy Institute (2007). *The vortex: The concentrated racial impact of drug imprisonment and the characteristics of punitive counties*. Washington, DC: Author.

Meyer, J. (2003). Improving men's health: Developing a long-term strategy. *American Journal of Public Health*, *93*(5), 709–711.

Piton Foundation. (2007). *The Piton perspective*. http://www.piton.org/Documents/ThePITONperspctiveSpring07_5–24.pdf

Sandman, D., Simantov, E., & An, C. (2000). *Out of touch: American men and the health care system. Commonwealth fund men's and women's health survey findings*. New York, NY: Commonwealth Fund. Retrieved from http://www.cccmwf.org/usr_doc/sandman_outoftouch_374.pdf

Satcher, D., & Rust, G. (2006). Achieving health equity in America. *Ethnicity and Disease*, *16* (2 Suppl. 3), S3–8–13.

U.S. Census Bureau, 2006–2008. *American community survey*. Denver County, Colorado. Retrieved from http://factfinder.census.gov/servlet/ADPTable?_bm=y&-geo_id=05000US08031&-qr_name=ACS_2008_3YR_G00_DP3YR2&-ds_name=&-_lang=en&-redoLog=false

Whitley, E. M., Everhart, R. M., & Wright, R. A. (2006). Measuring return on investment of outreach by community health workers. *Journal of Health Care for the Poor and Underserved*, *17*, 6–15.

Whitley, E. M., Samuels, B. A., Wright, R. A., & Everhart, R. M. (2005). Identification of barriers to healthcare access for underserved men in Denver. *Journal of Men's Health & Gender*, *2*(4), 421–428.

Williams, D. R. (2003). The health of men: Structured inequalities and opportunities. *American Journal of Public Health*, *93*(5), 724–731.

Chapter 15

The Impact of Invisibility

The Way Forward

Henrie M. Treadwell

Learning Objectives

- Understand the historical context of health disparities affecting African-American men.
- Gain a knowledge of health and health care issues affecting African-American men.
- Appreciate that the social determinants of health are integrally involved in setting the stage for poor health and that poor health is embedded in federal policy, or lack thereof.
- Gain an awareness of the relationship between the feminist movement and the health of African-American men.
- Appreciate that research in African-American men's health can improve and save lives.
- Appreciate that research in African-American men's health can lead to less expensive treatments and cost-saving prevention strategies.

• • •

The historical context and origin of disparities must be woven into any discussion of how this nation extricates itself from the abysmal health care system that costs more than any other in the world but that serves far too many and without quality, particularly if they are poor boys and men of color. Gunnar Myrdal's *An American Dilemma: The Negro Problem and Modern Democracy*

(1944) documented the lasting effects of slavery and continuing racism on the social and economic conditions, family structure and lifestyle, and political awareness of African Americans. However, the issue of health disparities did not seriously capture national attention until 1985, when Margaret Heckler, secretary of health and human services, released the *Report of the Secretary's Task Force on Black and Minority Health,* which detailed the many stark differences in health between blacks and whites (Kennedy, 2005). Efforts intensified in the 1990s, and under President Bill Clinton's leadership, several federal initiatives to address the disparities were launched, including Healthy People 2010, Health Disparity Collaboratives, Racial and Ethnic Approaches to Community Health (REACH), and Excellence Centers to Eliminate Ethnic/Racial Disparities (EXCEED). It is important to note that the Office on Women's Health (OWH) was established in 1991 within the U.S. Department of Health and Human Services (HHS); however, no Office of Men's Health has been established even though overall health outcomes for men are equally or more disparate than they are for women. Legislation to establish an office of Men's Health has been introduced in Congress since 2003. And, countervailing social policies such as the War on Drugs and the various changes to Temporary Assistance for Needy Families (TANF) and other programs have made it even more difficult to achieve parity in men's health (viz. restrictions in access to food stamps, housing, and so forth) if an individual has a felony-related drug conviction on their record. Although the Second Chance Act under the Bush administration has opened some opportunities for individuals to reestablish themselves after incarceration, that Act included no provisions to ensure access to health care.

In 2000, Congress advanced the minority health agenda as well and created the National Center for Minority Health and Health Disparities at the National Institutes of Health (NIH). The Agency for Healthcare Research and Quality (AHRQ) was mandated to conduct research on minority health and health disparities, and the National Academy of Sciences was directed to examine and report on the minority data collection practices of the Department of Health and Human Services (HHS). Despite these steps, data collection still does not provide a complete and integrated portrait of the depth of disparities in this nation. Those surveyed are generally already in a health-seeking mode. And, prison health data and public sector health data are not integrated. The picture is bleak and the conundrum: If we do not know the depth of disparity, how can we develop a plan to address and redress inequities, should the political will exist to do so?

The African-American man is a member of the U.S. family that is far too often overlooked and stereotyped and whose issues are dismissed, blamed on him, or "set-aside" for action on that day that has never come, while leaders purportedly move on to address other more pressing issues. What is more pressing in a democratic nation than the ability of a group of men to live without fear of poor health and other acts of **marginalization** that further destabilize well-being?

The summation of the social determinants of health and how these affect mental health, assist in the spread of the AIDS epidemic, propel substance use disorder, undermine trust in the system, and drive a financially sizzling prison industrial complex—in one tome by many notable researchers and theorists is a breakthrough for the nation's researchers and practitioners on the front lines. The breakthrough into meaningful change awaits the reawakening of a spirit of inclusion and an aversion to marginalization.

Poor Men, Access to Care, and the Global and U.S. Health Care System

In this period of constantly evolving national health reform, much of the raging debate is centered on the rising cost of health care in the United States. Most agree that a solution is warranted, but there are divergent opinions as to the exact type of reform that is needed. Frequently, the solutions posed without vocal opposition are those that fail to embrace the poor, particularly those of color. At bedrock of the failure to legislate fairly is the lack of a bipartisan agreement on health care as a right. The U.S. health care system is composed of a range of stakeholders and is privately administered with multiple payers and a multistate regulated system (McKinsey, 2008). The limitations of current morbidity and mortality reporting systems are that the data do not illuminate causality. The social forces (viz. the social determinants of health) that independently or in the aggregate become in and of themselves agents for the onset of illness and a lack of well-being, are obscured by a purely physiological approach to health protection and disease prevention. These social forces, such as racism; isolation and stereotyping of poor men of color; a judicial, legislative and ultimately criminal justice system operating without restraint or respect for the long-term damage inflicted on the individual and the individual's family; poor education; no employment, all coalesce to form formidable barriers that health access alone cannot ameliorate.

In the absence of viable alternatives to the current health care model, many turned to the Commission on the Social Determinants of Health (SDOH), established by the World Health Organization (WHO), which released a conceptual framework for Action on the Social Determinants of Health (2007). According to the WHO, leveling efforts across the dimensions of mental health, material circumstances, and individual behavior, not just health care, will have a much greater long-term impact on population health and well-being. The report did not address gender as a unique and often overwhelming social determinant of health in some societies, particularly those in which there has been historical isolation and marginalization. So although useful to a degree, the study does not go far enough to allow it to serve as crucible for alleviating the plight of African-American men in the United States.

The WHO's report on how gender equity can be addressed through health systems noted that the consequences of not addressing gender are likely to include persistent excess mortality among men, underuse and inefficient use of health resources, poor user satisfaction, and, for some countries, perhaps, a widening gender gap in health (Payne, 2009). The report recognizes the increasing appreciation of the health costs of wider social inequity and notes the significance of the social determinants of health. There is greater recognition in the global sphere regarding the importance of developing policies and strategies than there is in the policy and practice arena in the United States, perhaps due to the heterogeneity of the U.S. population and lingering social marginalization of some groups.

A Necessary Reflection: Individual Health and Health Care

Multilevel, national health, and social policy reform on virtually every platform of the human experience in the United States is required if we are to bring unbridled attention to a population whose future health and well-being is dependent on dramatic health and social policy change. In an early editorial, "Poverty, Race and the Invisible Man," the sad conclusion was that the plight of a poor African-American male is not acknowledged in the United States (Treadwell & Ro, 2003). These individuals have been, since entry into the country, a founding stone of economic development whether working as slaves and subsequently as sharecroppers in the fields or nation-building, or as the cogs in the wheels of the explosive, expensive, and profitable **prison industrial complex** (still picking cotton for virtually no pay), where they, by virtue of their incarceration, generate great sums of money and political power (via prison gerrymandering) (Plant-Chirlin, Rusch, & Wagner, 2010). Their invisibility when public policy is formulated to provide payment for health care, to guarantee employment at a living wage, or to shore up an educational system that has failed them has made these boys and men vulnerable to poor outcomes across every sector of U.S. society (Henry J. Kaiser Family Foundation, 2010).

The Health of African-American Men

There are approximately 17.3 million African-American men in the United States, a proportion that represents 48 percent of all African Americans in the United States (U.S. Census Bureau, 2002). The experiences of African-American boys and men are uniquely different than males of other ethnic groups.

African-American men have the poorest health indicators of all racial/ethnic groups, male or female. African-American males have the highest mortality rate and lowest life expectancy among men and women in all other racial or ethnic groups in the United States (National Center for Health Statistics [NCHS], 2010). It has been noted that the mortality rates of urban African-American men are comparable to those of men in developing countries (Murray, 2006). Black men suffer far worse health than any other racial group in the United States.

According to the Office of Minority Health (OMH; 2012), in 2007, the death rate for African Americans was higher than whites for heart diseases, stroke, cancer, asthma, influenza and pneumonia, diabetes, HIV/AIDS, and homicide. According to data collected by Experian Simmons (2010), the top five ailments currently affecting African-American males are: hypertension/high blood pressure, backache, diabetes, high cholesterol, arthritis, and acid reflux—ailments that are precursors or indicators of the top mortality causes within this population.

In 2006, African-American men were 1.3 times as likely to have new cases of lung and prostate cancer, compared to non-Hispanic white men, and African-American men are twice as likely to have new cases of stomach cancer as non-Hispanic white men. This group has lower five-year cancer survival rates for lung and pancreatic cancer, compared to non-Hispanic white men and, in 2006, African American men were 2.5 times as likely to die from prostate cancer, as compared to non-Hispanic white men (OMH, 2006).

In terms of prevention, African-American adults are twice as likely as non-Hispanic white adults to have been diagnosed with diabetes by a physician. This statistic is particularly important, because diabetes is commonly known as the silent killer. Although type 1 diabetes remains relatively rare, type 2 diabetes is reaching epidemic proportions in the United States, with the rest of the developed world following close behind (DiabetesTheSilentKiller.com, 2010). Diabetes is a strong indicator for co-morbidity with other serious illnesses and an overall health status determinant. In 2002, African-American men were 2.1 times as likely to start treatment for end-stage renal disease related to diabetes, compared to non-Hispanic white men (OMH, 2002).

Similarly, strokes are an indicator of poor health management and occur 1.7 times more within the African-American adult population than in white adults. African-American males are 60 percent more likely to die from a stroke than their white adult counterparts (OMH, 2007). Even further, data have shown that African-American stroke survivors were more likely to become disabled and have difficulty with activities of daily living than their non-Hispanic white counterparts (Steiner et al., 2008).

A related, yet often overlooked area is oral health, which has been linked to many common illnesses. Recent studies point to possible associations between oral infections and diabetes, heart disease, stroke, and preterm, low-weight births (Geerts, 2002). In 2000, the 16th Surgeon General, Dr. David Satcher, released *Oral Health in America: A Report of the Surgeon General*, which formally presented a case for increased attention and prevention education on oral health awareness. The report was significant in bringing attention to this issue by documenting a significant disparity between racial and socioeconomic groups in regards to oral health and ensuing overall health issues. It is estimated that African-American men have a higher incidence and a higher rate of death from oral cancer (U.S. Department of Health and Human Services [HHS], 2000). Oral diseases are preventable; however, oral health is often taken for granted, but is an essential part of everyday life. Recent studies conducted by the California Children and Families Commission's Oral Health Education and Training Project showed that barriers to oral health and dental health may include: cultural discordance with dental providers, lack of knowledge about oral health and eligibility for benefits, access to care and economic restrictions, and lack of resources to cover services when advanced disease or complex care is needed (Isman, 2002). The cost of inaction in this area is high, resulting in poor attributable health outcomes and even an increased risk of oral cancer, particularly among minorities.

In addition to the high proportion of African-American men who are currently imprisoned and incarcerated, African-American men are highest at risk for many illnesses, several of which are preventable with appropriate care, management, and public health access. In 2007, 49 percent of African Americans in comparison to 66 percent of non-Hispanic whites used employer-sponsored health insurance. Also in 2007, 23.8 percent of African Americans in comparison to 9 percent of non-Hispanic whites relied on public health insurance. Finally, in 2007, 19.5 percent of African Americans in comparison to 10.4 percent of non-Hispanic whites were uninsured (OMH, 2007).

Social Determinants of Health and the African-American Man

African-American men are particularly vulnerable to stress due to historical and ongoing racial discrimination and related issues, namely low socioeconomic status and incarceration (Xanthos, 2009). In their study on African-American men's perceptions of health, Ravenell and colleagues (2006) found that across all groups of African-American men, stress was cited as having a significant negative impact on both physical and mental health. African-American men are especially susceptible to psychosocial stress since they have limited peer-accepted outlets for pain (Franklin, 1998; Xanthos, 2009). Common sources of stress among African-American men include racial discrimination, low socio-economic status, and incarceration, which are interrelated and mediators of aforementioned outcomes within the population (Xanthos, 2009). Franklin notes that although reluctance to share vulnerabilities is not uncommon for men generally, African-American men have a tendency to project an image of "emotional invulnerability." Although it may seem like a useful coping mechanism in dealing with life in an often hostile society, this behavior creates further stress and pressure and can lead to unhealthy behaviors for short-term gratification (Franklin, 1998; Xanthos, 2009). Social determinants that pave the pathway from cradle to prison are known though not addressed by local or national policy makers. According to the U.S. Department of Labor, the unemployment rate for African-American men is more than twice the unemployment rate among white, Hispanic, and Asian men. To a man, the ability to work and provide for his family is the underlying essence of his identity and defines his role in the family unit. The inability to find work and/or retain employment, due to lack of skills, qualifications, or support, can have long-term detrimental effects on the African-American family unit, on the self-esteem of the boy or man, and on the actual ability to pursue a path to support his dependents.

According to the 2009 U.S. Census Bureau report, the average African-American family median income was $32,584 in comparison to $54,461 for non-Hispanic white families (DeNavas, Proctor, & Smith, 2009).

In 2009, the U.S. Census bureau reported that 25.8 percent of African Americans in comparison to 9.4 percent of non-Hispanic whites were living at the poverty level. As of October 2010, the unemployment rate for African Americans was twice that for non-Hispanic whites (15.7 percent and 8.8 percent, respectively). This finding was consistent for both men (16.3 percent compared with 8.9 percent) and women (12.7 percent compared with 7.3 percent) (Bureau of Labor Statistics [BLS], 2010).

Finally, the African-American man gets much of his health care in prison because there is no virtually guaranteed comprehensive primary health care and payment system for him unless he manages to get himself arrested. Systems that fail to prevent illness and then to treat disease are simply upping the financial cost of the system overall. A sick young man may become an ill adult who then becomes a senior with chronic conditions that preclude working, walking, or performing the daily routines of life and then requires nursing assistance or in-home care, not to mention home-delivered meals.

Social Movements: The Feminist Movement and the African-American Male

There are many researchers who feel that the status of the African-American male is indicative of the national priority placed on the health and overall wellness of this group, when compared to other groups. Although this may be particularly evident in 2010, as shown by the disparities in geographic, demographic, educational, psychological, and health statistics outcomes, this lack of priority may have begun decades ago at the onset of the **feminist movement**. Prior to that cultural turning point, African Americans were seen as second class and denied many of the liberties afforded to Caucasian Americans. The civil rights movement made great strides to bring equality to all Americans, particularly in the areas of workforce and education. The purpose of this chapter is not to present the societal underpinnings of the civil rights movement, but it is important to note that African Americans, both men and women, were seen as the national minority even up to the 1970s. Other events in the United States, notably the civil rights movement, contributed to the rise of the feminist movement. During the early 1960s, the civil rights movement gathered momentum, aided by new antiracist legislation, and reached a major goal in 1964 with the passage of the Civil Rights Act. Many feminists interpreted the ban on racial discrimination, established by the Civil Rights Act, to apply to gender discrimination as well (Carden, 1974). The student movement was also at its height in the 1960s, leading many younger citizens to question traditional social values and to protest against U.S. military involvement in Vietnam. Feminist groups followed the example set by these movements, adopting the techniques of consciousness raising, protests, demonstrations, and political lobbying in order to further their own agenda.

The feminist movement (1960s–1980s) brought about the next cultural shift that may have been the reason behind the lack of support overall for the establishment of an Office of Men's Health. The movement was concerned with gender inequality in laws and culture based largely on the assumption that *all* men had societal rights that were not afforded to all women because of discrimination and an imposed cultural value system. The gender roles of women in the household, society, and even sexuality were amplified. Although the feminist movement made many strides in reducing many of the barriers presented to women, the fallacy in the movement's assumptions is that *all* men were equal while women fought for balance of power. Thus, African-American boys and men and their plight and unequal status were not included or recognized in this hierarchical conversation.

Time Out for Talk: Time for Action

Evidence of the plight of the African American can be seen through the lens of disintegrating neighborhoods, and children living in poverty being raised by single women. The loss of family, community, and neighborhood infrastructure is chronicled in many places and lamented from time to time. Solutions, problem-solving, and national commitment to a change process requires a closer look at gender and color and how these factor into the lives and livelihood of poor men.

Invisible No More

Now we see him, this poor man of color, who has been marginalized from opportunity, options, work, education, his role as a father, and from his place as leader in his community. He is the main actor, the catalyst for profit in only one industry in the United States: the criminal justice system. As many come to grips with the social catastrophe that current policy and practice are developing, there is a growing sense of hope and a growing sense of urgency. The reality of where we are as a nation (health disparities statistics) versus where we would like to be (access to primary health care and prevention for all) is that there has not been enough commitment by health care providers and leadership across all sectors to the identification and eradication of the issues that cause poor health among African-American men. The failure to work toward health care for all is clear evidence of the lack of value placed on the poor men of color in our society. To be clear: There is a fiscal crisis; but there is always money for war. And, there is a critical need for research on the social determinants of health among African-American men. Many editorials and studies have been written with suppositions proposed, but systematic studies of the men affected by the sociopolitical and sociocultural context have not been performed in a scientific manner by culturally inclusive teams that present a point-to-point correlation that can be embedded into policy and quality of care criteria and acted on by the health care system, in collaboration with other systems (viz. education, employment, family income, criminal justice). The historic marginalization of all African Americans and particularly African-American men in health care research and discovery (unless the risk is great as in the Tuskegee study) is minimized unless there is profit. Even in the wake of such vulnerabilities and during a time of anticipated national health care reform, which may yet carve them out of the progress if Medicaid reform is not fully enacted, there are opportunities to address health disparity issues, including research that will inform effective policy decisions and provide options to reduce the burden of socioeconomic factors on health outcomes.

Policy Recommendations

This chapter has set forth specific status indicators of the African-American male, but the greater purpose is to provide a base on which a solid platform for health justice can occur. Questions to be posed include:

- Whether some geographic regions are more supportive of African-American boys and men and, if so, what are the factors that create a successful community for this population? What factors are negative? What are the factors in "place" that nurture and support?

- What are the underlying issues for African-American men that appear to thwart their completion of high school and seek postsecondary education in higher numbers?
- What are the factors that are integral in the march to incarceration?
- If not incarcerated, what are the realistic care options for poor men without insurance?
- What public health care options have been implemented to maintain a continuum of care following incarceration?
- What are the public health interventions that work aggressively to reduce the incidence of disease among this population (e.g. obesity, oral health care, behavioral health care)?
- What can we learn about the psychological factors that are imposed on vulnerable African-American men that affect their sense of confidence, self-perception, and motivations as an adult?
- What must be done to erase or mitigate the trauma that has been inflicted on the thousands of African-American boys and men that have been disproportionately adjudicated and incarcerated with disproportionate sentences?

Although these questions are only examples of the many areas of needed research, without such answers, effective solutions will not be found. Public health prevention programs and community initiatives should be targeted and tailored for the intended audience, which will increase the probability of individual-level adherence to behavior recommendations (Kukafka, 2005) and, ultimately, long-term improvements in health outcomes. Research to illuminate issues and address forthrightly historical and contemporary discrimination and marginalization is essential and must be funded by health, education, criminal justice, and other local, state, and federal agencies.

Participatory, Evidence-Based Programs and Research

The primary *Call to Action* is for community-based participatory research that identifies key influencers within the African-American male social network and that produces evidence that can guide system reform with accreditation implications, and human interactions that are inclusive of all regardless of gender, color, and socioeconomic circumstances. Little research has explored the relationship in the African-American male community between social influences (e.g., social networks, social support, social norms, civic affiliations) and health as it relates to modifying factors that may contribute to overall health disparities (Emmons, Barbeau, Gutheil, Stryker, & Stoddard, 2007).

Within the African-American male population, much of the **social network analysis** and research is within the context of sexually transmitted disease (STD) and HIV/AIDS research, or more benignly on illnesses related to prostate health. In addition, much of the research is conducted by those who are not representative of the cultural context in which poor men of color live. The workforce of those doing the research and providing care must be addressed as a part of any problem. The direction of research can be driven by redirecting the funding from the usual suspects, the traditional institutions that command most of the research dollars, and aligning these in partnership with communities that understand the issues because they have "lived" in the social milieu which causes disparate outcomes (Treadwell, Braithwaite, & Taylor, 2009). Mathematical modeling efforts (e.g., to determine risk estimates) have incorporated network structure into the evaluation of transmission dynamics and these social network dynamics have been used to evaluate disease control efforts within the target group (i.e., concurrent, as opposed to sequential, sexual partnerships, in epidemic propagation) (Rothenberg et al., 1998). In order to address inequalities across a broad range of areas, social network analysis and research should be expanded to consider the effects that an African-American male's social network has on his behavioral choices, psychological decision-making patterns, and overall esteem and self-perception. By examining how key social influence and contextual mediating variables relate to health behaviors, we can learn more about the types of unique interventions that are needed to promote sustained health behavior change and improved well-being within the African-American male population.

Mental Health and Substance Use Disorder

The second *Call to Action* is for research particularly in the areas to improve mental health and the tsunami of increasing substance use disorder. Findings from appropriately funded and implemented work will provide the tools needed to empower the African-American male population and their supporters (through collective action) to organize and change existing hierarchies. In this context, a hierarchy is not only defined by a distal, system attribute, but by those things that may bind and prevent those with the motivation to act from truly succeeding. Essentially, more dialogue, case studies, and evidence-base are needed to shape concrete steps that facilitate a change in the circumstances in which African-American men find themselves. Greater engagement in clinical trials would be in order, providing that issues of trust and health insurance to pay for care following engagement in the clinical trial are available (Perez & Treadwell, 2009).

Reenergizing the American Dream

Amid the reality of the staggering health disparities that exist for African-American men when compared to other groups, there are many that may dismiss this epidemic by simply believing the African-American boy and man should have the self-will to change his situation. Often invisible, African-American men have a unique plight in this country that may inhibit the use of such logic. The setting itself defies the logic of changing things yourself as social forces are aligned to defeat self-will alone. Therefore, changing their plight is not a simple matter of will. Rather the plight is interwoven within a complex social structure where race, fairness, employment opportunity, being pushed out of school too soon, a predatory criminal justice system, and other factors make escape to the very top of the heap extremely difficult for far too many (Steele, 1998). Learning theories emphasize that adopting a new, complex pattern of behavior, like changing from a sedentary to an active lifestyle, normally requires modifying many of the small behaviors that compose an overall complex behavior (Skinner, 1953). According to the Social Cognitive Theory, behavior change is affected by environmental influences, personal factors, and attributes of the behavior itself (Bandura, 1989). A central tenet of social cognitive theory is the concept of self-efficacy. A person must believe in his or her capability to perform the behavior (i.e., the person must possess self-efficacy) and must perceive an incentive to do so (e.g., changing one's situation must bring more benefit than not changing) and also value the outcomes or consequences that he or she believes will occur as a result of performing a specific behavior or action. According to Bandura, outcomes may be classified as having immediate benefits or long-term benefits, but because these expected outcomes are filtered through a person's expectations or perceptions of being able to perform the behavior in the first place, self-efficacy is believed to be the single most important characteristic that determines a person's behavior change.

Centuries of abuse and neglect and separation policies designed intentionally to marginalize have taken their toll and have abraded self-efficacy not only among the boys and men themselves. The total social construct that promulgated these policies has wreaked its toll on the entire society. A key research gap is in studies that assess the strategies and tools needed to rebuild sustainable self-efficacy in the African-American man and the notion of inclusion within the society. For example, an African-American man that is unemployed or that cannot find work to support his family may recognize the long-term value in obtaining an education in order to have access to more employment opportunities. But when many in his family and peer group have not been successful in finding a way up the ladder, he may give up and conclude that the social forces arrayed against him are just too formidable. Unable to "man-up" to the costs of supporting a family because he cannot find a job, he may choose flight from some routine responses, rather than be reminded every single day that he cannot compete against the brunt of social marginalization and isolation. Likewise, an African-American man that has a chronic illness may understand the long-term value in exercising and eating a healthy diet in order to manage his illness, but he may choose to continue a poor diet and inactive lifestyle because these activities provide a sense of habitual "escapism" from the institutional barriers that cause a more acute pressure, threatening his sanity and increasing his stress-level on a daily basis. This same man may have diabetes and a felony-related drug conviction that may ban him for life from food stamps in some states. Without money, a job, but with a debilitating chronic disease, he may conclude that society does not care if he survives or even want him to survive. It is difficult to determine how a positive message can be gleaned from marginalization that threatens life while continuing to have a positive perspective. The social determinants of poverty, a felony-related drug conviction, no stable place to live, and lack of even basic access to health care and food are powerful and perhaps, to some, persuasive evidence that his life has little value to his nation. A compelling thought is that one has a bed in prison but is homeless in his own neighborhood. The logic escapes reason. Research that unravels the entanglement in so many negative factors and that weaves together the fabric of community caring could educate the public and the policy maker while supporting health. Research that also follows the money in the criminal justice scenarios might also illuminate the degree to which a profit motive continues the scale of mass incarceration being witnessed.

A National Policy Commitment for African-American Men

The final *Call to Action* is to support the creation and funding of a national, federal-level Office of Men's Health. In 1991, Congress created the Office of Women's Health within the Department of Health and Human Services (HHS). Across the nation, dedicated efforts to improve the health and well-being of poor men of color and, indeed, all men, are needed; gender equity and equality would seem to mandate greater attention. Although the need for improvement in health services and health status is not equally distributed across the population in the United States, improvement for the most needy groups will improve the health of all. Men's Health Month in June in the United States has done little to improve the health of poor men of color (most do not even know that June is men's health month) as a payment system that guarantees access to health care does not exist for him and he has no way of following up on negative results obtained at a health fair that may be offered during that month. No organized federal entity is present to provide sustained leadership and national directives to improve men's health.

In 2009, U.S. Representative Tim Murphy introduced a bill that would raise the public's awareness of health problems affecting men, and ways to detect and prevent them (Men and Families Health Care Act of 2009, H.R. 2115). Congressional and grass-roots support of this effort will show a national commitment to prevention and health promotion in men, which will help curb this expenditure growth and create effective social norms by breaking through the stigma associated with men who avoid seeking care or who encounter barriers when they seek health care. The time has come for the creation of a federal Office of Men's Health. A recognized federal focus can act as the galvanizing force to bring into alignment all aspects of the social spectrum that can catalyze formation of a system of care that includes all men, and that has, at the same time, the reduction of human suffering and out of control spending on preventable chronic illness.

Looking ahead, using the framework developed by the Commission on Social Determinants of Health (SDOH) (2007) will provide some insight into the key areas of research that should be supported to gain insight into strategies that are uniquely successful to reach, and ultimately reduce disparities in African-American men. According to the SDOH framework, health inequalities flow from patterns of social stratification, from the systematically unequal distribution of power, prestige, and resources among groups in society. Inequalities in power, prestige, resources, and even in what is "valued" within a culture are the underlying causes of health inequity and disparity. Ideally, a restoration of the balance of "power" should reduce inequalities and disparities in the population. Research is needed to identify strategies that will empower, adequately educate, and restore the equity in the distribution of common social and health justice enabling resources across the population. Due to the lack of process guidelines and knowledge base that instructs (or directs) action to restore power (over, to, with, and within) African-American men, this chapter brings forward a call to action for research in these critical areas.

Perhaps more can be learned from the International Society of Men's Health (ISMH), the only international organization dedicated to the unmet need of improving the health of men of all ages (Shabsigh, 2010). Through its work on building consensus, ISMH is building a best practice statement on men's health maintenance, early detection, and prevention of disease and starting a process toward the improvement of men's health in addition to health policy and education. Although the determinants of health are yet to be integrally built into this nascent work, significant platform presentations at the World Congress of Men's Health in Nice, France, in October 2010 included issues of incarceration, mental and behavioral health, and systematic advocacy for men's health. The expansion of the programs and content of meetings will bring to global audiences the issues that concern all men, including the poor and underserved. The dialogue alone will do much to refocus the national and international health agenda from one focused principally on maternal and child health to the father of the child as an important person in the life of the family and as the greatest hope for improving the overall social and economic potential for all. The maternal and child focus, the major export from the health care system to the rest of the world, has saved the lives of many infants but offers nothing to baby boys who grow up to be men and find too little, too late for them in health care services and policy.

Summary

Men have significantly higher death rates in nine of the 10 top leading causes of death, higher rates of smoking and overweight/obesity, are more often uninsured, and are far less likely to receive routine preventive care. Understanding the audience will help to guide intervention planning, determine the exact demographic needs and preferences, and provide better clarity of who the African-American man is aside from health disparity data and incarceration rates. When assessing next steps in the health care debate, and indirectly in the health disparities arena, it is imperative that the unique characteristics, preferences, and beliefs of African-American boys and men are given consideration as strategies are introduced. Even further, it is an even greater imperative that the unique needs and voice of the "poor" African-American boys and men are also heard and validated. Essentially, the question is: Why should federal and nongovernmental agencies fund research in African-American men's health? This chapter has summarized the literature to show that:

- The social determinants of health are integrally involved in setting the stage for poor health and the setting for this poor health is embedded in federal policy, or lack thereof.
- Certain diseases and conditions exclusively affect African-American men, are more prevalent in African-American men, or affect African-American men differently than other groups.
- Research in men's health includes more than just reproductive health (e.g., prostate cancer).
- Research in African-American men's health can improve and save lives.
- Research in African-American men's health can lead to less expensive treatments and cost-saving prevention strategies.

Moving forward, it is the aim of this chapter to encourage more community-based/evidence-based practice and research that will identify effective solutions to reduce health disparities that disproportionately affect the African-American male population. It is clear that African-American men are affected by socioeconomic, physical, and mental health burdens that place the population at greater risk of failure, family fragmentation, and alternate health outcomes. Consequently, we need policies and programs that address the issues causing and related to social determinants of health affecting this population. Additionally, funding bodies must show a greater willingness to fund research and programs that address the social determinants of health among African-American men (Xanthos, 2009). Ultimately, the aim is to spark constructive dialogue and educate and encourage the nation (e.g., health care system stakeholders) to take action to address this often overlooked, yet critical public health issue. Invisibility of this population comes at great cost to the taxpayer, even if and when people prefer to look away.

Key Terms

invisibility

marginalization

prison industrial complex

social network analysis

Discussion Questions

1. After reading about the status of the African-American male, what are the system-level barriers that most impact health outcomes for the African-American male?

2. In what ways do you feel that the national health care reform will impact these issues?

3. What recommendations would you make to bring more attention to the issues affecting African-American men among policy makers?

References

Bandura, A. (1989). A social cognitive theory of action. In J. P. Forgas & M. J. Innes (Eds.), *Recent advances in social psychology: An international perspective* (pp. 127–138). Amsterdam, The Netherlands: Elsevier.

Bureau of Labor Statistics of the U.S. Department of Labor. (2010, December). *Monthly labor review* (Vol. 133, No. 12).

Carden, M. (1974). *The new feminist movement.* New York, NY: Russell Sage Foundation.

Commission on Social Determinants of Health. (2007) *A conceptual framework for action on the social determinants of health, discussion paper for the commissioon on social determinants of health DRAFT April 2007.* Retrieved from http://www.who.int/social determinants/resources/csdh framework action 05 07.pdf

DeNavas, C., Proctor, B., & Smith, J. (2009). *Income, poverty, and health insurance coverage in the United States: 2009.* U.S. Census Bureau, Current Population Reports, pp. 60–238.

DiabetesTheSilentKiller.com. (2010). *Diabetes—The silent killer.* Retrieved from http://www.diabetesthesilentkiller.com

Emmons, K., Barbeau, E., Gutheil, C., Stryker, J., & Stoddard, A. (2007). Social influences, social context, and health behaviors among working-class, multi-ethnic adults. *Health Education & Behavior, 34*(2), 315–334

Experian Simmons (2011). *Experian Simmons 2010 U.S. household consumer trend and benchmark report.* Retrieved from http://www.experian.com/assets/simmons-research/white-papers/2010-us-household-consumer-trend-benchmark-report.pdf

Franklin, A. (1998). The invisibility syndrome in psychotherapy with African American males. In R. L. Jones (Ed.), *African American mental health* (pp. 395–413). Hampton, VA: Cobb & Henry.

Geerts, S., Nys, M., Charpentier, J., Albeirt, A., Legrand, V., & Rompen, E. (2002). Systematic release of endotoxins induced by gentle mastication: Association with periodontitis severity. *Journal of Periodontology, 73*(1), 73–78.

Henry J. Kaiser Family Foundation. (2007). *The health status of African American men in the United States, social determinants of health.* Retrieved from http://www.kff.org/minorityhealth/upload/7630.pdf

Kennedy, E. (2005). The role of the federal government in eliminating health disparities. *Health Affairs, 24*(2), 452–458.

Kukafka, R. (2005). *Tailored health communication.* New York, NY: Springer.

McKinsey Global Institute. (2008). *Accounting for the cost of US health care: A new look at why Americans spend more.* Retrieved from http://www.mckinsey.com/mgi/reports/pdfs/healthcare/US_healthcare_report.pdf

Murray, C. J., Kulkarni, S. C., Michaud, C., Tomijima, N., Bulzacchelli, M. T., Iandiorio, T. J., & Ezzati, M. (2006). Eight Americas: Investigating mortality disparities across races, counties, and race-counties in the United States. *PLoS Medicine, 3*(9): e260.

Myrdal, G. (1944). *An American dilemma: The negro problem and modern democracy* (Vol. *1 & 2*) New York, NY: Harper & Row.

National Center for Health Statistics. (2010). *Health, United States, 2009, with special feature on medical technology.* Hyattsville, MD: Author. Retrieved from http://www.cdc.gov/nchs/data/hus/hus09.pdf

Office of Minority Health. (2002). *Diabetes and African Americans.* Retrieved from http://minorityhealth.hhs.gov/templates/content.aspx?ID=3017

Office of Minority Health. (2006). *Cancer and African Americans.* Retrieved from http://minorityhealth.hhs.gov/templates/content.aspx?ID=2826

Office of Minority Health (2007). *African American profile.* Retrieved from http://minorityhealth.hhs.gov/templates/browse.aspx?lvl=2&lvlID=51

Office of Minority Health. (2012). *Stroke data/statistics.* Retrieved from http://minorityhealth.hhs.gov/templates/browse.aspx?lvl=3&lvlid=10

Payne, S. (2009). *How can gender equity be addressed through health systems? Policy brief 12.* World Health Organization 2009 & World Health Organization, on behalf of the European Observatory on Health Systems and Policies, 2009. Retrieved from http://www.euro.who.int/__data/assets/pdf_file/0006/64941/E92846.pdf

Perez, L., & Treadwell, H. (2009, February). Determining what we stand for will guide what we do: On community priorities, ethnical research paradigms, and human experimentation in prisons. *American Journal of Public Health.*

Plant-Chirlin, J., Rusch, T., & Wagner, P. (2010). *Advocates commend census bureau for enhancing states' access prison population data in 2010.* Brennan Center for Justice at NYU School of Law. Retrieved from http://www.brennancenter.org/content/resource/advocates_commend_census_bureau_for_enhancing_states_access_prison_pop/

Isman, B. (2002). *Potential barriers to oral health and dental care.* Retrieved from http://www.first5oralhealth.org/rural_smiles/downloads/chapter1/Potential%20Barriers.pdf

Ravenell, J., Johnson, Jr., W., & Whitaker, E. (2006). African-American men's perceptions of health: A focus group study. *Journal of the National Medical Association, 98*(4), 544–550.

Rothenberg, R., Pottertat, J., Woodhouse, D., Muth, S., Darrow, W., & Klovdal, A. (1998). Social network dynamics and HIV transmission. *AIDS, 12,* 1529–1536

Shabsigh, R. (2010). Men's health in*2010*: "Turning the corner"! *Journal of Men's Health, 7*(3), 183–184.

Skinner, B. F. (1953). *Science and human behavior.* New York, NY: Free Press.

Steele, S. (1998). *A dream deferred: The second betrayal of black freedom in America.* New York, NY: HarperCollins.

Steiner, V., Pierce, L., Drahushk, S., Nofziger, E., Buchman, D., & Szirony, T. (2008). Emotional support, physical help, and health of caregivers of stroke survivors. *Journal of Neuroscience Nursing, 40*(1), 48–54.

Treadwell, H., Braithwaite, R., & Taylor, S. (2009). Closing the gap. In H. Treadwell, R. Braithwaite, & S. Taylor (Eds.), *Health issues in the black community* (pp. 581–586). San Francisco, CA: Jossey-Bass.

Treadwell, H., & Ro, M. (2003). Poverty, race and the invisible man. *American Journal of Public Health, 98,* S142–S144.

U.S. Census Bureau. (2002). *U.S. Summary: 2000.* Retrieved from http://www.census.gov/prod/2002pubs/c2kprof00-us.pdf

U.S. Department of Health and Human Services. (2000). *Oral health in America: A report of the surgeon general.* Rockville, MD: U.S. Department of Health and Human Services, National Institute of Dental and Craniofacial Research, National Institutes of Health.

Xanthos, C. (2009). *Feeling the strain: The impact of stress on the health of African-American men.* Community Voices, Morehouse School of Medicine, Atlanta, Georgia.

Chapter 16

Criminal Justice and Other Public Policies as Determinants of Health and Well-Being for African-American Men

Leda M. Pérez

Learning Objectives

- Understand the history of the marginalization of African-American men in the United States.
- Learn about how some public policies have been shaped and how these have contributed to poor health and social outcomes in African-American men over time.
- Understand how public policies—particularly those developed in relation to the criminal justice system—can be direct determinants of health and well-being in African-American men.
- Learn about alternative public policies that may improve health and social outcomes in low-income African-American men and their communities.

• • •

This chapter provides a brief history of how some public policies have developed and how these have influenced social and health outcomes for African-American men and, by extension, their communities. As we examine some of the policies that have arisen over time, careful attention must be provided to how these have affected low-income African-American men, ultimately shaping their relationship with the **criminal justice system**. As this chapter shares, there is a direct connection between current policies and the disproportionate number of African-American men in jail or prison, a phenomenon that later creates survival challenges for those formerly incarcerated. The objective of this chapter is to share alternative policies—particularly those that include the necessary attention to the **social and economic determinants of health**—to ensure that the numbers of African-American men in prison decrease; **recidivism** (return to jail or prison because of another conviction) rates reverse; and, that the underserved communities from which many of these men hail thrive.

In the first part of this chapter, the role of persistent racism, including the development of social policies with origins in slavery, segregationist, and separatist legislation, are examined. The second part focuses on the social policies that have developed inequitably, including health policies that have resulted in limited, if any, access to health care for men. The final part provides recommendations for how to improve the social and economic determinants of health for vulnerable African-American men and their communities, highlighting some specific policies to shift the **equity** pendulum toward better protections and care.

Brief History of the Marginalization of African-American Men in the United States

This section draws heavily from Douglas A. Blackmon's work, *Slavery by Another Name: The Re-Enslavement of Black Americans from the Civil War to World War II*. Blackmon (2008) provides an in-depth historical account of how many African-American men were kept in slavery through social policies that developed in the period immediately following the emancipation of slaves in the mid-nineteenth century through World War II.

Criminalization of Being Black

As Blackmon recounts, there was an economic imperative to maintain slavery. In complicity with local southern governments and the economy of the country as a whole, a kind of "industrial" slavery flourished as the south transcended the cotton business and began rebuilding through the exploration of mining and other industrial activities. This work demanded cheap labor, but with slavery abolished it became necessary to secure a low-cost labor force. Blackmon argues that one way in which this was accomplished was through the development of new codes. Whereas "slave codes" had existed during slavery to manage the conduct of slaves and slave owners, so, too, was a "black code" developed in the aftermath of slavery. Essentially what the latter did was to criminalize being black, particularly for black men.

One example of how this was done can be observed through the vagrancy laws established in the late nineteenth century. "Vagrancy," the condition of not being able to "prove" one's employment, essentially assured that without proper proof or the legitimate voucher of one man for another (read: white man as a voucher), the risk of going to jail was near certain. Although vagrancy was not established as exclusively for black people, it became clear that this social policy was established to entrap mostly black men. In this period, the majority of black men could not "prove" employment either because they had no documentation or because they might have been landholders themselves. Through this criminal justice system, it became legal for people to be brought back in chains to the very farms where they had served as slaves. They were imprisoned, sold, and forced into labor camps. According to Blackmon, records make it abundantly clear that thousands upon thousands of claims made against these men in the South had no basis in fact. Yet they served the time. Hard time.

The Beginning of a Prison-Centered Trajectory

As a nascent legal system began to grow in the South, it was common practice that a well-known, local businessman or market owner might have also served as the Justice of the Peace. What ensued was a situation in which a number of local men, posing behind the law, succeeded in growing a jail population, which was later leased to the growing mining and steel industry. A lasting effect is that large numbers of African-American women were left alone to raise their children.

Later, in the early part of the twentieth century, policies such as Aid to Dependent Children (ADC), a precursor to **Aid to Families with Dependent Children (AFDC)** and **Temporary Assistance for Needy Families (TANF)**, were established with the intent to support mothers who had been abandoned, divorced, never married, or whose husbands were unable to work (Williams, 2006, p. 4). However, as African-American women also became eligible for assistance, many states began to restrict eligibility by including the "man in the house" and "substitute father" provisions, suggesting that in order for women and children to be eligible for support, men could not be present in the household (Williams, 2006, p. 4).

At the same time, as Blackmon's work recounts, in the immediate post-emancipation period through World War II, bogus courts were established with the sole purpose of trying innocent men in order to feed a demand for cheap labor sold out through the incipient prison system of the first half of the twentieth century. This, together with the social welfare policies that were extended to black women in the late 1940s, including the provisions that made it impossible for there to be a "man in the house," helped to reinforce a trajectory of marginalization for many African-American men and women. These policies set a path of poverty as well as familial and community instability. Men were increasingly going to prison, or were self-separating from their homes and families so that their partners and children would qualify for some kind of public support given that many of the jobs available to both black men and women were limited and poorly paid. The laws insisting on the absence of a man in the house were later outlawed by the United States Supreme Court but these exclusionary policies did not come without their damaging effects in the moment and over time.

African-American Men and the Social and Economic Determinants of Their Health

As the previous section suggests, there were historical factors that shaped the highly "distressed" (Young, 2006) situation that is prevalent in many low-income, black communities of the United States, exacting some of the heaviest blows on men. It is no coincidence that there are high numbers of African-American men serving time in U.S. jails or prisons; nor is it happenstance that they also die more than any other race or gender from preventable diseases.

A Ready Pathway toward Prison

Pew's 2008 study reports that of the 2.3 million Americans in jail or prison, 1 in 15 African-American men 18 and older are in prison vis-à-vis 1 in 36 Hispanic men or 1 in 106 white men, also 18 and older (Warren, 2008, p. 8)! What accounts for this steady rise of mostly young, African-American men in the prison system? Some have suggested that the main drivers include the high rates of unemployment, barriers to quality education and social services, and the heavy impact of the **War on Drugs** on young, black men (Edelman, Holzer, & Offner, 2006).

Drug possession in the United States is criminalized instead of treated. As a result, people with substance abuse issues or those who are involved in the mental health system have higher chances than others of being incarcerated. Nearly three-quarters of prison inmates with **mental illness** also have co-occurring **substance abuse** issues (Blumstein & Beck, 1999), yet these remain untreated and are instead shifted into the prison system, where little **rehabilitation**, if any, occurs (Perez, 2010).

Other related issues include strict probation guidelines and the insufficient resources available through the courts to help formerly incarcerated people with appropriate communications and guidance from probation and/or **parole officers**. It is unsurprising, therefore, that a common reason for recidivating is a violation of parole or probation. Finally, given the comparatively poor resources in communities of color and the low educational attainment of young African-American men as compared to whites and other communities of color (Henry J. Kaiser Family Foundation, 2006), together with the high-unemployment or underemployment rate for this group, the trade of drugs for money, or other illegal forms of employment, are often more viable alternatives to working poorly paid jobs.

There is compelling research that suggests that **health insurance** may act as a protective factor against recidivism (Van Olphen, Freudenberg, Fortin, & Galea, 2006). Likewise, other research has suggested that resources in the community such as **supportive housing** may keep people from returning to prison (Community Voices Freedom's Voice Conference Proceedings, 2010). But in the absence of health care and social supports, low-income African-American men most often receive some kind of health care in jail or prison (Young, 2006). For those who are not in prison and who do not have employer-sponsored insurance coverage—either because they work part time or because they are employed by a small business that cannot afford to provide coverage—primary or preventative care is a distant possibility at best.

For those returning to their communities from prison, the situation is even more complex, as many employers will not hire people with criminal records. Moreover, for those convicted of a drug offense, public housing is not an option as the latter restricts residents with this criminal history. Thus, the basic elements required for survival—shelter, income, and health care—are simply not present for people, especially men, coming home from prison unless they have special familial support, which is unlikely as most people are returning to already distressed communities. The result is that most people recidivate, by some estimates as much as 71 percent within a three-year period (Community Voices Freedom's Voice Conference Proceedings, 2010)! And the cycle begins again.

Sicker Than the Rest

African-American men have the highest rates of HIV/AIDS and die more often of cardiovascular disease and cancer than any other racial/ethnic group in the nation (Henry J. Kaiser Family Foundation, 2007). And, as noted above, they are also disproportionately represented in jails and prisons, as well as in the parole system (Henry J. Kaiser Family Foundation, 2006; Pew, 2009).

Today, an African-American man is more likely to receive health care in jail or prison versus in a public or private health facility in his community (Warren, 2008). For those who have been in prison, there exists the possible exposure to infectious diseases including hepatitis C and HIV/AIDS. Beyond this, and perhaps less understood, is the role of posttraumatic stress arising from the prison experience, possibly including rape, violence, marginalization, and the absence of support structures and education (Young, 2006).

The reasons for these high rates of morbidity and mortality have their roots in history and the social and health policies that have developed over time. One of the reasons for why men are not receiving care in clinics or health centers in the United States is directly related to public health insurance policy (i.e., **Medicaid**), which provides coverage to low-income women and children, but, excluding few exceptions, does not include men. Poor men who do not receive insurance through their jobs, or who may be chronically unemployed or underemployed, are not covered unless they can prove a disability or mental illness. Thus, men's health has not been addressed as a matter of policy, and the result is that the lack of comprehensive family-focused policies and systems continue to perpetuate the exclusion of men as valued members of our families and communities (Treadwell, Ro, & Perez, 2011). With the passage of the Patient Protection and Affordable Care Act (PPACA) in March 2010, single men with incomes below 133 percent of the federal poverty level may qualify for Medicaid beginning in 2014. How this legislation is implemented in the different states remains to be seen, as half of the country is legally contesting the requirement that all people must carry health insurance.

It's about the Policy

As the previous sections suggest, there were a number of historical decisions—decisions of public policy—that determined the fate of many African-American men, particularly among the poorest. Today, in many ways, those arcane policies have been recycled under other guises.

Persistently Poor Communities

African Americans are among the poorest in the nation. Nearly 40 percent of black children in the United States were living in poverty in 2007 (National Poverty Center, 2008). Moreover, nearly six decades after *Brown v. Board of Education*, which desegregated schools so that all children would have an equal opportunity for a quality education, much is left to be desired. In many cases, public schools in the United States vary in quality given their geographic location. The poorest neighborhoods most probably will not have the same access to quality teachers, educational materials, supplies, and the safe and healthy environments to be found in higher-income areas. One of the possible results of this is that fewer than 8 percent of African-American men have graduated from college, as opposed to 17 percent of white men and 35 percent of Asian men (Henry J. Kaiser Family Foundation, 2006).

The low levels of college attendance, high levels of unemployment or under-employment, and imprisonment of African-American men pose serious threats to the health and well-being of families and communities. One chilling conse-quence is that approximately 2 million young children have parents in prison. The environments in which many of these children are being raised are insecure and unsafe, with fathers in prison, mothers also increasingly incarcerated, and grandparents stepping in where possible in the context of blighted neighbor-hoods where some have alleged that "it is easier to get a gun than a tomato," or anything remotely healthy. At the same time, the cycle of poor education in poor communities continues. Though in recent years, the test score gap has narrowed, black children still lag behind their white counterparts. Although the quality of schools and teachers is an important indicator for success, the treatment—the attention to the well-being—of children in schools and in their home environ-ments should also not be overlooked (Jencks & Philipps, 1998).

Health insurance is not a right in the United States unless one is impris-oned. Even then, it is a not a "right," but a matter of law that one should have access to medical care in prison should the need arise. As noted before, this situation is especially dire for poor men of color who, with few exceptions, will not qualify for any **public assistance**. However, for those who do qualify, under the provisions made for those men with a disability and/or mental health issue, problems arise for those who go to jail or prison.

Despite a call by the **Center for Medicare and Medicaid Services (CMS)** that states employ the practice of suspending versus terminating Medicaid ben-efits for prisoners, many states still do not heed this policy. The result for many people who go to prison with Medicaid benefits is that these are terminated on their incarceration, and the logistics of reintegrating benefits for these popula-tions once released are quite cumbersome, if not insurmountable (Perez, Ro, & Treadwell, 2009).

Beyond not being able to easily recoup Medicaid benefits in some states as people exit prison, housing is not readily available for those with prior drug convictions and, in many states of the country, voting rights are rescinded, effectively silencing this population's voice. All of these elements ultimately contribute to the persistent poverty that can be seen in many communities across the nation. These factors are based on public policy decisions—Medicaid benefits policy, housing policy, and employment policies—which impact not only on one life, but on many.

War on Drugs

In just the past 25 years, the prison population has grown by 274 percent (Pew, 2009). Much of this expansion can be attributed to the War on Drugs and highly punitive sentencing policies that have been implemented hand in glove.

Uneven Territory and Justice

A July 2007 Sentencing Project report suggested that the War on Drugs has produced ethnic and racial disparities in terms of both the sentences handed down for drug offenses as well as the geographic distribution of prisoners (Mauer & King, 2007). Sentencing laws have been neither equitable nor even. Federal cocaine statutes, for example, have disproportionately affected low-income men of color as a result of the prosecution of low-level offenders. One clear example of this can be seen with regard to the disparity in sentencing for the possession of crack versus powder cocaine.

The current federal law mandates far more severe sentences for low-level offenses involving crack cocaine than powder cocaine, even though the former is not necessarily more addictive or dangerous than the latter: A first-time conviction for possessing just 5 grams of crack—which has the weight of two sugar packets—brings a five-year sentence. It takes possession of 500 grams of powder cocaine to bring a mandatory five-year sentence (Defenders Online, 2009).

This policy has, in effect, contributed to the disproportionate number of poor, young African-American men in prison. **Sentencing reform** advocates have insisted for decades that such a policy has only served to ensure that the most economically depressed people—most often, poor men of color—would surely see prison time. Legislation intended to reform this policy and eliminate the five-year **mandatory minimum sentence** associated with the same was introduced in late 2009. Though there is hope on the horizon, as of this writing, the bill has not yet become law.

Another important issue is related to geography. Despite that most low-income African-American men hail from urban communities, they are serving prison sentences in distant rural areas. The results of such a decision means that these prisoners are often far away from their families and communities, ensuring little family support during their incarceration period as well as a limited opportunity for employment once released (Pew, 2009). Furthermore, moving urban prisoners to rural areas means that the census will not count them in their communities of origin, effectively reducing potential resources that could accrue to these neighborhoods were all of their original residents counted.

Uneven Representation

Directly related to the low-income status of most of the African-American men who have served time or are currently serving sentences is that their limited resources help to contribute to the disparate outcomes within the justice system. Because they are disproportionately poor, they are also more likely to rely on an overburdened defense system and live in communities with limited access to treatment and alternative sentencing policies (Pew, 2009).

The Way Forward

Much has been written and said about the issues raised here, and due to the abundant research and evidence that has been brought to bear, there is now greater understanding of what is at stake (see Urban Institute, Pew, the Sentencing Project, Bazelon Law Center). Likewise, work that has persisted in raising awareness of ethnic/racial health and social disparities is of utmost importance to underscoring that the United States has still not achieved the American Dream for all, and that although all men may be "created equal," all men are not "treated equally." Of even more importance, perhaps, is the fact that this inequity has passed from generation to generation of African-American men, not only impacting those on the margins but increasingly affecting entire communities. The economic, social, and environmental imperative for closing the equity gap can be seen on a number of levels.

For a number of consecutive years, the Pew Center has provided compelling evidence regarding the inordinate amount of resources spent on the current prison system. Some of the cost drivers include prison health as well as the amount of time for which prisoners are incarcerated for low-level offenses. According to Pew's 2009 "One in 31" report, the U.S. spent $51.7 billion on corrections in 2008 alone! In response to these growing costs, some states have opted to slash programs and social services, in some cases at the expense of the very populations in most need of the same. Ironically, as suggested here and elsewhere, it has been the absence of appropriate programs and resources in communities that have helped to create a pathway toward prison for young, low-income African-American men.

On a social and environmental level, unless the "distress" in low-income, low-resource communities is addressed upfront, the same trajectory will continue. Not only resources, but opportunities, must be equally available in all neighborhoods regardless of economics. This means decent housing, living wage jobs, good schools, safe neighborhoods, health care, and healthy food.

Because of the history laid out here, the high numbers of incarcerated or formerly incarcerated African-American men, and the collateral effects of these experiences on families and communities, much is required to shift the pendulum toward equity. This final section provides some of those policy and program alternatives that must be considered to change the status quo and to ensure that all communities have an equal chance of prospering.

Community Support and Treatment

Despite all of the challenges, there is good news. Sustained academic and activist efforts have resulted in the introduction of new legislation such as the **Second Chance Act** (2009) and the **Sentence Reform Act**. Second Chance is committed to ensuring that employment opportunities and resources are available for those coming home from prison. Sentence Reform, should it pass, will effectively change current sentencing policy, which has succeeded in incarcerating high numbers of African-American men for low-level drug offenses, also ensuring lengthier sentences for the same (i.e., possession of crack versus powder cocaine). Given the present context that has helped focus attention on the collateral effects of imprisonment on community health and wellness, two compelling program and policy alternatives may be gaining ground. One is to treat people for their illness (e.g., mental health, substance abuse, or both) rather than to incarcerate them. The other is to change the way in which the system presently functions, transitioning into community-based corrections.

Treatment versus Incarceration

Although it costs much less to provide substance abuse and mental health treatment in community versus in corrections, people continue to be incarcerated for drug-related and/or mental health issues. Despite this, drug use is not diminishing nor is harm-reduction occurring in communities. In other words, the cycles have not been broken. Yet there is compelling research that suggests that treating people in a community-based setting as opposed to prison is not only an economically superior alternative for states and communities whose budgets can no longer support the high costs of prison, but may also provide the needed support for individuals, families, and communities (Community Voices Freedom's Voice Conference Proceedings, 2010; see also Bazelon Center for Mental Health Law).

Beyond providing much-needed **comprehensive community-based treatment**, judges also have a paramount role to play in ensuring that people obtain care versus prison. Through judicial discretion in the sentencing process, judges can "craft" sentences that take into account the context of the offense and the person (Pew, 2009). Some states (Maryland) already provide judges with options for directing people to the health department for care versus the department of corrections. Others, such as Louisiana, Mississippi, and Delaware, have reviewed mandatory minimum sentencing (Pew, 2009). On mental health, judges such as Stephen Leifman in Florida, Stephen G. Goss of Georgia, and others around the country have played key roles in supporting **Crisis Intervention Treatment (CIT)** as well as promoting **Assertive Community Treatment (ACT)** and **Forensic Assertive Community Treatment (FACT)** as jail diversion strategies for people living with mental illness. (These programs all work to help divert people with mental health and/or substance abuse issues away from the corrections system and into care.)

Community-Based Corrections

Building on the knowledge that there are currently 5 million people on parole, a nearly fourfold increase in the past 25 years, Pew (2009) makes a compelling argument for transitioning the corrections system into the community in an effort to depopulate prisons and provide people with the appropriate guidance, which will help to reduce recidivism and strengthen communities. At present, prisons receive the lion's share of the funding, but Pew's assertion that providing more resources to **community-based corrections** is sensible if there is real interest in providing the community-based support that, as previous research suggests, may be the defining difference in keeping people out of prison. Moreover, the economic argument is hard to ignore: "the daily cost of supervising a probationer in fiscal year 2008 was $3.42; the average daily cost of a prison inmate, $78.95, is more than 20 times as high" (Pew, 2009, p. 2). Beyond the strength of the economic argument, the promise of keeping people out of prison and in their communities with their families and neighbors is also noteworthy. As described by Pew:

> Despite the meager funding and ballooning workload, there have been significant advances in community supervision. Sophisticated risk assessment tools now help determine which offenders require the most supervision and what sort of monitoring and services they need. Global positioning systems, rapid-result drug tests and other technology can track offenders' whereabouts and behavior. Offender supervision, treatment and **re-entry programs** are incorporating solid research on how to cut recidivism. . . . Taken together and implemented well, these approaches can produce double-digit reductions in recidivism and save states money along the way. If policy makers want these results, though, they will have to invest in the overburdened system of community corrections. (p. 2)

Level the Playing Field

Although the civil rights movement drove a significant wedge in the heart of segregation and separation, and although the first African-American president nears the end of his first term in office, there is still a significant road to travel to effectively reverse existing policies that ensure poverty, segregation, and stunted development for many communities of color. And much remains to be done to remedy the damage caused by the **structural violence** inflicted on generations of African-American men.

Place Matters: Environment

As Angela Glover Blackwell and others have rightly observed, "place matters"—when violence is more common than nutritious food, or playgrounds do not exist; when the kinds of teachers employed to educate and inspire can find no inspiration themselves; when a parent, or both, are in prison, the outcomes should be of no surprise. Among youth, especially, there are growing concerns because of the issues presented here and the collateral damages that accrue to them. African-American boys make up a disproportionate share of those who are at risk. Although programming may be part of the answer, interventions are deeply challenged in the context of blighted and stressed communities.

Decent housing and clean and safe neighborhoods are indispensable to economic, health, and social outcomes in communities. Access to health care and quality education also matter. But without the necessary sustainable investments for community well-being, including not only affordable, but planned housing that includes mixed-income options; not only job opportunities, but real workforce development; unfettered access to quality education, safe streets, and nutritious food, it becomes impossible to reap the presumed "equal opportunity" because people are not starting from an equal place. There is nothing novel about this. We know that where we live will determine everything from the quality of education to the ability to access reliable public transportation, to the illnesses contracted. If the tide is to change, the appropriate investments must be made. Community residents must, undoubtedly, do their part. But, without the appropriate foundation, it will be impossible to do so.

Removing Barriers to Work and Developing Creative Approaches to Employment

Together with decent and safe housing, the ability to work and care for oneself and one's family is a foremost indicator of well-being. Yet, a number of barriers to work exist for low-income African-American men.

• *Improving the quality of education.* Formidable barriers exist for African-American men as a result of their comparatively lower educational levels. Although the right to education is universal in the United States, quality is not, and still too many poor communities suffer the consequences of unequal resources for the education of their children. The answer in education lies not only in the resources available, but also in the environment in which a child is educated, both in school and at home. Ensuring that "place" is conducive to education is critical to how and whether children learn. Young boys—particularly African-American boys from impoverished families, many who have parents serving time in prison—must be given careful consideration. Efforts to ensure a positive trajectory in school through "**restorative justice**" approaches versus harsh punishments for poor behavior must be emphasized (see http://www.restorativejustice.org/university-classroom/01introduction for a definition of restorative justice).

Without this, the "cradle-to-prison" trajectory cannot be broken. Moreover, early childhood programs, parenting programs, and the prevalence of safe spaces for play and living are the integral foundation to education.

• Eliminate criminal history questions on employment applications. Formerly incarcerated men are commonly confronted with policies that permit employers to request the criminal histories of job applicants, making it exceedingly difficult (if not impossible) for people reentering their communities to recoup their lives and livelihood. A serious problem with this practice is that criminal records are often inaccurate. For example, while someone's record may only indicate an arrest, and not a conviction, it may still act as a formidable barrier to employment. It is therefore critical that standards be established for employers to follow so that they can conduct case-by-case assessments of individuals with criminal pasts. Another possibility for changing current policy is to simply remove this question from job applications. Some cities have already done so (San Francisco, Berkeley, Boston, Cambridge, and Minneapolis, to name only some. See "Ban the Box" and "All of Us or None," http://www.allofusornone.org/campaigns/ban-the-box).

• *Ensure proper identification for those leaving corrections.* Another barrier for formerly incarcerated people is that they often leave corrections without proper identification, making it impossible for them to obtain employment or benefits. In some states, driver licenses are confiscated for those with drug-related convictions, a real barrier to employment for many, especially those in rural communities who may be heavily dependent on driving to and from work. Policies such as this must be overturned, as they make it impossible for people to proceed toward sustainable employment.

• *Provide tax incentives for employers who hire formerly incarcerated people.* Programs that provide tax incentives for employers who hire formerly incarcerated exist. Creative approaches such as this that establish partnerships between employers and the government in a real effort to facilitate employment for those who have been in prison can help to ensure that formerly incarcerated men will remain employed and productive.

• *Provide skill development and job training.* For those men who have been in corrections, it is critical to ensure that navigable pathways exist for job training and workforce development. Those serving time in prison must be able to develop skills while incarcerated so that they will be prepared to support themselves when they reenter their communities. Researchers and advocates working on reentry programs and policies insist that efforts must begin the day someone enters prison:

> If people need treatment and they don't get treatment but they get a job,
> they won't have that job for long. If people don't have a place to live, but

you get them a job and they can't take a shower and get cleaned up and go to work, they won't be going to work for very long . . . it is the integrated model that works for people who are coming home . . . Safe transition centers, vis-à-vis work release centers, that provide opportunities for people to connect with family; to connect with work; and, to connect with educational opportunities prior to release and to do that in a setting where one can continue post-release.

(B. Diane Williams, President/CEO Safer Foundation of Chicago, Illinois, Community Voices Freedom's Voices Conference Proceedings, 2010)

Resources must be available and targeted within communities in order to develop a skilled work force among young, African-American men. This begins in schools and continues through other programs, including those of the twenty-first century meant to bridge the digital divide; to develop needed and marketable skills that will simultaneously help create a skilled workforce while lifting communities out of poverty.

For example, in an effort to link health access with job development, health advocates around the country have promoted **community health workers** (CHWs). CHWs can help link people to needed health and social services, while simultaneously developing an innovative path to work for themselves. Although recent legislation now acknowledges these workers as part of the U.S. workforce, CHWs were historically viewed as volunteers, indigenous to the communities they served and, if paid, often compensated very little. Through CHW training programs offered in different cities and states, efforts are being made to develop a higher level of skill and capacity for these workers, while at the same time employing a valuable method for connecting hard-to-reach people to health care services and support. In some places CHWs have worked to reach men through peer outreach, often formerly incarcerated men as well as those who have touched the substance abuse and/or mental health systems (see Denver Health Community Voices).

Conclusion

This chapter has provided a review of historical, social, and health policies and the impact of the same on African-American men and on their communities. In addition, discussion regarding possible alternative social and health policies that incorporate the needs of those imprisoned and those reentering their communities was included. In doing so, this chapter has placed emphasis on the social, economic, and political determinants of health as foundational to crafting policy that is effective in meeting the needs of a historically marginalized and underserved population, African-American men.

Summary

Creative strategies and approaches such as those suggested here can make a difference in helping low-income African-American men obtain needed care and providing a pathway to work and decent wages for those with limited skills and/or those who are reintegrating into society. Without this support, it may be impossible for some men to lead stable lives. Resources and support must exist in communities such that alternative pathways to prison are established early. All efforts devoted to working against a "cradle to prison" pipeline must ensure that the necessary investments are made in education, parenting, nutrition, housing, and safe neighborhoods regardless of a family's income, but because it is what is necessary in order for the country to progress as a whole. At the same time, unless some of the policies discussed here change, they will only serve to reinforce the upward spiraling prison trajectory.

A key possibility for improving resources in communities may finally come as the census is now revisiting the manner in which it is counting communities. Until recently, a common practice was to count prisoner populations sent to rural communities, thus inflating the numbers of people in those areas. In essence, this practice has hindered the resources available to poor, urban communities. With the census now committed to discerning the accurate number of a population without disingenuously including the number of prisoners in the area, a real accounting may be finally possible and the pathway for appropriate resources may be paved.

Key Terms

Aid to Families with Dependent Children (AFDC)

Assertive Community Treatment (ACT)

Center for Medicare and Medicaid Services (CMS)

community-based corrections

community health workers

comprehensive community-based treatment

criminal justice system

Crisis Intervention Training (CIT)

equity

Forensic Assertive Community Treatment (FACT)

health insurance

mandatory minimum sentences

Medicaid

mental health

parole officers

public assistance

recidivism

reentry programs

rehabilitation

restorative justice

Sentence Reform Act

social and economic determinants of health

structural violence

substance abuse

supportive housing

Temporary Assistance for Needy
    Families (TANF)

The Second Chance Act

War on Drugs

Discussion Questions

1. Why is social and health policy important for community development?

2. Why are some current social and health policies relevant to the health of African-American men?

3. Why should policy makers consider the role that social and economic determinants of health play when developing policy?

4. What kinds of interventions might help to create healthier lives for African-American men?

5. What kind of support and resources are necessary for African-American men reentering their communities from prison?

6. What kinds of reforms might be considered in order to reduce the incarceration of African-American men and invest in marginalized communities?

References

Blackmon, D. A. (2008). *Slavery by another name: The re-enslavement of black Americans from the Civil War to World War II.* New York, NY: Random House.

Blumstein, A., & Beck, A. J. (1999). Population growth in US prison, 1980–1996. *Crime & Justice, 17.* Retrieved from http://consensusproject.org/downloads/fact_about-the-problem.pdf

Defenders Online. (2009, May 27). Retrieved from http://www.thedefendersonline.com/2009/05/27/sentencing-disparity-crack-cocaine-v-powder-cocaine/

Edelman, P., Holzer, H. J., & Offner P. (2006). *Reconnecting disadvantaged young men.* Washington, DC: Urban Institute Press.

Henry J. Kaiser Family Foundation. (2006). Retrieved from http://usjamerica.files.wordpress.com/2010/01/7541.pdf

Henry J. Kaiser Family Foundation. (2007, January). *Key facts: Race, ethnicity and medical care.*

Jencks, C., & Philipps, M. (1998). The black test gap: Why it exists and what can be done. *Brookings Review.* Retrieved from http://www.jstor.org/pss/20080778

Mauer, M. (2003). The crisis of the young African American male and the criminal justice system. In O. Harris & R. Robin Miller (Eds.), *Impacts of incarceration on the African American family* (pp. 199–218). New Brunswick, NJ: Transaction.

Mauer, M., & King, R. S. (2007). *Uneven justice: States rates of incarceration by race and ethnicity.* The Sentencing Project.

National Poverty Center. (2008). *Poverty facts*. Retrieved from http://www.npc.umich
.edu/poverty/#4

Perez, L. M., Ro, M. J., & Treadwell, H. M. (2009, April). Vulnerable populations,
prison, federal and state Medicaid policies: Avoiding the loss of a right to care. *Journal
of Correctional Health Care*, 15(2), 142–149.

Perez, L. M. (2010). *Strengthening families during incarceration and homecoming*.
Community Voices Freedom's Voice Conference Proceedings, National Center for
Primary Care, Atlanta, Georgia.

Treadwell, H. M., Ro, M. J., & Perez, L. M. (Eds.). (2011). *Community voices: Health
matters*. New York, NY: Jossey-Bass.

Urban Institute. (2009). Retrieved from http://usjamerica.files.wordpress.com/2010/
01/7541.pdf

Van Olphen, J., Freudenberg, N., Fortin, P., & Galea, S. (2006). Community reentry:
Perceptions of people with substance use problems returning home from New York
City jails. *Journal of Urban Health: Bulletin of the New York Academy of Medicine*,
83(3). doi: 10.1007/s11524–006–9047–4

Warren, J. (2008). *One in one 100: Behind bars in America 2008*. Pew Center on States.
Retrieved from http://www.pewcenteronthestates.org/uploadedFiles/
8015PCTS_Prison08_FINAL 2-1-1_FORWEB.pdf

Williams, N. (2006). *Where are the men? The impact of incarceration and reentry on
African American men and their children and families*. Community Voices, National
Center for Primary Care, Retrieved from http://www.communityvoices.org/Uploads/
wherearethemen2_00108_00144.pdf

Young, A. M. W. (2006, May). *The Overtown men's health study*. Collins Center for
Public Policy.

Chapter 17

Social Determinants of Health and Black Men

The Culture of Empowerment and the Policy Process

Adewale Troutman
Nandi Marshall

Learning Objectives

- Understand the social determinants as they relate to population health.
- Explain the concept of empowerment as a health improvement strategy.
- Recognize the dynamics of the AMEN program as a vehicle for personal and community health improvement among African-American men.

• • •

It has been recognized that there is a dramatic difference between the health of communities of color and the majority white population of the United States. Further, it is black (African-American) men who as a group have the worst health of any demographic group in the United States. Efforts to close the gap of excess death have to date proved ineffective at best. Evidence suggests that in fact the gap is increasing. These facts suggest a different approach to the ongoing tragedy of premature death and inequitable incidence and prevalence of both acute and chronic conditions. That approach while paying attention to individual behavior needs to focus on the **social determinants of health**, the so-called causes of the causes.

Part of this new approach to closing the gap needs to focus on the unique dilemma of the health of black men. There is a clear relationship between the current health status of black men in America and a long history of intentional marginalization and demonization of that group. Black men therefore have been separated from their power. The history of black men in the United States has created an "**Invisibility Syndrome**" among black men.

Addressing the social determinants of health as drivers of the health of populations, particularly black men, will yield positive results. Further attention to the social determinants can provide a mechanism to empower black men. That process and the results of this focus can assist men in creating **health equity**. One example of this process, presented in this chapter, is the **African American Male Empowerment Network** or AMEN. It is important to note that although individual activity is seen as important in the **empowerment** process, recognition is given to the fact that it is social change, systems change, and structural renovation through the policy process that must prevail to change the health status of black men.

Social Determinants of Health and Black Men: The Culture of Empowerment and the Policy Process

It has been well documented that of all demographic groups in the United States, black men have the worst health and a significantly shorter life expectancy that their counterparts (Heckler, 1985). In the landmark study, *What If We Were Equal? A Comparison of the Black White Mortality Gap in 1969 and 2000* (Satcher et al., 2005), the authors pointed out that contrary to the 60,000 excess deaths/year figure, published in the 1985 Secretary's Task Force on Black and Minority Health, using 2002 data that number had risen to 83,570 deaths in the African-American community alone. The study further identified African-American men, particularly those between 45 and 62, as having experienced a significant increase in death rates. The World Health Organization's report, *Closing the Gap in a Generation,* states that "life expectancy is 17 years shorter for black men in Washington, DC, than for white men in nearby Montgomery County" (World Health Organization [WHO], 2008). Even as the death rate among African-American women narrowed, the rate among men continued to rise. In addition the study showed that black men had not experienced the same improvements in income as their white counterparts. Research showed that black men earned only earned 78 percent of what white men earned. Disproportionate rates of homicide and HIV among black men further added to the inequity. Among the reasons for these facts are the effects of the social determinants of health as identified in the writings of the World Health Organization (2006), the research of David Williams (2003), and the research of Marmot and Wilkinson (2008). They cite such areas as occupation, educational attainment, unemployment, addiction, and early childhood development. One must add racism in all its forms (Jones, Hatch, & Troutman, 2008), income gaps, place (neighborhood), and other factors. We must also recognize the long history of slavery, oppression, social exclusion, racism, lynching, and what has become a pattern of marginalization and vilification of black men across the country.

At the same time there seems to be a link between low educational attainment, mirrored by increasing rates of incarceration and unemployment. Recent studies out of Harvard, Columbia, and Princeton show "the huge pool of poorly educated black men is becoming even more disconnected from the mainstream of society" (Mincey, 2006). With this before us, we must add the presence of powerlessness, real or perceived, to the long list of social determinants of health.

We know that health is a complex interaction of multiple determinants. The World Health Organization defines health as the presence of physical, psychological, social, and economic well-being, not merely the absence of disease or infirmity. This would strongly suggest that what we now define as the Social Determinants of Health are the key drivers of the health of populations. The WHO, in its recently released report from the Commission on the Social Determinants of Health, recognizes that these differences are not just between countries but within countries, particularly when looking at communities of color (WHO, 2008). We would submit that this is particularly relevant for black men, whose history suggests that focusing on empowerment, healing, and the social determinants of health and policy development is a viable means of establishing health as defined by WHO. Ultimately, this is an issue of **social justice**, **human rights**, and the need for a health equity movement.

This chapter will (1) examine the social determinants of health as they relate to the unique position of black men in America; (2) discuss empowerment as a vehicle for obtaining good health among black men; (3) examine one strategy for black male empowerment (the African American Male Empowerment Network—AMEN); and (4) delineate the policy process, the role of cultural competence, and its potential to assure a healthy community of black men.

Anderson J. Franklin, PhD, opens his book *From Brotherhood to Manhood* with the following quote from Ralph Ellison's classic work *Invisible Man*: "I am an invisible man. No I am not a spook like those who haunted Edgar Allen Poe; nor am I one of your Hollywood movie ectoplasms. I am a man of substance, of flesh and bone, fiber and liquids—and I might even be said to possess a mind. I am invisible, understand simply because people refuse to see me. . . . When they approach me they see only my surroundings, themselves or figments of their imagination—indeed everything and anything except me." According to

Ellison, then, black men are invisible. Dr. Franklin goes further to delineate the following effects of the "Invisibility Syndrome" on black men. They are frustration, increased awareness of perceived slights, chronic indignation, pervasive discontent and disgruntlement, anger, immobilization or increasing inability to get things done, questioning ones worthiness, disillusionment and confusion, feeling trapped, conflicted racial identity, depression, substance abuse, and loss of hope (Franklin, 2004). In short, Dr. Franklin's analysis points to a population that is unempowered, is in need of healing, and demonstrates the effect of many of the social determinants of health, including stress and the effects of the location of black men as a group on the social gradient. It is of significance that Dr. Franklin's work cuts across all socioeconomic groups within the black male community with consistency in findings.

Empowerment

We believe that the long history that has led to the current deteriorating health of black men supported by the work of Dr. Franklin has led to one description of that demographic group as being an unempowered population. Recognize that an unempowered male population means by definition that similar issues will exist among black families and consequently black communities. It would be helpful here to describe one approach to defining what is meant by empowerment. This will assist us in determining how to proceed to rectify this problem. Gutierrez and Ortega (1991) in their study to establish empowerment divided it into three categories, which we find extremely useful in establishing policy priorities. They are listed here with their definitions.

Categories of Empowerment

1. *Personal empowerment*—Ways to develop feelings of personal power and self-efficacy, defined as a conscious awareness of one's ability to be effective, to control actions or outcomes (Zulkosky, 2009). Self-efficacy speaks of self-confidence in one's ability to achieve goals.

2. *Interpersonal empowerment*—Includes "the development of different skills, including helping people to help others and *learning how to influence the political process*."

3. *Political empowerment*—Focuses on social action and social change, the process of transferring power between groups. Implied in this definition of empowerment is the issue of control over the forces that influence our lives.

Recent work on the social determinants of health and stress (Marmot, 2008) strongly suggest that the absence of that control may be a major factor in poor health and the ongoing gap in excess deaths among communities of color in the United States. This would be particularly telling as it relates to the health of black men in U.S. society. Gutierrez and Ortega (1991) make one further distinction in this definition. Parallel to personal efficacy, they establish political efficacy as the feeling that the individual can impact the political process in order to bring about social change.

The supposition therefore is that black men to different degrees, but still stretching across the entire demographic, have similar issues. There is a relative lack of the ability to achieve goals, the ability to help others, and a relative lack of control over the forces that control their lives and ability to affect the political process. Powerlessness then can be seen as an important determinant of health. Any examination of social determinants will include such factors as employment, housing, social exclusion, unemployment, and educational attainment to name a few (Marmot, 2008). This powerlessness can also be manifested through neighborhood segregation and wider societal discrimination (Wallerstein, 2002). Wallerstein continues by stating that living in an environment of physical and social disadvantage, in an environment lacking social capital and a relative inequity, is a major risk factor for poor health. Wallerstein proceeds to quote Syme (1988), whose findings are consistent with subsequent work that "Lacking control over one's destiny becomes a core social determinant."

We must be careful to stay out of the trap of allowing an analysis of this lack of power to focus exclusively on the individual. This would emphasize the western philosophy of rugged individualism and the supremacy of **Market Justice** as the driving force in U.S. society. Market justice attributes the realizing of both benefits and burdens to the responsibility of the individual. This gives them a reason to deny social factors in that determination. In fact, public health has done such a thorough job in focusing on individual lifestyle behaviors in determining health that we now need to refocus our attention to those social factors that control our ability to make those choices.

In the introduction to this chapter we stated that this was in the final analysis an issue of social justice, human rights, and creating health equity. To further this understanding it is appropriate to offer definitions of these concepts and principles to lead us through the remainder of the analysis. One definition of health equity is that it is "the attainment of the highest level of health for all people. Achieving health equity requires valuing all individuals and populations equally, and entails focused societal efforts to equalize the conditions for optimal health for all groups, particularly for those who have experienced historic injustices or socioeconomic disadvantage."

Human Rights Health Inequity and Social Justice

In contrast, health inequity is the presence of systemic, unfair, and unjust differences in health outcomes and mortality that is sustained over time and generations and beyond the control of individuals. Social justice "demands an equitable distribution of public goods, institutional resources and life opportunities." It is the elevation of the principles of justice (fairness, equal opportunity) to the broadest definition of society. "It is an assertion that reminds us that health and well-being . . . intimately reflect the workings of the body politic for good and for ill" (Krieger & Birn, 1998). Human rights are those rights established for all as a result of our humanity and nothing else. It is independent of civil law, which can vary from jurisdiction to jurisdiction.

Community Capacity and Empowerment

Expanding our attention to **community capacity** and community empowerment will bring us closer to a realization that all social dynamics are critical to health. Community capacity focuses on active participation, leadership, rich support networks, *understanding of history*, values clarification, and lastly access to power (Wallerstein, 2002). The realization of the role of history has long been an issue among the black community for both men and women. For instance, in the lead author's opinion, one of the objectives of the Black Studies Movement (the creation of black studies departments at universities and colleges all over the United States) was partly based on the correction of and the completeness of the teaching and study of the history, culture, and politics of blacks in this country and abroad (Africa and the Diaspora). This focus on history was partially seen as a means of empowering a population by arming them with that history (Merelman, 1993). Dr. Troutman bases this on his own study of black history and his career as a member of the early black studies departments at the State University of New York at Albany, Nassau Community College, and the City College of New York. Whether we can discern any difference in the measure of empowerment in black men who engaged in this experience is not known. The research is scant in this area and should be seen as an area of new information.

Community Empowerment

In this time period when we are increasingly turning our attention to the social determinants of health for understanding and answers it seems that our colleagues in these departments may have something unique to add to our analysis. The role of history will be an important element of the AMEN approach to building black male empowerment through a small group empowerment strategy. As we examine the AMEN process and its attention to black men we must also keep our eyes on the prize of **community empowerment**. This is particularly relevant to the discussion of empowering black men. Community empowerment is further defined as "a social action process by which individuals, communities and organizations gain mastery over their lives in the context of changing their social and political environment to improve equity and quality of life" (Wallerstein, 2002). Empowered black men will make better decisions about their health, their families, and their communities. They will cease to be invisible and will change the social and political environment in which they live, work, and play.

African American Empowerment Network (AMEN)

Dr. Franklin documents in his book *From Brotherhood to Manhood* his decades of experience in working with black men in small groups to address issues of empowerment. One view of the environment necessary to build empowerment lists four characteristics. We offer you four of them here. They are (1) small group setting; (2) a common belief system; (3) opportunities to acquire skills; and knowledge; (4) experience in the target community or group (Angelique, 2002). Freire, famous for his work *Pedagogy of the Oppressed*, goes further in identifying a process of creating awareness about society, oppression, and history (Freire, 1970).

The Clinton "Race Initiative"

In 1999, as a result of President Clinton's race initiative, agencies within government were directed to establish a mechanism to address race in America. Health and Human Services through the Centers for Disease Control created an initiative entitled Racial and Ethnic Approaches to Community Health or REACH 2010. The Fulton County Department of Health and Wellness was successful in obtaining one of those highly competitive grants. This community collaborative project had among its partners the local chapter of the Association of Black Psychologists. This segment (AMEN) of the project was aimed at black men and was based on the principles set by Dr. A. J. Franklin. The description and the data below are from unpublished work of Dr. Adewale Troutman, lead author of this chapter. As previously stated, the belief was that black men were un-empowered and in need of an empowerment strategy. The premise was that empowered men make better choices about their health, their family's health, and are more likely to be engaged in and make better choices in their communities as active community-empowered individuals. Many of the principles of Angelique's empowering environment turned out to be part of the project design.

African-American Male Empowerment Elements

The network was made up of small groups of black men in weekly group meetings. These meetings were facilitated by black male behavioral health professionals. The initiative was based on a definition of the empowered male that included emotional stability, understanding the principles of self-determination in health, confidence, commitment to family and community, and saw health both from the standpoint of the WHO definition and as the balance of mind, body, and spirit.

The meetings were facilitated through a multisection curriculum created by the Atlanta chapter of the Association of Black Psychologists. It had four parts: spiritual health, mental health, physical health, and social health. Each part had multiple modules, some of which were mandatory and many others that were left to the group to choose from. The spiritual health section included questions from the department's Behavioral Risk Factor Surveillance System spiritual health module (created by the Fulton County Department of Health and Wellness). In addition it focused on self-acceptance, an introduction to meditation, African history, defining African-American malehood, and affirming the self. The mental health section focused on making good choices and problem solving, personal development, depression, and anger management. It also covered stress management, Tai Chi, Qi-gong, and empowerment through music. The physical health section discussed such critical issues as HIV/AIDS, substance abuse, cancer, and diabetes. The groups also discussed nutritional empowerment, hypertension, and smoking cessation through acupressure. The social intervention modules included domestic violence, community organizing, financial planning, and practical legal advice.

AMEN Results

The following results reflect the experience of some 428 participants. Despite the belief that it would be extremely difficult to keep a group of black men together for months of group meetings, where a primary focuses was on emotional healing and empowerment, the retention rate was 75.2 percent. Focus group feedback in response to discussion around the most meaningful topics included anger management, stress management, meditation, affirming the self, HIV/AIDS, and defining African-American manhood. Further, when asked to define the most important thing that the men gained from the experience, they said they developed a sense of hope and empowerment. The participants said that they overcame a fatalistic view of life and affirmed significant habit changes, including more frequent physicals, improved nutrition, drinking more water, and engaging in more physical activity.

In 2008 a paper was published in the *Health Education Journal* by Stephens et al. entitled "Cardiovascular Risk Reduction for African American Men through Health Empowerment and Anger Management." This paper used the same group process and AMEN format years after its inception worked with men in the Atlanta Empowerment Zone. In the zone the poverty rate is 57.4 percent and it suffers from the ills of many urban center cities around the nation. The authors postulated that unexpressed or concealed anger among African-American men would contribute to the incidence of cardiovascular disease (early heart attack) in these men. Men were exposed to the anger management curriculum component then followed up with two sets of measurements. The following are the specific five goals for that curriculum: (1) Increasing awareness of anger as an emotional stressor that if not managed appropriately can increase risk of CVD; (2) assisting participants in recognizing that anger is a normal emotion; (3) assisting them in identifying their anger triggers; (4) assisting them in identifying healthy versus unhealthy anger management skills; and finally (5) assisting participants in developing their own behavior change plan. In conclusion the authors recognize that "Research has . . . revealed associations between several psychosocial factors and heart disease. These factors include chronic stress, anger, depression, inadequate social support, anxiety, hostility and socioeconomic status (occupation, education and income)" (Stephens et al., 2008). It should be noted how close this list is to the list of Social Determinants of Health as delineated by WHO in *The Solid Facts*, as well as the WHO Commission on the Social Determinants of Health report "Closing the Gap in a Generation: Health Equity Through a Focus on the Social Determinants of Health."

The authors recognize that current definitive data on the beneficial effects of anger management in reducing CVD are not available, but this study, when viewed in the light of the need to address the social determinants of health and the evidence from the AMEN project, is compelling. The study concludes that "empowerment interventions that focus on health empowerment models which are culturally, racially and ethnically appropriate are needed and effective" (Stephens et al., 2008). The AMEN project has been replicated by the Metro Louisville Department of Public Health and Wellness through its men's health initiative.

Policy Recommendations and the Policy Process

Ultimately, it must be understood that the health of black men is particularly sensitive to the social determinants of health. Examination of socioeconomic status, effects of racism, educational attainment, incarceration rates, and unemployment among black men, to name a few, point to the importance of structural change to address this issue. It is structural change, systems reform, and the policy process focused on the social determinants of health that stand the best chance of bringing about health equity and eliminating once and for all the gap in excess death experienced by the black community and black men in particular.

Policy development requires several things. This includes the presence of an evidence base and adequate data to measure where you are and to measure your success when you get where you are going. The importance of an evidence base for the social determinants is crucial in the efforts to bring about health equity. This challenge is based on the importance of public perception. It is crucial in the development of a policy agenda and of value to policy makers. It will also assist the efforts of the public health workforce in its understanding of social determinants as the main driver of health status and health inequities in particular.

Developing an Evidence Base

The following principles for developing the evidence base on the role of the social determinants of health is presented in the National Institute for Health and Clinical Evidence publication, "Constructing the Base on the Social Determinants of Health: A guide" (Bonnefoy, Morgan, Kelly, Butt, & Bergman, 2007). They are: (1) a commitment to the value of equity; (2) taking an evidence-based approach; (3) methodological diversity; (4) gradients and gaps; (5) causes: determinants and outcomes; (6) social structure and social dynamics; and (7) eliminating bias. In recognition of the importance of this work, the WHO Commission on the Social Determinants convened a group of experts to work on the parameters of the MEKN or the Measurement and Evidence Knowledge Network. Among the many challenges is the task of determining the effect of specific determinants on health status and outcomes in order to devise strategies and policies to bring about health justice.

Policy and Health Equity

What are the policies that will move us toward health equity through a focus on the social determinants of health for black men and communities of color in general? How do we get them on the policy agenda? Bonnefoy et al. (2007) point out that although the evidence base is important, it alone will not move the policy agenda to address the issues we are concerned about. They state that there must be problem recognition, formulation of solutions, including transferability of evidence into appropriate social strategies. In addition there must be appropriate scalability into different contexts and settings and last, political will. The authors recognize that the policy process is not well understood by either the population at large, black men in general, or the public health workforce in particular. The institutions that are expected to lead, namely local public health, must find their way forward to recognize the interactions of the social determinants of health on the populations they serve. To add to this dilemma, there are significant forces in this country that reject the influence of the social determinants and instead continue to push the philosophy that states health is all about personal choice. Further, they state that social forces play no role in the health of populations. In the case of black men that would indicate that black men choose to go to prison rather than college, choose to die younger, choose to work in the most dangerous and unstable jobs, choose to be the targets of racist policies and practices, and choose to be at the bottom. "African American men abide at the lower end of the income continuum" (Bonhomme & Young, 2009).

Health in All Policies

It is clear that personal choice, although important, gives way to the potential to bring about healthy societies and healthy black men in particular through the policy process and a focus on social determinants. Policy is the tool with which to make that change. There is solid evidence that health can be influenced by policies of other sectors. Health has important effects on the realization of the goals of other sectors, such as creating a just system of education, employment, and the elimination of structural racism. Taking the injustice out of the criminal justice system and creation of economic wealth can also be influenced by examining intersectoral policies. We propose that **Health in All Policies (HiAP)** is a strategy to help strengthen this link between health and other policies. HiAP addresses the effects on health across all policies such as agriculture, education, the environment, fiscal policies, housing, and transport. It seeks to improve health and at the same time contribute to the well-being and the wealth of the nations through structures, mechanisms, and actions planned and managed mainly by sectors other than health. Thus HiAP is not confined to the health sector or to the public health community, but is a complementary strategy with a high potential toward improving a population's health, with health determinants as the bridge between policies and health outcomes (Ministry of Social Affairs in Health, 2006). The key to HiAP is that it requires a deliberate effort to be promoted and adopted (Ministry of Social Affairs in Health, 2006). For example, in Europe the main theme of the Finnish European Union (EU) Presidency in 2006 was HiAP (Ministry of Social Affairs in Health, 2006). Through the existence and sustainability of HiAP in Finland, their population's health is constantly improving. It is important to note that the success of HiAP in the previous example is due to the shared value of well-being and health across the societal sectors (Ministry of Social

Affairs in Health, 2006). A stronger statement of political will calls for health equity in all policies and focuses on such diverse arenas as early childhood development, education, fair employment, social protection, and political empowerment, to name a few (Marmot, 2008).

Health inequity is a fact of life in this country. It is reflected in chronic and acute disease data. It is reflected in the social gradient, housing access, unemployment, and incarceration rates, among others. The very nature of the structure of institutionalized processes cries out for policy contributions to resolve the inequities.

Commission to Build a Healthier America (Educational Attainment)

We know that according to the Robert Wood Johnson Commission to Build a Healthier America (2009) report, "People with higher education are likely to live longer." Further, the report documents the fact that educational attainment is inversely proportional to high graduation rates. In June 2009, according to the commission, unemployment rates for those who had not graduated high school was 15.5 percent, 9.8 percent for high school graduates, and 4.7 percent for college grads (Robert Wood Johnson Commission to Build a Healthier America [RWJ], 2009). Educational attainment is linked to a greater sense of control, social standing, self-perception, and presence of social support. Mincey states that in 2004, 72 percent of black male dropouts in their twenties were unemployed. As it relates to incarceration rates in 1995, 16 percent of those without college were in jail or prison and the black male high school dropout rate in inner cities was greater than 50 percent (Mincey, 2006). Incarceration of black men takes them out of the educational scene during their most productive years and cripples them as it relates to competitiveness when they get out and reenter society (Raphael, 2006). In light of these and many other facts, examples of policy interventions that may have value are included here.

Policy Characteristics

Policies may be short-term or long-term. Another way of looking at them is as either upstream or downstream. This refers to addressing a problem after it manifests itself (downstream) or defining the causes of the causes and applying policy change at that point (upstream). Note that an unbalanced focus on the short-term policies will only create a healthier underclass, which is unacceptable. They may be distributive, regulatory, or redistributive. Undoubtedly some combination of all the above will be needed to bring about health equity. Remember that this must be seen in the light of a health equity in all policy approaches. Educational policy reform, including the consideration of male-only separate education, has been considered and should not be over-looked. The disproportionate rate of poverty would indicate the need for an assets-development policy focusing on financial literacy, home ownership, self-sufficiency, job skills, and so forth. Reentry policies for black men coming back into society that reestablishes their rights to full citizenship would address many of the problems faced by those with criminal records. Policies that enforce the AMEN methodology of empowering black men should be con-sidered. "I argue that the existence of the social gradient strengthens the case for income redistribution in favor of the poor" (Deaton, 2002). The authors agree with Gollust, Lantz, and Ubel in *The Polarizing Effect of News Media about the Social Determinates of Health* that a cabinet-level response to the existence of health inequities, particularly these that affect black men, is needed to develop policy responses at the highest level of government. Other policy areas include the expansion of black men in the professions, such stan-dard policies as a living wage, fair housing, neighborhood redevelopment, and so on. The need for community empowerment is crucial for success. Therefore capacity building around the policy processes, both development and imple-mentation/advocacy that fully engages black men, will have significant posi-tive effect in creating health equity. All policies must meet the test of cultural consciousness/cultural sensitivity. It must take into account the practices, beliefs, and traditions of those who are the focus of that policy. Adequate research has yet to be done, for instance, to identify those practices among black men that would support positive movement and those that would block the success of a policy agenda.

Summary

The health of African-American (black) men is the worst of any demographic group in the United States. This demonstrates the absence of health equity and is a social justice and human rights issue. The roots of this fact are historic, social, political, economic, structural, and to a degree cultural. Health is—according to the World Health Organization—a mix of physical, social, psycho-logical, and economic well-being, not just the absence of disease. This makes the case for determinants of health that are outside of the individual. In fact, recent work of the WHO Commission on the Social Determinants of Health and the Robert Wood Johnson Commission for a Healthier America both focus their attention on the social determinants of health, looking to the causes of the causes, looking upstream for the answers. Choices are determined by the choices available. That demonstrates the structural foundation of health ineq-uities. Solutions to this unacceptable scenario are to be found in the policy arena. Health equity in all policies should be the driving force that leads to cab-inet-level response. Attention must be paid to the relevance of culture and community engagement as partners in addressing creative policies designed to reverse what has seemed to be an intractable problem. A focus on the social determinants of health can be a significant part of a strategy designed to empower black men. Empowerment of black men can increase their sense of control and their ability to make better decisions for their own health and the health of their families and their communities. Empowered men can organize to address the social inequities in society that support the existence of health inequities.

Key Terms

African American Male Empowerment Network

community capacity

empowerment (personal, interpersonal, political, community)

Health in All Policies (HiAP)

human rights health equity

invisibility syndrome

market justice

social determinants of health

social justice

Discussion Questions

1. What is the role of personal and community empowerment in eliminating health inequities among black men?
2. What is the role of empowerment strategies in addressing the social determinants of health among African-American men?
3. What is the role of policy in addressing the social determinants of the health of African-American men?
4. What historic forces have played a role in the creation of the current state of health among black men and the black community?
5. Describe the principles inherent in the "Health in All Policies" movement. Why is it so much further along as a viable approach to equity in other parts of the world then it is in the United States?

References

Angelique, H. L., Reischl, T. M., & Davidson, W. S. (2002). Promoting political empowerment: Evaluation of an intervention with university students. *American Journal of Community Psychology, 30*(6), 815–833.

Bonhomme, J., & Young, A. M. W. (2009). The health status of black men. In R. L. Braithwaite, S. E. Taylor, & H. M. Treadwell (Eds.), *Health issues in the black community* (pp. 73–94). San Francisco, CA: Jossey-Bass.

Bonnefoy, J., Morgan, A., Kelly, M., Butt, J., & Bergman, V. (2007). *Constructing the evidence base on the social determinants of health: A guide*. Retrieved from http://www.who.int/social_determinants/knowledge_networks/add_documents/mekn_final_guide_112007.pdf

Deaton, A. (2002). Policy implications of the gradient of health and wealth. *Health Affairs, 21*(2), 13–30.

Ellison, R. (1995). *Invisible man* (2nd ed.). New York, NY: Random House.

Franklin, A. J. (2004). *From brotherhood to manhood: How black men rescue their relationships and dreams from the invisibility syndrome*. Hoboken, NJ: Wiley.

Freire, P. (1970). *Pedagogy of the oppressed*. New York, NY: Herder and Herder.

Gollust, S. E., Lantz, P. M., & Ubel, P. A. (2009). The polarizing effect of news media messages about the social determinants of health. *American Journal of Public Health, 99*(12): 2160–2167.

Gutierrez, L. M., & Ortega, R. (1991). Developing methods to empower Latinos: The importance of groups. *Social Work with Groups, 1*(2), 23–43.

Heckler, M.M. (1985). *U. S. Task Force on Black and Minority Health. Report of the Secretary's task force on black and minority health*. Washington, DC: U.S. Department of Health and Human Services.

Jones, C. P., Hatch, A., & Troutman, A. (2009). Fostering a social justice approach to health: Health equity, human rights and an antiracist agenda. In R. L. Braithwaite, S. E. Taylor, & H. M. Treadwell (Eds.), *Health issues in the black community* (pp. 555–580). San Francisco, CA: Jossey-Bass.

Krieger, N., & Birn, A.E. (1998). A vision of social justice as the foundation of public health: Commemorating 150 years of the Spirit of 1848. *American Journal of Public Health, 88*, 1603–1606.

Marmot, M., & Wilkinson, R. G. (Eds.). (2008). *Social determinants of health* (2nd ed.). New York, NY: Oxford University Press.

Merelman, R. M. (1993). Black history and cultural empowerment: A case study. *American Journal of Education, 101*(4), 331–358.

Mincey, R. (Ed.). (2006). *Black males left behind*. Baltimore, MD: Urban Institute Press.

Ministry of Social Affairs and Health. (2006). *Health in all policies: Prospects and potentials*. Retrieved from http://www.euro.who.int/__data/assets/pdf_file/0003/109146/E89260.pdf

Raphael, S. (2006). The socioeconomic status of black men: The increasing importance of incarceration. In A. J. Auerbach, D. Card, & J. M. Quigley (Eds.), *Public policy and the income distribution* (pp. 319–358). New York, NY: Russell Sage Foundation.

Robert Wood Johnson Foundation. Commission to Build a Healthier America. (2009). *Education matters for health*. Retrieved from http://www.commissiononhealth.org/PDF/c270deb3-ba42-4fbd-baeb-2cd65956f00e/Issue%20Brief%206%20Sept%2009%20-%20Education%20and%20Health.pdf

Satcher, D., Fryer, G. E., McCann, J., Troutman, A., Woolf, S. H., & Rust, G. (2005). What if we were equal? A comparison of the black-white mortality gap in 1960 and2000. *Health Affairs, 24*(2), 459–464.

Stephens, T., Braithwaite, H., Johnson, L., Harris, C., Katkowsky, S., & Troutman, A. (2008). Cardiovascular risk reduction for African-American men through health empowerment and anger management. *Health Education Journal*, *67*(3), 208–218.

Syme, S. (1998). Social epidemiology and the work environment. *International Journal of Health Services*, *18*, 635–645.

Wallerstein, N. (2002). Empowerment to reduce health disparities. *Scandinavian Journal of Public Health*, *30*(59), 72–77.

Williams, D. R. (2003). The health of men: Structured inequalities and opportunities. *American Journal of Public Health*, *93*(5), 724–731.

World Health Organization. (2008). Commission on the Social Determinants of Health. *Closing the gap in a generation: Health equity through action on the social determinants of health*. Retrieved from http://www.who.int/social_determinants/thecommission/finalreport/en/index.html

Zulkosky, K. (2009). Self-efficacy: A concept analysis. *Nursing Forum*, *44*(2), 93–102.

Afterword
Social Determinants and African-American Men

Where Do We Go from Here?

David Satcher

This book's focus on the social determinants of health among African-American men is long overdue. It should help to move us forward in the quest for health equity and the elimination of disparities in health.

The science is clear—between countries and within countries, there are differences in health status and health outcomes related to socioeconomic factors such as education and income. The World Health Organization (WHO) Commission on Social Determinants of Health (CSDH), on which I served from 2005 to 2008, concluded that targeting/attacking differences in social determinants of health, including the power base, was the most cost-effective approach to eliminating disparities in health and achieving global health equity. In the commission's report, *Closing the Gap in a Generation*, a call was made for all governments and civil organizations globally to take action to improve the lives of "the world's citizen."[1]

Also, as United States Surgeon General and Assistant Secretary for Health, I had the opportunity to lead in the development of *Healthy People 2010*, whose overarching goals were to increase years and quality of healthy life and eliminate racial and ethnic health disparities.[2] *Healthy People 2020* continues this goal and incorporates a greater focus on social determinants of health.[3]

The CSDH defined "social determinants of health" as the conditions into which one is born, grows, learns, works, ages, and ultimately dies, and the power to impact these conditions.

This book's contributing writers have clearly outlined the role of social determinants of health in the lives of African-American men in the United States. The African-American male has the worst health outcomes of any groups on measures such as cardiovascular disease, cancer, mortality, HIV/AIDS, and life expectancy. The plight of African-American males in the United States is deeply rooted in U.S. history, especially slavery, segregation, and continued discrimination and racism.

A clear focus on the social determinants of health as they impact African-American males in the United States provides the greatest promise for progress in this arena. The health of these men affects the health of African-American families.

Indeed there are also gender differences in mortality rates among African-Americans. Although we are closing the gap in life expectancy between African-Americans and whites, there remain significant differences in life expectancy between African-American men and white men and between African-American women and African-American men as well. In 1970, life expectancy for white males was 68 years while it was 60 years for African-American males. It was 75.6 years for white females and 68.3 years for African-American females. As reported in the U.S. Census Bureau's 2011 Report, in 2007, life expectancy for white males was 75.9 years, African-American males, 70 years, white females 80.8 years, and African-American females, 76.8 years.[4] So while African-American men have gained some 10 years over the past 40 years, their life expectancy remains almost six years shorter than that of white men and close to seven years shorter than African-American females. Meanwhile African-American females have closed the gap to four years when compared to white females, down from seven years' difference in 1970.

Socioeconomic differences between African-American men and women are significant.[5] Some factors contributing to these differences are: (1) income gains among African-American women, moving toward closing the income gap, from around 66 percent of white women's earnings in 1960 to 89 percent in 2000, while African-American men earned only 78 percent of white men's earnings in 2000; (2) Medicaid has provided women with better access to care—coverage for prenatal care and family planning. Sixty-two percent of African-American births are covered by Medicaid, compared to 23 percent of births to white, non-Hispanic mothers; (3) men have generally been ineligible for Medicaid coverage unless blind, disabled, or elderly; (4) health access expansions have consistently excluded nonelderly, nondisabled adult men; (5) the average African-American male barely lives long enough to become eligible for Medicare; and (6) a spike in gun-related homicide deaths starting in 1983 and peaking in 1994 to 1995 disproportionately impacted African-American males.

Problems have often been promoted and sustained by social and political policies that fail to adequately address the health needs of this population. Further, health conditions, both mental and physical, are exacerbated by lifestyle, which is largely shaped by the social environment. Many men who are poor, uneducated, and unemployed find themselves incarcerated.

African-American men and other men of color have been incarcerated at rates disproportionate to their representation in the general population.

The fact that most African-American men are estranged from health care services is reflective of how the system presents itself in their eyes. The African-American man is least likely to see himself, his culture, and his influence in the current system. Also, many men have to be convinced of the benefits of attending to their physical, mental, and oral health. They must feel comfortable with doctors and must release the cultural and societal impositions of toughness and machismo.

One approach to targeting social determinants of health that impact the health of African-American men is the McKinlay Model where we look *downstream* with a continual focus on education, health care, and justice; *midstream*, community nurturing from conception onward; and *upstream* where policies that speak directly to the plight of African-American men are developed.[6] At every level African-American males must be better targeted and more involved.

This writer proposes that while continuing to work with African-American males, relative to optimizing opportunities for education, health care, and healthy behaviors, we must provide physical and social environments that promote health and prevent disease. It is important that more research focus on social determinants of health and testing interventions to ascertain their effectiveness. Services earmarked toward improving health care outcomes for this population should be integrated across several fronts and the problems of the homeless and mentally ill must be addressed in ways that prevent these populations from being further marginalized by incarceration. Poverty and all of its ramifications must be addressed relative to African-American males.[7]

The consciousness of those who can make a difference—policy makers, educators, researchers, and health care providers, must be raised to the severity of this problem and the urgent need to address it. The bad news is that poor health outcomes, minimal education, unemployment, and incarceration have kept men, particularly African-American men, from contributing as productive members of society and heads of their families. The good news is that this book—*Social Determinants of Health among African-American Men*—will play a significant role in raising awareness of the plight of African-American men, by targeting the many fronts on which African-American men experience disparate treatment and addressing not only the role that social determinants of health play in creating those conditions but also the role that social determinants of health can play in providing solutions that will allow us to see improvements in health outcomes for African-American men.

It is encouraging that included in the Patient Protection and Affordable Care Act (Health Reform Act) is a commitment to a prevention agenda. The Prevention Council, chaired by the Surgeon General, will have representation from all of the governmental agencies including education, labor, commerce, and justice, to name a few. This is a major step forward and a hopeful sign for beginning to address the social determinants of health and the health of African-American men.

Notes

1. CSDH. (2008). *Closing the gap in a generation: Health equity through action on the social determinants of health.* Final report of the Commission on Social Determinants of Health. Geneva, World Health Organization.
2. U.S. Department of Health and Human Services (2000, November). *Healthy people 2010: Understanding and improving health* (2nd ed.). Washington, DC: U.S. Government Printing Office.
3. U.S. Department of Health and Human Services. (2010, November). Office of Disease Prevention and Health Promotion. *Healthy People 2020.* Washington, DC: U.S. Government Printing Office.
4. U.S. Census Bureau. (2011). *Statistical Abstract of the United States.*
5. Satcher D., Fryer G. E. Jr., McCann J., Troutman A., Woolf, S. H., & Rust, G. (2005). What if we were equal? A comparison of the black-white mortality gap in 1960 and 2000. *Health Affairs, 24*(2): 459–464.
6. McKinlay, J. B. (1995). The new public health approach to improving physical activity and autonomy in older populations. In E. Heikkinen (Ed.), *Preparation for aging* (pp. 87–103). New York, NY: Plenum Press.
7. Wilensky, G. R., & Satcher, D. (2009). Don't forget about the social determinants of health. *Health Affairs, 28*(2): w194–w198.

Index